MW01106068

ALLERGIES
SOURCEBOOK

Volume Nineteen

ALLERGIES
SOURCEBOOK

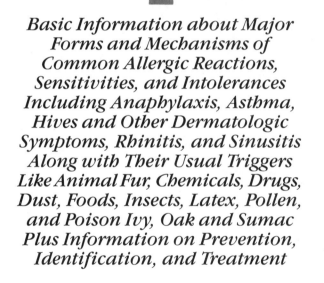

*Basic Information about Major
Forms and Mechanisms of
Common Allergic Reactions,
Sensitivities, and Intolerances
Including Anaphylaxis, Asthma,
Hives and Other Dermatologic
Symptoms, Rhinitis, and Sinusitis
Along with Their Usual Triggers
Like Animal Fur, Chemicals, Drugs,
Dust, Foods, Insects, Latex, Pollen,
and Poison Ivy, Oak and Sumac
Plus Information on Prevention,
Identification, and Treatment*

Edited by
Allan R. Cook

BIBLIOGRAPHIC NOTE

This volume contains individual publications issued by the National Institutes of Health (NIH), its sister agencies, and sub-agencies. Numbered publications are: NIH 77-540, 80-388, 82-703, 82-1046, 83-490, 91-2414, 93-493, 93-529, 93-3469, 94-2751, and FDA 90-1161, 91-1166. The unnumbered publications are: the NIH pamphlets "How to Create a Dust-Free Bedroom," "What You Need to Know About Asthma," and "Allergic Diseases;" NIH Healthline pamphlet "Poison Ivy: It's Still out There;" National Heart, Lung, and Blood Institute Data Fact Sheet "Asthma Statistics, May 1992," and the Department of Agriculture bulletins No. 1972 and 246. Also included are reprints from the *FDA Consumer*, May 1996, January/February 1995, October 1993, December 1993, September 1992, May 1990, May 1989, June 1986, November 1986, December 1984/January 1985; *EPA Journal* 19:4 October/December 1993; *Mortality and Morbidity Weekly Report*, April 19, 1994; *NCRR Reporter*, September/October 1994; and *Research Resources Reporter* March/April 1993 and May/June 1992. In addition, the volume includes copyrighted articles from American Academy of Dermatology, *American Family Physician*, and Asthma and Allergy Foundation.

Edited by
Allan R. Cook

Peter D. Dresser, Managing Editor, Health Reference Series
Karen Bellenir, Series Editor, Health Reference Series

Omnigraphics, Inc.
Matthew P. Barbour, Production Manager
Laurie Lanzen Harris, Vice President, Editorial
Peter E. Ruffner, Vice President, Administration
James A. Sellgren, Vice President, Operations and Finance
Jane J. Steele, Vice President, Research

Frederick G. Ruffner, Jr., Publisher

Library of Congress Cataloging-in-Publication Data

Allergies sourcebook / edited by Allan R. Cook.
    p.   cm. — (Health reference series ; v. 17)
    Includes bibliographical references and index.
    ISBN 0-7808-0036-2 (lib. bdg. : alk. paper)
    1. Allergy—Popular works.   I. Cook, Allan R.   II. Series.
RC584.A3446 1996
616.97—dc20   96-30992
                                              CIP

∞

Printed in the United States of America

Table of Contents

Preface ix

Part I: Introduction: Allergies and the Immune System

Chapter 1—Basic Mechanisms of Allergic Diseases 3
Chapter 2—Understanding the Immune System's Role in
             Allergic Reactions 31
Chapter 3—Research Directions for Allergic Diseases 37
Chapter 4—The Socioeconomic Impact of Allergies and
             Asthma in the United States 45

Part II: Types of Allergic Reactions

Chapter 5—Allergic Rhinitis 61
Chapter 6—Asthma: A Severe Allergic Reaction 77
Chapter 7—Sinusitis: A Painful Response to Allergies
             and Infections 95
Chapter 8—Dermatologic Allergies 105
Chapter 9—Allergic Drug Reactions 115
Chapter 10—Chemical Photosensitivity: Common Products
             Can Make You Allergic to Sunlight 133
Chapter 11—Occupational/Environmental Asthma and
             Related Allergic Respiratory Diseases 139

Chapter 12—Pediatric Allergies 155
Chapter 13—Allergic Emergencies 163
Chapter 14—Holiday Allergies: 'Tis the Season! 173
Chapter 15—Allergic and Immunologic Aspects of Other
          Diseases 179

Part III: Food Allergens

Chapter 16—Food Allergies and Intolerances 195
Chapter 17—A Fresh Look at Food Preservatives 209
Chapter 18—From Shampoo to Cereal: Seeing to the
          Safety of Color Additives 217
Chapter 19—Deadly Foods: Even a Trace Can Trigger
          Anaphylaxis 227
Chapter 20—Lactose Intolerance: Soured on Milk 233
Chapter 21—Allergy to Foods Containing Concealed
          Milk Proteins 241
Chapter 22—Childhood Atopic Dermatitis: A Result of
          Food Hypersensitivity 245
Chapter 23—Scientists Net Major Shrimp Allergen 253
Chapter 24—Cooking for People with Food Allergies 257
Chapter 25—The New Food Label: Better Information
          for Special Diets 297

Part IV: Airborne Allergens

Chapter 26—Something in the Air: Pollen, Mold, and
          Dust Allergens 309
Chapter 27—Indoor Allergens 327
Chapter 28—How to Create a Dust-Free Bedroom 331
Chapter 29—Allergies to Dogs and Cats: Man's Best
          Friends? 335
Chapter 30—Populations at Risk from Particulate Air
          Pollution—United States, 1992 341

Part V: Contact and Proximity Allergens

Chapter 31—Insect Allergies.. 349

Chapter 32—Insect Sting Allergy and Venom
          Immunotherapy 363

Chapter 33—Poison Ivy, Poison Oak, and Poison
          Sumac: They're Still Out There 367

Chapter 34—Poison Ivy, Poison Oak, and Poison
          Sumac: Identification, Precautions,
          Eradication 375

Chapter 35—Chemical and Other Environmental
          Sensitivities 391

Chapter 36—Contact Dermatitis: Solutions to Rash
          Mysteries 397

Chapter 37—Atopic Eczema/Atopic Dermatitis 407

Chapter 38—Hand Eczema 411

Chapter 39—Latex Allergies: When Rubber Rubs the
          Wrong Way 415

Chapter 40—Cosmetic Allergies: When Beauty Aids
          Turn Ugly 425

Part VI: Asthma

Chapter 41—Asthma Myths and Statistics: Two Views
          of Respiratory Distress 437

Chapter 42—Allergic Mechanisms in Asthma 445

Chapter 43—Asthma by Age Group.. 451

Chapter 44—The Role of Eosinophils in Allergic Lung
          Reactions 459

Chapter 45—Research for the Future: Asthma and
          Allergic Diseases 465

Part VII: First Aid for Allergy Symptoms

Chapter 46—Easing the Itch of the Great Outdoors 475

Chapter 47—It's Spring Again and Allergies Are in
          the Bloom.. 479

Chapter 48—Topical Nasal Sprays: Treatment of Allergic
          Rhinitis 489
Chapter 40—"Over-the-Counter" Medications: Do They
          Work for Allergies? 503
Chapter 50—Immunotherapy: Avoiding Allergies Is
          Worth a Shot 507
Chapter 51—Adverse Effects from Asthma and Allergy
          Medication 517

Part VIII: Glossary of Common Medical Terms

Chapter 52—Glossary of Medical Terms 525

Index 557

Preface

About This Book

Allergies, in one form or another, afflict some 50 million Americans, or 1 out of every 5. One out of every eleven doctor's office visits involves treatment for allergic reactions, which vary from annoying rashes or sniffles to life-threatening respiratory distress. The patients are of all ages, and the allergic reactions differ accordingly, but the treatment varies little: allergy medication can relieve the symptoms, bring temporary relief, and allow the body to repair minor damage caused by the allergic reaction, but unless the cause of the reaction, the allergic trigger, is discovered, the symptoms will return as soon as the patient ceases taking the medication. Coping with the long-term effects of allergy means identifying the underlying cause of the reaction and avoiding or limiting that trigger.

This book contains basic information for the layperson on the connection between the immune system and allergic reactions; common allergies, their triggers, and methods of treating, avoiding, and coping with them; and an analysis of the economic implications of allergic and immune disorders. Patients, friends, family members, and the interested general public will find this volume a good place to begin to understand the complexities of allergic reactions. However, some topics are handled in more detail in other volumes of this series: the *Immune System Disorders Sourcebook,* the *Respiratory Diseases and Disorders Sourcebook,* the *AIDS Sourcebook,* the *Arthritis Sourcebook,* and the *Skin Disorders Sourcebook.*

How To Use This Book

This book is divided into parts and chapters. Parts focus on broad areas of interest and chapters on specific topics within those areas.

Part I: *Introduction: Allergies and the Immune System* gives an overview of how allergies work and examines the mechanism of human immunity, describing the specific components and functions of the immune network. It also examines the costs of allergies, both economic and human.

Part II: *Types of Allergic Reactions* describes the most common forms of allergic reactions and offers general recommendations on treatment, coping and avoidance.

Part III: *Food Allergens* describes the particular triggers associated with food allergies. It also explains the difference between allergies, intolerances, and sensitivities. One chapter includes detailed recipes designed to help the food-sensitive patient design healthy and interesting meals.

Part IV: *Airborne Allergens* describes the various allergic irritants often transmitted through the air, including dust, pollen, dander, spores, and fungi. Along with treatment suggestions, the section includes information on predicting difficult seasons and identifying sources of the allergens, and it offers suggestions on how to maintain a relatively dust-free home environment for the dust-sensitive.

Part V: *Contact and Proximity Allergens* describes the triggers of allergy commonly transmitted by physical contact or near contact, including poison ivy, poison oak, and poison sumac; insect bites and stings; chemicals; and metals and fabrics. The section also discusses some common conditions resulting from these allergens, including eczema, dermatitis, and other contact rashes.

Part VI: *Asthma* considers the severe allergic mechanisms and implications of asthma with one section focusing particularly on older patients. It also briefly considers recent advances in respiratory disorder research.

Part VII: *First Aid for Allergy Symptoms* discusses some of the more common allergy medications and their side-effects.

Part VIII: *Glossary of Common Medical Terms* provides a listing and short explanations of some common medical terms used throughout this volume.

Index: gives page references and cross-references for key words and phrases used in the various articles.

Acknowledgements

The editor gratefully acknowledges the assistance of the many people who helped produce this volume and the private organizations which agreed to grant permission to reprint their articles: the Asthma and Allergy Foundation, and the American Academy of Dermatology. Special thanks to Margaret Mary Missar for her patient search for the documents that make up this volume, Karen Bellenir for her technical assistance and advice, Bruce the Scanman and special assistant Mike for their electronic alchemy, and Valerie Cook for her sharp-eyed text verification.

Note from the Editor

This book is part of Omnigraphics' *Health Reference Series*. The series provides basic information about a broad range of medical concerns. It is not intended to serve as a tool for diagnosing illness, in prescribing treatments, or as a substitute for the physician/patient relationship. All persons concerned about medical symptoms or the possibility of disease are encouraged to seek professional care from an appropriate health care provider.

Part One

Introduction: Allergies and the Immune System

Chapter 1

Allergic Diseases

Basic Mechanisms of Allergic Diseases

What is an Allergy?

When Clemens Freiherr von Pirquet coined the term "allergy" early in this century, he meant it to embrace any altered reaction of the immune system, whether the reaction was helpful or harmful. Today we speak of immunity, which is a protective, enhanced resistance, and allergy, which is a harmful increased susceptibility to a specific substance.

The Importance of Immunity

Without the body's vigilant and finely tuned immune system, there would be no human race. We live in a world populated by a host of potentially deadly germs: viruses, bacteria, and parasites. We survive because, over millions of years, the body has evolved a complex defense system capable of recognizing invading germs and destroying or controlling them. We call this sophisticated biological mechanism our immune system.

The existence of human immunity was recognized by the ancients. Centuries before the birth of Christ, scribes recorded the fact that survivors of a plague were protected against a second outbreak. But

NIH Publication *Medicine for the Public*, April 1991 and extracts from NIH Publication 80-388.

it was not until the 15th century that the immune system was manipulated. Chinese and Arab physicians began infecting people with pus from smallpox patients, a risky procedure. Sometimes, it produced a mild form of smallpox and protected against the serious illness; sometimes, it caused severe smallpox and death.

Late in the 18th century, an English physician named Edward Jenner noted that milkmaids who contracted cowpox from cows rarely developed smallpox. In 1796, Jenner inoculated an 8-year-old boy with fluid from a milkmaid's cowpox pustule, and the boy developed cowpox. Months later Jenner inoculated the boy with smallpox. The youngster did not develop the deadly disease. Jenner's work established the principle of vaccination, which is now used to protect us against such dreaded diseases as polio, diphtheria, typhoid, whooping cough, and tetanus.

But it wasn't until Louis Pasteur advanced the germ theory of disease in the 19th century that scientists began looking for the specific components of the immune system. The 20th century has seen an explosive growth in our understanding of the immune system, and its relationship to asthma and allergic diseases.

The fundamental concept of immunity is the body's ability to recognize foreign material—viruses, bacteria, pollens, dust, etc.—and react against the intruders. In other words, the body can tell "self" from "nonself." This ability to detect and destroy such things as viruses and bacteria helps protect us from disease. But this same system can produce many types of harmful reactions, for example, an allergy, the rejection of human transplanted tissue, or, in autoimmune diseases, destruction of the body's own tissues.

Four Types of Allergic Reactions

The allergic person may suffer a number of harmful reactions, ranging from mild to life-threatening. The mechanisms of these reactions are varied. But, generally, they are grouped into four types.

Type I. Called anaphylactic-hypersensitivity reaction or immediate hypersensitivity, this is the immune response that has become synonymous with the word allergy. Hay fever, some asthma and hives, some food and drug reactions, insect-sting reactions, and anaphylactic shock (a very severe, potentially fatal reaction) all fall into this class. The reactions occur within minutes after exposure to the antigen (allergen). The common denominator among these reactions is the antibody immunoglobulin E (IgE), which mediates the reactions.

4

Types of Allergic Reactions

		Mechanism	Examples
Type I	Immediate hypersensitivity or anaphylactic	IgE antibody on mast cell reacts with antigen resulting in release of mediators	Hay fever; allergic reaction to insect sting; allergic shock
Type II	Cytotoxic	IgG antibody reacts with cell membranes or antigen associated with cell membrane	Transfusion of incompatible blood types
Type III	Arthus	Antigen and antibody bind together to form immune complexes which deposit in walls of blood vessels or kidneys	Serum sickness; some drug reactions
Type IV	Delayed hypersensitivity or cell-mediated	T cells interact directly with antigen	Poison ivy; graft rejection

Table 1.1. Types of Allergic Reactions.

Type II. This is also an immediate reaction, in which IgG reacts against a cell membrane or an antigen associated with a cell membrane. The body's complement system—a series of interacting proteins—also plays an important role. An example of this reaction occurs when a patient is given a transfusion of an incompatible blood type.

Type III. In this type of reaction, sickness occurs several hours or even days after exposure to antigen. The reactions result from immune complexes: large molecules of antigen and antibody bound together. In this case, IgG binds antibodies and the resulting immune complexes are deposited in the walls of blood vessels. The complement system is also involved in producing the disease state. Some allergic drug reactions and serum sickness—a reaction to an injection of an animal serum—are type III reactions.

Type IV. This type of reaction reaches its peak two or three days after exposure and, thus, is sometimes referred to as delayed hypersensitivity. In it, T cells interact directly with the antigen. This interaction initiates a complex process of cell production and the release of certain chemicals which bring more cells into the reaction to fight the invader. The body's reaction to poison ivy and some aspects of its rejection of transplanted organs are type IV reactions.

Allergens and Immunoglobulin E

By far the most common of the allergic reactions are the type I reactions. The key to understanding them is IgE. Of the five major antibodies, or immunoglobulins, IgE is normally found in the lowest concentration in the blood. What protective role it plays remains unknown.

Little is known about the factors that control IgE production in humans. Animal studies, however, have demonstrated the existence of T cells, which, depending upon the message they receive, can either help or hinder the production of IgE antibodies. IgE is the major antibody responsible for the classic "allergy" symptoms of hay fever.

In susceptible individuals, allergies begin with exposure to certain antigens. These may be grass or tree pollens, molds, dusts, animal danders, drugs, or other substances. An antigen that produces an allergic reaction is called an **allergen.**

The immune system reacts to such allergens by producing IgE antibodies. These attach to the surfaces of certain cells called **mast cells** or **basophils.** A single mast cell or basophil may have 500,000 IgE antibodies sitting on it. Mast cells are abundant in the respiratory and gastrointestinal tracts, and the skin, while the basophils are found in the blood.

Each IgE antibody is specific, meaning that it will only react to the single allergen against which it was made. Thus, an IgE antibody against oak pollen will react against **proteins** from a grain of oak pollen, but not against grass or ragweed proteins. When an IgE antibody encounters its specific allergen, the antibody—which is sitting on a mast cell—reacts with the allergen. This reaction signals the mast cell to release powerful chemicals, including **histamine.** It is these chemical mediators that cause the symptoms of allergy, such as wheezing, sneezing, runny eyes, itching, abdominal pain, or diarrhea.

Amplifying the Immune System

An allergic reaction produces inflammation, a basic response of the body to injury. Often characterized by redness of the skin, warmth, swelling, and pain, inflammation results from a complex series of events involving cells and chemicals that are intended to protect the

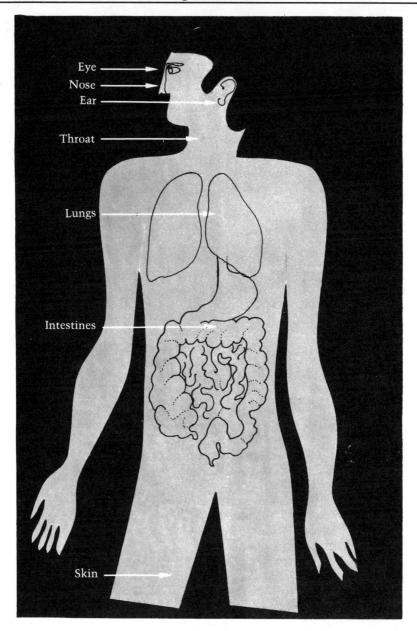

Figure 1.1. *The sites of the body where allergic reactions most frequently occur are: the eyes; the ears; the respiratory tract—nose, throat, and lungs; the gastrointestinal tract—stomach and intestines; and the skin. Shock— collapse of the vascular system—can also occur but is not illustrated.*

body. The chemicals can be classified into two groups. The first are substances released by mast cells, including histamine, that are particularly important in IgE-mediated allergic reactions. The second are larger molecules and include enzymes found in the complement system.

The exact role played by all of the chemical mediators remains to be determined. Histamine, however, causes itching, constriction of smooth muscle in the bronchial tubes, and increases the leakiness of blood vessels. **Slow reacting substance of anaphylaxis (SRS-A)** is the most powerful known constrictor of human bronchial smooth muscle. **Eosinophil chemotactic factor of anaphylaxis (ECF-A)** attracts a type of blood cell, called an **eosinophil,** to the allergic-reaction site.

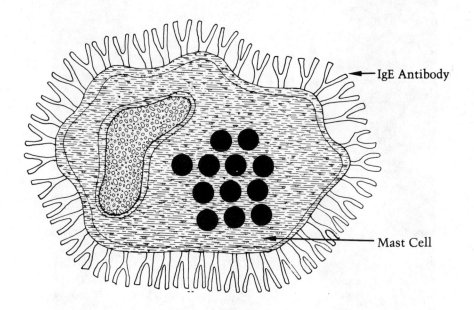

IgE Antibody

Mast Cell

Figure 1.2. *The first step in developing an allergy is exposure to certain pollens, dusts, molds, or other substances. The body reacts or becomes allergic to these substances, called allergens, by producing a protein known as IgE antibody, which is responsible for allergic reactions. Up to 500,000 IgE antibodies can attach to the surface of two types of cells known as mast cells or basophils. The basophils are found in the blood, while the mast cells are found primarily in tissues such as the respiratory tract, the gastrointestinal tract, and the skin.*

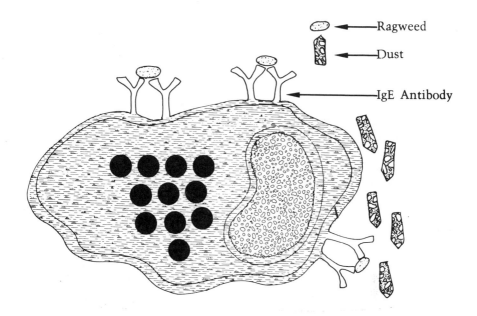

Ragweed

Dust

IgE Antibody

Figure 1.3. *Each IgE antibody will react only with the allergen against which it was made. This means that an IgE antibody made against a ragweed pollen will only react with another grain of ragweed pollen. This is why it is important to know those substances to which one is allergic. When an allergic person again encounters this allergen, it binds to the IgE antibodies that are already sitting on the surface of the mast cells or basophils.*

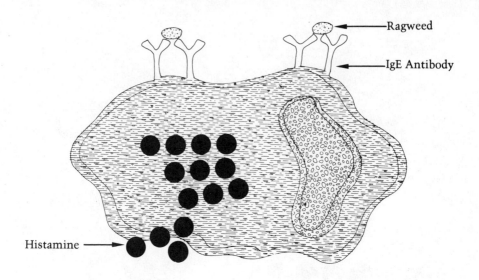

Ragweed

IgE Antibody

Histamine

Figure 1.4. This combination of allergen and antibody is a signal to the mast cells and basophils to release the little packets of chemicals that they contain, including histamine. These powerful chemicals or mediators, as they are known, can then cause the various symptoms of allergy, such as wheezing, sneezing, runny eyes, itching, abdominal pain, retching, or diarrhea.

The search for additional chemical mediators involved in the inflammation process has recently implicated other substances. An unstable form of oxygen, called the **superoxide radical,** is generated by mast cells in the lungs of humans in response to both immunologic and non-immunologic stimulations. It is too early to say what role this chemical plays, but there is some evidence it may be a cause of the deterioration of the **mucous membrane** seen in severe asthma.

Prostaglandins are a group of fatty acids that are involved in the regulation of a number of body reactions. IgE-mediated reactions generate several prostaglandins. Although their role in asthma and allergies, if any, remains unclear, they may cause some of the tissue reactions observed in the allergic disorders.

Other chemicals that may be involved in allergies are: platelet activating factor, a substance that causes the cells (platelets) responsible for blood clotting to clump together and may amplify the allergic reaction; enzymes released by mast cells that may generate

Mediators Released From Human Mast Cells and Basophils

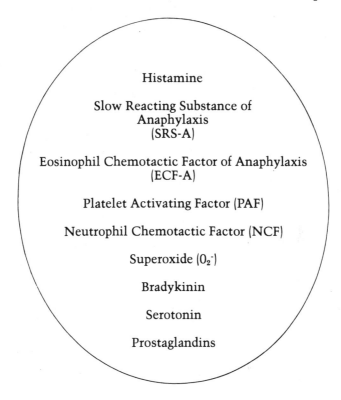

Histamine

Slow Reacting Substance of
Anaphylaxis
(SRS-A)

Eosinophil Chemotactic Factor of Anaphylaxis
(ECF-A)

Platelet Activating Factor (PAF)

Neutrophil Chemotactic Factor (NCF)

Superoxide (O_2^-)

Bradykinin

Serotonin

Prostaglandins

Figure 1.5. Mediators are released when an allergen reacts with IgE antibody on the surface of a mast cell or basophil. These chemicals lead to tissue injury either by their direct effects on blood vessels, certain nerve fibers, and smooth muscles in the lungs, or by attracting other damage-producing cells to the site of the allergic reaction.

bradykinin, a potent blood-vessel dilator; and **serotonin**, which can contract smooth muscle and stimulate mucus secretion.

Once chemical mediators are released, they have a relatively short life. Recent research has provided some understanding of how the body destroys these chemicals. For example, histamine is destroyed by two enzyme systems and SRS-A appears to be destroyed by another enzyme in the body.

Human blood also contains four systems of high-molecular weight proteins that play vital roles in inflammation and some allergic disorders. The most important is the complement system.

The complement system was first recognized in the late l9th century. Originally, it was thought to be a single substance that was needed to "complete" the killing of a bacterium coated with an antibody. It is now known to consist of a series of approximately 20 proteins. The complement system both aids in the removal of certain nonself materials and produces inflammation.

The complement system may be activated in two ways, called the "classic" and "alternative" pathways. The classic pathway was discovered first, but the alternative appears older in terms of evolution and probably predates the development of the immune system.

The Pathways of Complement Activation

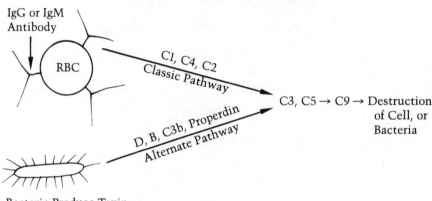

IgG or IgM Antibody

RBC

Cl, C4, C2
Classic Pathway

C3, C5 → C9 → Destruction of Cell, or Bacteria

D, B, C3b, Properdin
Alternate Pathway

Bacteria Produce Toxin

Figure 1.6. The complement system consists of a series of interacting enzymes which can be activated in either of two ways. In one, known as the classical pathway, the system is turned on when antibody reacts with an antigen such as a red blood cell (RBC), forming an immune complex. This complex binds C1, the first enzyme in the series, and the cascade reaction begins. In the alternate pathway, certain substances—such as the toxins (poisons) produced by bacteria—trigger the latter part of the cascade. The effect of both pathways is the same: damage to the membrane of the cell or bacteria, resulting in its destruction.

The classic pathway of the complement system is turned on when either IgG or IgM antibody binds to an antigen such as bacteria to form an immune complex. This immune complex then binds the first of the complement system's proteins, an enzyme designated C1. Then C1 binds and activates another enzyme. This cascading process continues through a series of enzymes, each being bound and activated in turn. Finally, enzyme C9 and some of the system's other components form a complex molecule that punches a hole in the surface membrane of the bacteria, killing the organism.

In the alternative pathway, certain substances—such as a toxin produced by an invading cell—can trigger only the latter part of the complement system. But the effect is the same. The invading material is attacked and destroyed. Defects in the complement system are associated with **autoimmune diseases.** Immune complexes and the activation of complement, which in turn cause acute and chronic inflammations that damage healthy tissue, play a role in a number of disorders. These include **rheumatoid arthritis, glomerulonephritis** (a kidney disease), and **pulmonary fibrosis** (a scarring of the lungs).

The complement system also interacts with the enzyme systems responsible for the clotting of blood, the dissolving of blood clots, and the formation of potent chemicals called kinins that dilate blood vessels. Collectively, these three systems are called the **Hageman factor (HF) systems.** While the HF systems are important in inflammation, their roles in various disease processes remain undetermined. The components of the three have only recently been isolated. Now, with newly developed research techniques, scientists should be able to determine more accurately the role of the HF systems in disease.

Genetics and the Allergic Response

You may inherit a tendency to be allergic. This fact has been known since the early part of the 20th century from a number of family studies. People with allergic diseases usually have a close relative who also suffers some allergic problem (see the chapter on Pediatric Allergies).

But heredity alone doesn't explain allergies. Authorities generally agree that allergies are controlled by a combination of genetic and nongenetic factors. Understanding the genetics of the immune system and the allergic response will be important in fully understanding the allergic mechanism, and in improving the diagnosis, treatment, and prevention of allergies.

Recent studies of identical and fraternal twins provide strong evidence that a person's total level of IgE is largely genetically determined. A single major gene apparently determines IgE levels, with a high IgE concentration inherited as a recessive trait.

In recent years, researchers have searched for genetic markers, certain identifiable inherited characteristics, that would predict before symptoms appear who is at high risk of developing a disease. If such markers could be found for asthma and the allergic diseases, people at high risk might be identified early enough in life to reduce the severity of these disorders.

The search for genetic markers has focused on the body's **histocompatibility (HLA) antigens.** These antigens exist on the surface of our cells and tell the immune system whether a cell is self or nonself. There are many HLA antigens, although some are more prevalent than others.

Histocompatibility antigens serve as genetic markers for certain diseases; that is, researchers have found a striking association between some HLA types and these diseases. In the case of **ankylosing spondylitis** (a form of arthritis that attacks the spine), if a patient carries an HLA antigen which is a genetic marker for this disease, he or she is at higher risk of developing it than someone who does not carry the antigen.

Several HLA antigens that may indicate an increased risk of allergic reaction to ragweed pollens have been identified. But attempts to find genetic markers for asthma have produced no conclusive findings.

Who Gets Allergies?

Allergies are incredibly common. More than 50 million Americans—one out of five—suffer from allergic diseases. One out of every eleven office visits to the doctor is for an allergic disease.

Inheritance has a major influence on allergy. If one parent has allergies, the odds are that one in three of the children will have allergies. If both parents have allergies, then all the children will probably have allergies.

Aside from inheritance, it is not known why some people get allergies and others do not. Some believe that hormonal influences, viral infections, smoking, and a number of other influences affect whether one develops allergies. No one knows all the reasons why people with equal likelihood to develop allergies become allergic to different things, or why some have hay fever and others have asthma.

Second, a person has to be exposed to an allergen, a foreign protein that causes allergy. Ragweed pollen is the major cause of allergy in the United States. It is an unusual allergen that is found in high concentrations only in this country. Most people who move to the United States are exposed to ragweed for the first time. Many have never had allergies previously in their families for centuries, yet they develop allergies within two or three years of living in the United States. A large part of why they develop allergies is exposure to ragweed, which is an incredibly potent allergy-producing plant.

Each ragweed plant produces about one billion pollen grains during an average allergy season. Those pollen grains are very small—microscopic. They float in the air and may be carried out to sea as many as 300 or 400 miles. So it does not matter if people do not have ragweed plants in their backyards; they are clearly exposed to ragweed every place in the United States except for the arid southwest and southern California, where ragweed does not grow. Other major allergens include grass pollens, tree pollens, dust, molds, and animal dander. Worldwide, however, the major allergen is the dust mite. All temperate climate areas in the world have dust mites, which live in carpeting, mattresses, and upholstery. They have to have temperatures above 60 degrees to reproduce. Most people keep the temperature in their homes above 60 degrees all year. Dust mites also need a relative humidity above 50 percent.

People are not actually allergic to the dust mite; they are allergic to its feces. The fecal balls are sticky, heavy materials that bind to carpeting or upholstery. One of the worst ways to bring dust mite allergens into the air is to vacuum the floor; this blows the dust up into the air, where it floats for a couple of hours and makes up the motes in a beam of sunlight.

How Do Allergies Work?

There are three components to allergies:

* **mast cells**, which contain chemicals like histamine;
* **antibodies**, a specific type of protein made by the immune system, known as IgE; and
* **allergens**, which trigger the reaction.

Mast cells are the allergy-causing cells and are found in every tissue throughout the body, though they are most heavily concentrated in those tissues that are exposed to the outside world—the skin, linings of the nose and lungs, gastrointestinal tract, and reproductive system.

15

The IgE antibody, which actually causes allergy, sits on the surface of these mast cells. A mast cell has about 1,000 histamine-containing granules in its cytoplasm, and on its surface are between 100,000 and 1 million receptors for IgE. When the IgE encounters the allergen, it triggers the mast cell to release granules from its cytoplasm. Those granules contain histamine and other chemicals. These mediators that are released then interact with the tissues, causing the allergic symptoms.

With ragweed, for example, the pollen grains from the plant are male gametes equivalent to sperm. They carry the male genetic code from a male ragweed plant to a female ragweed plant. Since the pollen grains are wind-borne and do not have a particular way of finding a female plant, many excess pollen grains are produced in the hopes that one or another will find a female plant and fertilize it.

On the surface of a pollen grain are enzymes that help the pollen grain enter female plants. Unfortunately, people breathe in pollen grains that are floating in the air. When a pollen grain gets on the skin that lines the inside of the nose, those enzymes are released from the pollen grain and work their way through the mucus in the nose. The enzymes sensitize the person by initiating the production of IgE antibodies, which then sensitize mast cells that are in the nose. It generally takes about two to five seasons of allergen exposure before a person makes enough IgE to result in allergy symptoms.

Everyone makes some IgE. Only people with genetic predispositions toward allergies make large quantities. IgE, like other antibodies that the body produces, is part of the body's defense mechanism. Some antibodies, like IgG, get rid of Streptococcus and help cure those infected with a strep throat. Other antibodies get rid of cold viruses. The IgE antibody is directed against parasites. Its function is to protect the body against parasitic infections. There are few parasites in the United States, but the IgE antibody system reacts against the enzymes from the surface of pollen grains as if they were parasites and elicits an allergic response. The body is misdirecting an extremely important immune response at pollens, dust, dander, and molds.

Most antibodies last in the body about three weeks, but IgE may sit on its receptor on mast cells and sensitize the mast cells for years. For example, someone who had an adverse allergic reaction to penicillin as a child could still be allergic to the drug as an adult. The IgE antibody the person made as a 6-year-old child would still be present in the 40-year-old adult. It is sitting on the mast cells, which are long-lived cells, and it conveys incredibly long-lived sensitivity to allergens.

In one research study, we looked at mast cell histamine release under the electron microscope. We sensitized a mast cell to IgE, making it allergic to grass, trees, ragweed, and certain breeds of cats and dogs. We then took this mast cell and exposed it to an extract of ragweed. Over a 15-minute period, many of the granules in its cytoplasm disappeared. Fifteen minutes later, the granules were all gone.

Although the mast cell had no visible secretory granules in its cytoplasm, it was alive and well; over the next 6 to 24 hours it would reconstitute all the granules that had disappeared. After releasing histamine from its granules, a mast cell can once again do damage to the person the next day when he or she breathes in ragweed.

The chemicals that are released from mast cells are the mediators that cause allergies. At last count, there were 28 separate chemicals released by mast cells that orchestrate allergic responses. The allergic symptoms a person experiences depend on the tissue in which the mediators are released. For example, if these chemicals are released in the nose, the person will get hay fever, allergic rhinitis. If they are released in the chest, the person will get asthma or coughing. Chemicals released in the skin will produce hives or eczema, in the intestine will produce food allergy or diarrhea, and in the brain may result in a migraine. There is a whole spectrum of problems that these mediators can cause.

Allergic reactions often take place very quickly. Those who experience allergy may go outside on a bright, sunny, windy morning during the ragweed season and within 15 minutes begin to have allergic reactions. This reaction is referred to as immediate hypersensitivity. When mast cells release their chemicals, they cause immediate reactions.

Some people also experience late-phase reactions. When mast cells release their chemicals, they cause an inflammatory response. The site of the allergic reaction gets red, swollen, hot, and tender, causing a more prolonged response. A person may go out at 8 a.m. and experience a late reaction at 4 p.m. Such reactions may last one day, two days, one week, or one month from a single allergen exposure. They are part of the underlying problem for chronic asthma, rhinitis, eczema, hives, and other allergic diseases.

How Are Allergies Diagnosed?

Allergy is diagnosed through skin testing, which shows an immediate reaction to allergens. The procedure traditionally involves introducing a minute amount of allergen into the skin. The tip of the needle is used to puncture the skin, causing an interaction between the allergen and a mast cell.

When doctors administer skin tests, they are introducing allergen into the skin and causing the same reaction that the patients experience in their noses or lungs during the allergy season. In the past, doctors used to take small needles and inject them under the skin surface and put a minute amount of allergen in the skin. Within 15 minutes a welt formed, like a mosquito bite, if the patient had a positive reaction. That was minimally uncomfortable, but it was still uncomfortable.

Today, doctors use a needle to put a drop of allergen on the skin without breaking the skin surface. They "tent" the skin by putting the needle through the droplet and lifting up the skin without breaking the skin surface. It is essentially painless, yet it is very sensitive and specific.

Diagnosis, preferentially, is done by skin testing. Skin tests are fast; they take about 5 minutes to administer and can be read within 15 minutes. They are very sensitive, relatively cheap, and cause minimal discomfort, but require some medical expertise.

A second way to diagnose allergy is with a blood test that looks for IgE antibodies. This test is relatively expensive, slightly less sensitive, requires a blood drawing, and does not require expertise. It is done frequently by non-allergists who want to see if the patient has allergies. In proper hands, both tests are equally informative.

Allergic Rhinitis

Allergic rhinitis (hay fever) is a disease of incredible proportion. Thirty-five million Americans—17-percent of the population—experience allergic rhinitis. It is the single most common chronic disease experienced by human beings. As a single entity, 1 out of every 40 doctor office visits (1.5 percent) are due to allergic rhinitis.

Allergic rhinitis is caused by exposure to airborne allergens. The process of allergic rhinitis takes place in the nose. Pollen grains, dust, and dander are trapped by hairs in the nose and are trapped in the mucus that lines the inside of the nose. The allergens release soluble proteins that reach the mucous membranes, causing allergic rhinitis.

The skin that lines the inside of the nose is a succulent tissue full of glands and blood vessels. The submucous glands in this living tissue produce the mucus in the nose. In fact, that is why the lining is called a mucous membrane; it specifically makes mucus. Although many people think of mucus as a bother, mucus is quite helpful.

18

Mucus is important because it humidifies and protects the mucous membrane. It contains antimicrobial factors that protect people from both bacterial and viral infections. When people get colds, it is despite the fact that they have mucus; if they did not have that mucus, they would have infections all the time.

What about nasal congestion? The body has cavities in the lining of the nose where blood can pool. The nose can become swollen with blood pooling in these sinusoids. When blood is diverted into these sinusoids, this tissue gets markedly enlarged and the person cannot breathe through his or her nose. Everyone experiences nasal congestion; every 45 minutes to 2 hours, one side of the nose congests and the other side constricts. People breathe preferentially through one side, resting the other side, and then alternating sides. One never breathes evenly through both sides of the nose because of this process of congestion. Of course, during allergic rhinitis it gets much worse and the allergy sufferer experiences more severe, chronic nasal congestion.

What can the mucous membrane do? It can congest by pooling blood in these sinusoids; it can become itchy or sneezy by stimulating some of the sensory nerves in the nose; and it can produce secretions. These are the processes that people experience when they have rhinitis—allergic rhinitis, vasomotor rhinitis, rhinitis from colds, or from eating hot and spicy foods.

The most common features of allergic rhinitis are sneezing attacks and itching of the nose, eyes, pharynx, and palate. Clicking the tongue on the top of the mouth is the way one scratches the soft palate, and the soft palate itches if one has allergic rhinitis. One also gets a runny nose or congestion of the nose.

To confirm a diagnosis of allergic rhinitis, the doctor performs a nasal examination and looks for changes in the mucous membrane. If the patient has allergic rhinitis, the mucous membrane becomes very pale because it is swollen. In fact, it takes on a whitish-blue tint. It is very wet with a watery secretion. A smear of the mucus would be loaded with a type of white blood cell known as an eosinophil, which is very characteristic of allergic diseases, and the patient would have an increase of eosinophils in his or her blood. If the doctor does a skin test or a blood test, called a **RAST test**, which measures an increase in the patient's IgE antibody, both would be positive.

There are two kinds of allergic rhinitis: seasonal and perennial. Seasonal allergic rhinitis characteristically occurs as spring/fall allergies. Springtime begins with tree allergies. Grass is another major springtime allergen.

In the eastern United States, there are few allergens in July and early August, and individuals with allergic rhinitis get better. Pollen from plants that bloom in the summer is spread by the insects, not by the wind, so that is a good time for most people unless they are allergic to molds. Seasonal allergies begin again when ragweed pollinates, starting from mid-August and lasting until the first frost.

Some people also have seasonal allergies to dust during the winter months when the house is closed up and the dust mite feces are richest in the air. But most people with dust allergy have perennial (year-round) symptoms.

Other things that cause year-round allergies are molds. Many people who live in humid areas have damp cellars in which molds form. These molds cause major problems for people with mold allergies.

The other common cause of year-round allergies is allergens from pets. Cats are the worst source of pet allergens, much worse than dogs. The source of allergen from cats is not their fur or skin; it is their saliva, or the proteins in their saliva. And what do cats do all day? They preen. They put saliva on their fur, the saliva dries, aerosolizes, and is the source for the allergen. Dogs—sloppy, friendly little animals that they are—only preen selected parts of their body and are much less likely to expose humans to salivary allergens.

Dogs are still a major source of allergy, especially if they slobber, but if one had to choose between the two, one would choose a dog over a cat. Ideally, allergy sufferers would not have any furred animals in the house because they all cause allergy. Cockroaches also are a major source of year-round allergens.

How Is Allergic Rhinitis Treated?

Seasonal allergic rhinitis generally has a better prognosis because it is not a year-round exposure. It is easier to treat and tends to be much less severe. By contrast, perennial disease tends to be much more difficult to treat and is harder to control.

When treating patients with allergic rhinitis, doctors try specifically to take away the causes of the disease. By using allergy avoidance, they get rid of the allergen and the patient is better. Other common treatments include antihistamines, allergy immunotherapy (allergy shots), a drug called cromolyn sodium, and topical corticosteroids.

To avoid pollen allergens, one must know when the pollen counts are highest. They are generally highest early in the morning, about

6 a.m., on a bright, sunny, breezy day. That is the time allergy sufferers should try to stay inside. If they ride in a car, they should use the car air conditioner. Allergy sufferers should use their house air conditioner, too. Air conditioning filters the air very well, taking out more than 99 percent of all the pollen- and allergen-producing material in the air. If people who are very sensitive during the ragweed, grass, or tree season must go outside in the yard, they should wear nuisance masks, which are like surgical masks and available in drug stores. They are comfortable and will reduce the likelihood of inhaling allergens.

Those with dust allergy should design their bedrooms accordingly. The worst things to have in the bedroom of an allergic person are venetian blinds, which are dust traps; down-filled blankets; feather pillows; heating vents with forced hot air; carpeting; dogs; cats; and closets full of clothing.

Instead of venetian blinds, people should have shades over the windows because they cannot trap dust. If curtains are used, they should be washable curtains that are cleaned periodically in hot water to kill the dust mites. A hardwood or linoleum floor is best, but a washable throw rug is acceptable if it is cleaned in hot water regularly. The bedding should be encased within allergen-proof encasements that are airtight to keep in dust mites, along with their feces. Pillows should be hypoallergenic and replaced every one to two years because when people sleep, they sweat and the sweat makes the pillows moldy over time. Blankets and bedding should be hypoallergenic, definitely not down filled. If at all possible, clothing should be kept in another room. Ideally, the closets would be empty in order to remain dust free. Heat registers should be covered with a filter. New products are appearing in the market that can kill dust mites in carpeting and may prove to be a boon to allergy sufferers.

Allergy shots are extremely effective. Eighty-five percent of the people who receive allergy shots to treat hay fever due to grass, ragweed, trees, and dust get better. It usually takes one to two years. Many people get better for years, and some even permanently. Allergy shots, which are the only known way to turn off allergic disease, reduce the production of IgE and cause the body to make another class of antibody called IgG, which actually protects people from allergic diseases. Shots are the only method available for long-lasting protection from allergies.

Patients with problems only two to four weeks of the year usually are treated with medications. Those with perennial disease are more likely to be put on allergy shots unless their condition can be controlled completely with allergy medications.

There are several medications available to treat allergic rhinitis. One is cromolyn sodium administered in the nose, which prevents allergic reactions from taking place. This drug actually stops the release of chemical mediators like histamine from the mast cell. It is often a very effective therapy. Unfortunately, it must be used about four times a day as a nasal spray.

A second major improvement in therapy of allergic rhinitis has been the use of topical nasal steroids. These steroids are not anabolic steroids. They are anti-inflammatory steroids that stop the late phase reaction. They reduce the number of mast cells in the nose, reduce mucus secretion and swelling, and have other beneficial actions. Because they are given topically, they have no effects elsehere in the body—only in the nose.

The other major medication used is antihistamines. Over the last five or six years, non-sedating antihistamines have become available. These antihistamines are just as effective as older antihistamines, but they do not cause sleepiness. However, they are considerably more expensive than some of the over-the-counter antihistamines.

Antihistamines work beautifully for immediate hypersensitivity. They reduce sneezing, itching, runny nose, and partially reduce the congestion of allergic rhinitis. Unfortunately, they have no effect on late phase reactions. Antihistamines and nasal steroids are effective combinations to treat allergic rhinitis.

Asthma

Fifteen million people—seven percent of those who live in the United States—have asthma. It is the number-one cause for school absenteeism among all chronic diseases. It is the number six cause for hospitalization of all diseases and the number one cause for hospitalization of children.

It is estimated that $4.5 billion is spent every year on medically related charges for the treatment of asthma. That includes hospital and doctor visits. This is an extremely important disease that kills as many as 4,000 Americans a year. Asthma is a disease of the airways, the tubes through which people breathe. The causes of airflow obstruction in asthma are swelling of the airways, excessive mucus production, inflammation of the airways with eosinophils and neutrophils, and airway smooth muscle contraction. Asthmatic airways are full of secretions, mucus containing eosinophils and neutrophils—white blood cells—that reflect the underlying inflammation. The epithelial cells that line the airways have been lifted off and the airways are denuded. The muscles contract, closing the airways, and the glands are very reactive and produce large quantities of mucus.

Asthma is an inability to breathe out. Normally when people breathe in, they lower their diaphragms, raise their ribs, and breathe in. It is an active process. To breathe out, they stop breathing in. Breathing out is passive. They breathe out because the lungs are made of elastic tissue, like a rubber band. When a person stops breathing in, the lungs try to assume their relaxed size and do so by letting the air out, if there is no obstruction.

Asthmatic airways have excess mucus, are swollen and inflamed, and have their muscles contracted. As people with asthmatic airways breathe in, they open up their chests and their lungs get bigger. As a result, the airways get bigger and they can move air around these obstructions. They have opened up the airways. When they stop breathing in to breathe out, these obstructions close, thereby trapping the air in the lungs.

Take a deep breath to the maximum and do not let it out for the next minute. Breathe at the top of your lungs and do not let out any air. That is what it feels like to have asthma. Asthmatics trap 2 liters of air in their chests, which is the amount of air in a basketball. They have to breathe at the top of their lungs. It is exhausting and feels terrible.

What Causes Asthma?

The most common cause of asthma is allergy. Of the children under 16 years old who have asthma, 90 percent are allergic. Of the people under 30 who have asthma, 70 percent are allergic. Of the people over 30, 50 percent have allergies.

Asthma also may be caused by infections such as bronchiolitis, which is a wheezing disease that effects children less than 2 years old and is caused by a viral infection of the airways. This disease leads to asthma; more than half the children who get bronchiolitis have asthma until they are at least 7 years old.

Adults with asthma also get infections that make their asthma worse. They will have colds that commonly develop into bronchitis. Because their lungs are inflamed, the lungs get irritated by a cold very readily and go into an asthmatic attack.

Drugs like aspirin cause asthma in 10 percent of asthmatics. Aspirin and aspirin-like drugs specifically cause asthma in a population of patients that have recurring sinusitis, or infections of the sinuses, and have nasal polyps.

Other drugs that may cause asthma or make it worse are beta-adrenergic blocking agents, which are used for treatment of such conditions as migraine, too rapid a heart rate, congestive heart failure, tremor, and glaucoma.

A third type of agent that may cause asthma is sulfiting agents, which are chemicals that are added to processed foods to keep them from turning brown. If a food should ordinarily turn brown and has not, it has sulfiting agents in it. This includes dried fruits, fruit juices, vegetables, and wines. As sulfites are eaten, they mix with acids in the stomach and become sulfuric acid, which is a gas. The gas travels up through the esophagus, is breathed in, and provokes asthma.

Industrial and occupational exposures also have a bad effect on asthma. On smoggy days, the air is loaded with exhaust from motor vehicles. This is a major source of pollutants, and people with asthma experience increased asthmatic symptoms as a result.

How Is Asthma Diagnosed?

An allergist will do spirometry to measure the patient's ability to blow air out of the chest. The patient takes a deep breath and blows into a machine called a spirometer. The doctor then measures how much and how quickly air was blown out. Most people blow all the air in their chest out within 3 seconds; 75 percent of the air is exhaled within 1 second. The point of maximum expiration is called the "peak flow."

Asthmatics have trouble blowing out the air. That is because of airflow obstruction during breathing out. As a result, they have a very hard time blowing out air and it takes much longer.

Over the past few years, the availability of inexpensive and accurate peak flow meters has made life easier for doctors. Patients can measure their own peak flow in the morning and evening. The patient blows into the flow meter and it measures the peak expiratory flow rate.

For home use it is reliable and inexpensive. A patient can use it before and after taking bronchodilators. It tells the doctor how much the airflow increased with the use of bronchodilators and can be used to regulate medications. It also tells the doctor when the patient is doing well, and warns when trouble is coming.

Airway hyper-responsiveness is increased reactivity of the airways, a "twitchiness" of the airways. Asthmatics have nonspecific airway responsiveness. They react when breathing in certain chemicals, including irritants and chemical mediators, or under certain physical conditions like exercise. The importance of airway hyper-reactivity is that it clearly separates those who do not have hyper-reactivity from asthmatics. Airway hyper-reactivity actually predicts who will develop asthma. Patients who have abnormal hyper-reactivity are very likely to be predisposed to developing asthma under the right conditions.

There is a range of abnormal airway hyper-reactivity among people with asthma, ranging from mild to severe, and doctors can use that range of near normal to very abnormal to determine which medications are required.

Airway hyper-reactivity gets worse with allergic reactions that cause late phase reactions. But airway hyper-reactivity can get better if the patient avoids allergens, goes on allergy shots, and uses inhaled cromolyn or corticosteroids. Recently, it has been recognized that one of the major targets for the treatment of asthma is airway reactivity.

How Is Asthma Treated?

In order to treat asthma and airway reactivity, doctors recommend that asthma patients avoid the allergens to which they are sensitive whenever possible. They put the patients on allergy shots if they have allergic asthma in hopes of reducing the allergic contribution to the asthma. They use inhaled cromolyn, which stops allergic reactions, and often use inhaled corticosteroids, which stop inflammation of the airways and reduce airway hyper-reactivity.

With all patients, doctors also use symptomatic treatment of asthma involving agents that relax the airways. These agents include beta-adrenergic agonists, theophylline, anti-cholinergics, and occasionally expectorants and mucolytics. These medications are employed to try to reverse the airflow obstruction, but they do not have any effect on the underlying causes of asthma.

Until recently, the therapy of asthma was based on the drug theophylline. This drug is an excellent, time-proven, time-tested, and very reliable bronchodilator that opens up asthmatic airways. It was the foundation of asthma therapy from 1970 to 1990.

In the 1980's beta-adrenergic agents became available. These medications relax the airways and make many people better. They became very important in asthma therapy, and have become the predominant drug used to relax airways.

In 1990, asthma therapy shifted so that all asthmatics are now treated with specific therapy aimed at the underlying causes of the disease: allergy avoidance, inhaled corticosteroids, perhaps allergy shots, and perhaps inhaled cromolyn. Nearly all patients use inhaled corticosteroids or cromolyn for the treatment of their airway inflammation. For control of airway obstruction, patients use beta-adrenergic agonists, as well as theophylline and ipratropium, which is an anticholinergic agent. Theophylline, however, has gone from being the foundation of treatment to a second-line therapy. It is added later and taken away sooner.

What about general treatments?

It is recommended that all asthmatics exercise. Some patients have exercise-induced asthma, so it sounds contradictory, but with the proper medications every asthmatic—particularly children—can and should exercise. Swimming is the preferred form of exercise; biking is the second preferred; and running is the least preferred. It is recommended that asthmatics do not smoke, and that people with asthmatic children stop smoking. Patients are advised to monitor their pulmonary function with a home peak flow meter and learn as much as possible about asthma.

Questions and Answers

Nobel Laureate Linus Pauling made mention of the fact that vitamin C has some effect on allergic reactions. What is the latest on that?

Scientifically it has not been proven that vitamin C has any effect, beneficial or detrimental, on allergies. It is not harmful, at least in reasonable doses, but it will not help the disease.

How are food allergies effectively identified and then treated?

Dr. Dean Metcalfe, here at the National Institute of Allergy and Infectious Diseases, screened adults for food allergy, and he found that when people came in and said, "I'm allergic to strawberries," they were likely to be allergic to strawberries. If people came in and said, "I'm allergic to food," they were almost never allergic to food. When people come in and can identify the food to which they are sensitive, we can confirm that by skin testing. In the case of a specific allergen, the skin tests are positive almost all the time. And, if we do a double-blind food challenge, it is frequently positive.

We have many examples where people have said, "I haven't been able to eat eggs for 25 years," and we skin tested them and the tests were negative. We did a provocation challenge, and the only response was they did not care for the taste of eggs. So, the skin test plus a good history is how we screen for food allergies.

Have you ever observed any ophthalmological effects from allergies such as double vision?

The eye is always involved in allergy, but the symptoms are generally itching, swelling, and redness. Eye movement and visual acuity are not affected.

What advice would you give to parents, both of whom suffer from allergies, regarding the introduction of foods for their infant children?

Our instructions are very simple. We would recommend, especially if you have two allergic parents, that solids not be introduced until the children are at least 6 months of age. We recommend exclusive breast-feeding through at least the first 6 months. There is some suggestion that very allergenic foods, like cow's milk and peanuts, should be avoided by the mother during breast-feeding because she can transfer some allergens in her breast-milk. But the opportunity for a child to become allergic to allergens in breast-milk is very limited versus drinking cow's milk. Thus, breast-feeding is highly recommended.

I have two questions. First, what are the possible side effects of allergy medications and how often do they occur? Second, I read that in some cases either asthma or hay fever, or some combination, can be due to emotional problems. Is there any information about that?

The side effects for drugs is a very broad question, very hard to answer, but I can tell you that the agents that we use today have been selected from many others because of their efficacy versus their very limited side effects. And the reason that theophylline is being used less today is because it has some side effects we wish to avoid.

It has often been claimed that asthma is a psychological disease. That is not the case. Asthma is a real, very important disease that can kill you. It may be worsened by psychological stresses, but it is not caused by stress. It is not psychological. The parents of asthmatics often feel very guilty that their child has asthma, and they wonder if it is their fault in some way that influenced their child's asthma. That is not the case.

I would like your comments on sinusitis. Is it associated with allergies?

Sinusitis is an infection of the sinus areas of the skull, which are between the eyes, on either side of the cheeks, in the forehead, and center of the head. They are frequently associated with allergies and the development of sinus congestion; sinus infections are frequent accompaniments of allergy.

What about the long-term effects of corticosteroids? Did I understand you to say that that was no problem?

Corticosteroids have major complications associated with them. In the past, we balanced the use of oral corticosteroids, which have systemic side effects, with the effects of the disease. When the disease was bad enough, we gave oral steroids and accepted the side effects if we had to. Now, with topical, inhaled steroids we have little or no systemic effects, so we get all the beneficial capabilities of steroids with none of the unwanted side effects.

Why do some medications like Benadryl, which you might give a child for hives, say, "Do not give to a child with asthma?" Is it dangerous to give a child Benadryl when he or she has hives and not asthma?

That is an interesting and good question. The classical (older) antihistamines, like Benadryl, if you read the label, are not supposed to be used in asthma. Testing in the early 1950s suggested that antihistamines made asthma worse. So there is a label insert that says they should not be used in asthma. We do not use any of the classical or older antihistamines for the treatment of asthma because they do not work very well. Despite the labeling, however, we do not believe they have any danger for people with asthma.

Some of the new, non-sedating antihistamines do have some efficacy in asthma, and they are being used cautiously for asthma treatment. These new antihistamines have no limitations on their use in asthma and may, indeed, be useful.

I wondered if there has ever been a program to eradicate ragweed.

Yes, there has been. A woman in the Pennsylvania area and her family had terrible ragweed allergies and she organized the community to eradicate ragweed. It did not make any difference because ragweed moves through the air for such a long distance.

Many of the over-the-counter antihistamines say, "Do not take it for more than seven days." If I want to take them longer, should I get a prescription from a doctor?

Antihistamines have been available since the 1940s and many people have taken antihistamines for more than 30 years. They have been among the world's safest drugs. That does not mean that you should use an over-the-counter antihistamine without caution. By and large, we would recommend that everyone would benefit from an appropriate diagnosis and proper therapy, which might include over-the-counter drugs, but might also include prescription drugs, which are really quite a bit more potent and maybe more specific.

—by Michael A. Kaliner, M.D. Head,
Allergic Diseases Section
Laboratory of Clinical Investigation
National Institute of Allergy and Infectious Diseases.

Chapter 2

Understanding the Immune System's Role in Allergic Reactions

The Body's Automatic Defense System

The immune system is a complex network of specialized cells and organs that has evolved to defend the body against attacks by "foreign" invaders. When functioning properly it fights off infections by agents such as bacteria, viruses, fungi, and parasites. When it malfunctions, however, it can unleash a torrent of diseases, from allergy to arthritis to cancer to AIDS.

The immune system evolved because we live in a sea of microbes. Like man, these organisms are programmed to perpetuate themselves. The human body provides an ideal habitat for many of them and they try to break in; because the presence of these organisms is often harmful, the body's immune system will attempt to bar their entry or, failing that, to seek out and destroy them.

The immune system, which equals in complexity the intricacies of the brain and nervous system, displays several remarkable characteristics. It can distinguish between "self" and "nonself." It is able to remember previous experiences and react accordingly. Once you have had chicken pox, your immune system will prevent you from getting it again. The immune system displays both enormous diversity and extraordinary specificity. Not only is it able to recognize many millions of distinctive nonself molecules, it can produce molecules and cells to match up with and counteract each one of them. And it has at its command a sophisticated array of weapons.

Taken from NIH Publication No. 93-529.

31

The success of this system in defending the body relies on an incredibly elaborate and dynamic regulatory-communications network. Millions and millions of cells, organized into sets and subsets, pass information back and forth like clouds of bees swarming around a hive. The result is a sensitive system of checks and balances that produces an immune response that is prompt, appropriate, effective, and self-limiting.

Self and Nonself

At the heart of the immune system is the ability to distinguish between self and nonself. Virtually every body cell carries distinctive molecules that identify it as self.

The body's immune defenses do not normally attack tissues that carry a self marker. Rather, immune cells and other body cells coexist peaceably in a state known as self-tolerance. But when immune defenders encounter cells or organisms carrying molecules that say "foreign," the immune troops move quickly to eliminate the intruders.

Any substance capable of triggering an immune response is called an antigen. An antigen can be a virus, a bacterium, a fungus, or a parasite, or even a portion or product of one of these organisms. Tissues or cells from another individual, except an identical twin whose cells carry identical self-markers, also act as antigens; because the immune system recognizes transplanted tissues as foreign, it rejects them. The body will even reject nourishing proteins unless they are first broken down by the digestive system into their primary, non-antigenic building blocks.

An antigen announces its foreignness by means of intricate and characteristic shapes called epitopes, which protrude from its surface. Most antigens, even the simplest microbes, carry several different kinds of epitopes on their surface; some may carry several hundred. However, some epitopes will be more effective than others at stimulating an immune response.

In abnormal situations, the immune system can wrongly identify self as nonself and execute a misdirected immune attack. The result can be a so-called autoimmune disease such as rheumatoid arthritis or systemic lupus erythematosus.

In some people, an apparently harmless substance such as ragweed pollen or cat hair can provoke the immune system to set off the inappropriate and harmful response known as allergy; in these cases the antigens are known as allergens.

Genes and the Markers of Self

Molecules that mark a cell as self are encoded by a group of genes that is contained in a section of a specific chromosome known as the major histocompatibility complex (MHC). The prefix "histo" means tissue; the MHC was discovered in the course of tissue transplantation experiments. Because MHC genes and the molecules they encode vary widely in the details of their structure from one individual to another (a diversity known as polymorphism), transplants are very likely to be identified as foreign by the immune system and rejected.

Scientists eventually discovered a more natural role for the MHC: it is essential to the immune defenses. MHC markers determine which antigens an individual can respond to, and how strongly. Moreover, MHC markers allow immune cells such as B cells, T cells, and macrophages to recognize and communicate with one another.

One group of proteins encoded by the genes of the MHC are the markers of self that appear on almost all body cells. Known as class I MHC antigens, these molecules alert killer T cells to the presence of body cells that have been changed for the worse—infected with a virus or transformed by cancer—and that need to be eliminated.

A second group of MHC proteins, class II antigens, are found on B cells, macrophages, and other cells responsible for presenting foreign antigen to helper T cells. Class II products combine with particles of foreign antigen in a way that showcases the antigen and captures the attention of the helper T cell.

This focusing of T cell antigen recognition through class I and class II molecules is known as MHC (or histocompatibility) restriction. [For a more in-depth discussion of the immune system, its components and its function, please see Omnigaphics' *Immune System Disorders Sourcebook* (1996).]

Allergic Disorders

The most common types of allergic reactions—hay fever, some kinds of asthma, and hives—are produced when the immune system responds to a false alarm. In a susceptible person, a normally harmless substance—grass pollen or house dust, for example—is perceived as a threat and is attacked.

Such allergic reactions are related to the antibody known as immunoglobulin E. Like other antibodies, each IgE antibody is specific; one reacts against oak pollen, another against ragweed. The role of

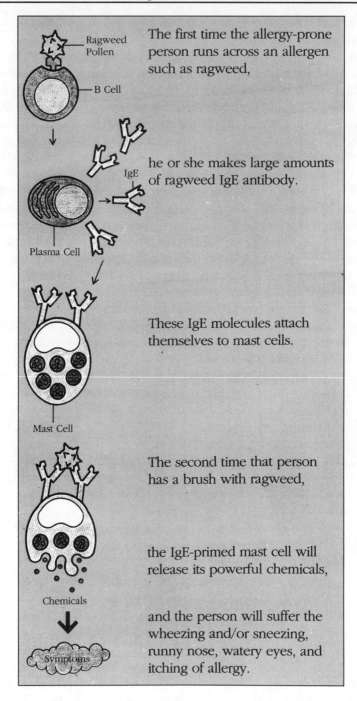

Figure 2.1. *An inappropriate immune response triggers an allergic reaction.*

IgE in the natural order is not known, although some scientists suspect that it developed as a defense against infection by parasitic worms.

The first time an allergy-prone person is exposed to an allergen, he or she makes large amounts of the corresponding IgE antibody. These IgE molecules attach to the surfaces of mast cells (in tissue) or basophils (in the circulation). Mast cells are plentiful in the lungs, skin, tongue, and linings of the nose and intestinal tract.

When an IgE antibody sitting on a mast cell or basophil encounters its specific allergen, the IgE antibody signals the mast cell or basophil to release the powerful chemicals stored within its granules. These chemicals include histamine, heparin, and substances that activate blood platelets and attract secondary cells such as eosinophils and neutrophils. The activated mast cell or basophil also synthesizes new mediators, including prostaglandins and leukotrienes, on the spot.

It is such chemical mediators that cause the symptoms of allergy, including wheezing, sneezing, runny eyes, and itching. They can also produce anaphylactic shock, a life-threatening allergic reaction characterized by swelling of body tissues, including the throat, and a sudden fall in blood pressure.

—by Lydia Woods Schindler

Chapter 3

Research Directions for Allergic Diseases

Allergic diseases are currently among the major causes of illness and disability in the United States. It is estimated that more than 20 million Americans suffer from allergic disorders. Allergic diseases such as allergic rhinitis, or "hay fever," may cause only mild discomfort. However, sensitivity to a substance such as penicillin or bee venom can lead to a severe, potentially life-threatening, allergic reaction known as anaphylaxis. What our immune system perceives as an allergen varies according to the individual. For example, although most people can eat seafood safely, some individuals suffer severe allergic reactions to certain types of shellfish. The details of this discrimination process remain a mystery. However, production of the antibody IgE is known to trigger the mechanism of allergic response (figures 3.1 and 3.2). After IgE has initiated this response, special cells produce substances that are ultimately responsible for the symptoms and discomforts of allergies. Although scientists have devised treatments for the symptoms of allergic responses, they do not yet totally understand several crucial aspects of this response. To develop innovative therapies and strategies for inducing immunologic tolerance, scientists need to elucidate the mechanisms of allergen recognition; the cascade of immunophysiologic events and its consequences on the entire immune system and, thus, the well-being of the host; and the environmental agents that are responsible for the development of allergic responses.

NIH Publication No. 91-2414.

Overview

Recent advances in molecular and cell biology, as well as current research in the disciplines of biochemistry, genetics, pharmacology, and immunology, have provided new insight into the etiology and pathogenesis of allergic diseases. This understanding is important because allergic diseases represent one of the major causes of illness and disability among the U.S. population. Allergic diseases range in severity from allergic rhinitis, which may produce symptoms of mild nasal discomfort, to asthma and anaphylaxis, which can be life-threatening. Food, drug, and occupational allergies, as well as urticaria (hives), angioedema, and atopic dermatitis, are among the many clinical conditions that have similar immunopathogeneses. Research that addresses selected mechanisms of allergic responses would enhance the ability of scientists to develop innovative therapeutic interventions for these and other allergic diseases.

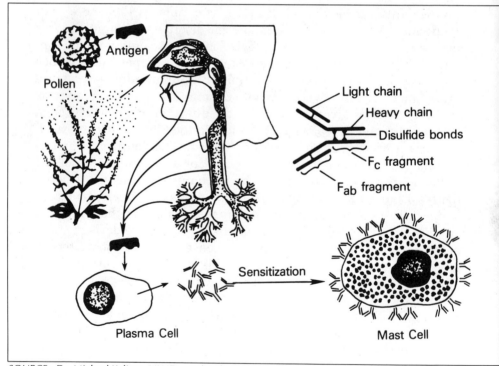

SOURCE: *Dr. Michael Kaliner, NIAID; used with permission.*

Figure 3.1. *Sensitization*

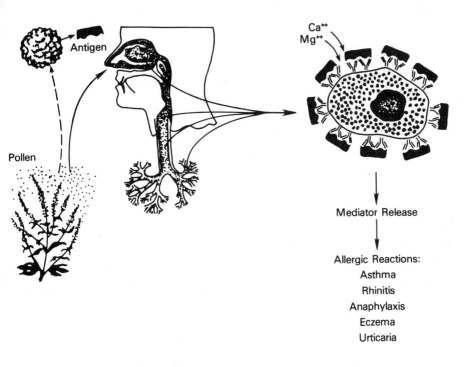

Mediator Release

Allergic Reactions:
Asthma
Rhinitis
Anaphylaxis
Eczema
Urticaria

Figure 3.2. *Allergic Response*

IgE Synthesis and Control

Production of IgE antibodies underlies all immediate hypersensitivity allergic disorders. These disorders typically result from the synthesis of specific IgE antibodies to relevant environmental allergens. Recent findings indicate that IgE synthesis is regulated by a series of interleukin molecules that facilitate or suppress IgE antibody production. These molecules offer the opportunity for disease intervention by inhibiting IgE production, thereby ameliorating symptomatic disease. In addition, the induction of specific immunologic tolerance remains an important goal for the alleviation of IgE-mediated disorders.

39

Research Opportunity

- Decipher the cellular mechanism that controls the synthesis of IgE in allergic and non-allergic subjects, and uncover opportunities for therapeutic intervention that use this mechanism.

Activation and Control of the Secretory Process in Allergic and Inflammatory Diseases

Traditionally, antiallergy therapy has focused on counteracting the effects of inflammatory mediators at their final site of action. Current evidence suggests that directly targeting the secretory process may be a more effective antiinflammatory strategy. This management approach to a wide variety of allergic and inflammatory diseases depends on precise knowledge of each step in the secretory process by which these cells are activated and controlled. Researchers need to emphasize the study of both intrinsic biochemical cascades and biological communication among inflammatory cells as well as between these and other cell types such as lymphocytes and neurons.

Research Opportunities

- Elucidate the biochemistry of secretory events in key inflammatory cells such as mast cells, basophils, and eosinophils.

- Develop the pharmacology of extrinsic modulation by endogenous substances as well as novel therapeutic agents.

Biochemical Cascades and Biological Communication Among Cells in Inflammation

Immunologists have learned that both immediate allergic reactions and allergic diseases involve an inflammatory response within the tissues, which is initiated by the interaction of IgE and the allergen at the cell surface of mast cells and basophils. However, allergic diseases also involve a late-phase inflammatory response in which the products of mast cells trigger the recruitment of other cell types, including neutrophils, eosinophils, lymphocytes, and monocytes. Further cell-to-cell communication leads to cell activation and secretion. These reactions involve a variety of substances, including cytokines, histamine-releasing factors, prostaglandins, leukotrienes, platelet-activating factor, kinins, cell adhesion molecules, chemotactic factors, and presumably other, uncharacterized factors. The process also is modulated by the secretory products of adjacent nerve endings. Variants of this inflammatory reaction underlie the tissue inflammation seen in allergic rhinitis, asthma, chronic urticaria, and atopic dermatitis. However, scientists still need to elucidate the specific role of these cell types, to identify the critical substances that are secreted by these cell types, and to describe the relationship of these events to specific allergic symptoms. Deciphering this cascade of events is critical to understanding allergic diseases and to developing an array of new therapeutic approaches.

Research Opportunity

- Uncover the cell-to-cell communication that leads to the development of the late-phase inflammatory response, including the role of cytokines, histamine-releasing factors, and neurohumoral modulation.

Innovative Therapeutic Interventions For Allergic Diseases

Recent advances in molecular biology have allowed scientists to determine the precise molecular mechanisms of critical cell function. These findings have provided new opportunities for developing highly selective interventions for allergic diseases. Regulatory molecules now can be synthesized in large quantities and used to modulate inflammatory pathways. Alteratively, synthesized antagonists or monoclonal antisera can be used to neutralize excess amounts of proinflammatory endogenous biochemicals. Both of these approaches have demonstrated clinical efficacy for treating malignancies and selected immunodeficiency states. Further research is needed to adapt these approaches to the therapy of allergic and inflammatory diseases.

Research Opportunity

- Employ recombinant molecules as therapeutic agents for allergic diseases. These agents should target critical interactions, including the binding of IgE to its receptor, the interaction of cytokines and their receptors, and the switch to IgE synthesis.

41

Selective and Defined Characterization of Immunogens

We are continually exposed to an increasing array of environmental agents that may cause disease. Immunologists have identified and characterized only a small number of these diseases, such as adverse reactions to certain foods and allergic responses to specific drugs. Little is known about the immune response to drugs, including virtually all antibiotics other than penicillin. Scientists also have insufficient knowledge of the metabolites of drugs to which allergic response may be directed; therefore, they lack diagnostic reagents. Furthermore, the precise means to identify "at-risk" individuals are limited.

Foods can cause allergic responses as well as several other types of adverse reactions. Scientists need to learn more about specific allergenic substances; the nature and control of the immune reaction to foods; and the role of foods as precipitants of, or contributors to, gastrointestinal reactions, atopic dermatitis, chronic urticaria, anaphylaxis, and asthma. A variety of substances in the work environment may interact with the body's proteins, become immunogenic, elicit an immune response, and cause disease. These manifestations of disease can be a consequence of either cellular or humoral immunity but typically are a combination of both. To improve our ability to diagnose and treat these types of allergic diseases, scientists need more information about the specific biochemistry of environmental agents and the response that they elicit in the host.

Research Opportunity

- Characterize the environmental agents responsible for the development of immune responses that lead to allergic and other environment-triggered diseases. Include the study of agents that are responsible for drug reactions, food allergy and intolerance, occupational lung disease, anaphylaxis, urticaria and angioedema, and atopic dermatitis.

Bibliography

Alam, R.; Welter, J.B.; Forsythe, P.A.; Lett-Brown, M.A.; Grant, J.A.. Comparative effect of recombinant IL-1, -2, -3, -4, and -6, IFN gamma, granulocyte-macrophage colony stimulating factor, tumor necrosis factor alpha, and histamine-releasing factors on the secretion of histamine from basophils. *Journal of Immunology* 142: 3431-3435, 1989.

Austen, K.F. The anaphylactic syndrome. In: *Immunological Diseases,* 4th edition, edited by M. Sampter, D.W. Talmage, N.M. Frank, K.F. Austen, and H.N. Claman. Boston: Little, Brown and Company, p. 1119, 1988.

Golden, D.B.K.; Marsh, D.G.; Kagey-Sobotka, A.; Addison, B.A.; Freidhoff, L.; Szklo, B.; Valentine, M.D.; Lichtenstein, L.M. Epidemiology of insect sting allergy. *Journal of the American Medical Association* 246: 240-244, 1989.

Hanifin, J.M. Epidemiology of atopic dermatitis. In: *Epidemiology of Allergic Diseases,* edited by H. Schlumberger. Basel, Switzerland: S. Karger, p. 116, 1987.

Ishizaka, K. Control of IgE synthesis. In: *Allergy Principles and Practice* (3rd ed.), edited by E. Middleton, Jr.; C.E. Reed; E.F. Ellis; N.F. Adkinson, Jr.; J.W. Yunginger. St. Louis: C.V. Mosby Co., p. 52, 1988.

Kaplan, A.P. Urticaria and angioedema. In: *Allergy,* edited by A.P. Kaplan. New York: Livingston, p. 439, 1985.

Proctor, E.F.; and Anderson, E.B., eds. *The Nose.* Amsterdam: Elsevier Biomedical Press B.V., 1982.

Proud, D.; Togias, A.; Naclerio, R.M.; Crush, S.A.; Norman, P.S.; Lichtenstein, L.M. Kinins are generated *in vivo* following nasal airway challenge of allergic individuals with allergen. *Journal of Clinical Investigation* 72: 1678, 1983.

Smith, P.L.; Sobotka, A.K.; Bleeker, E.R.; Traystman, R.; Kaplan, A.P.; Garainick, H.; Valentine, H.P.; Permutt, S.; Lichtenstein, L.M. Physiologic manifestations of human anaphylaxis. *Journal of Clinical Investigation* 66: 1072-1080, 1980.

Chapter 4

The Socioeconomic Impact of Allergies and Asthma in the United States

Overview

Allergic and immunologic diseases are among the leading causes of illness and disability in the U.S. population. More than one out of every ten persons is reported to have a condition related to immunologic illnesses. Table 4.1 lists more than 30 diseases that demonstrate immunopathology as their underlying mechanism. Several of these, such as asthma or rheumatoid arthritis, affect millions of individuals. Other immunologic conditions, such as scleroderma, combined immunodeficiency syndrome, or Wegener's granulomatosis, occur less frequently. However, when viewed collectively, even these less prevalent immunologic diseases constitute a significant disease burden within the U.S. population.

This chapter reviews how immunologic diseases affect the health of the U.S. population. The first section reviews current knowledge about the overall prevalence, morbidity, disability, and mortality associated with selected immunologic conditions. The second section presents a case study of the economic impact of a specific immunologic disease, asthma. The third section focuses on how immunologic diseases disproportionately affect two vulnerable subsets of the U.S. population: children/young adults and minorities.

This review is based on readily available data sources. Whenever possible, the information has been extracted from U.S. population-based surveys. Some of the surveys provide information on a variety

Taken from NIH Publication No. 91-2414. A special report to the NIAID Task Force on Immunology and Allergy.

Figure 4.1. U.S. hospitalizations for selected immunologic diseases and conditions.

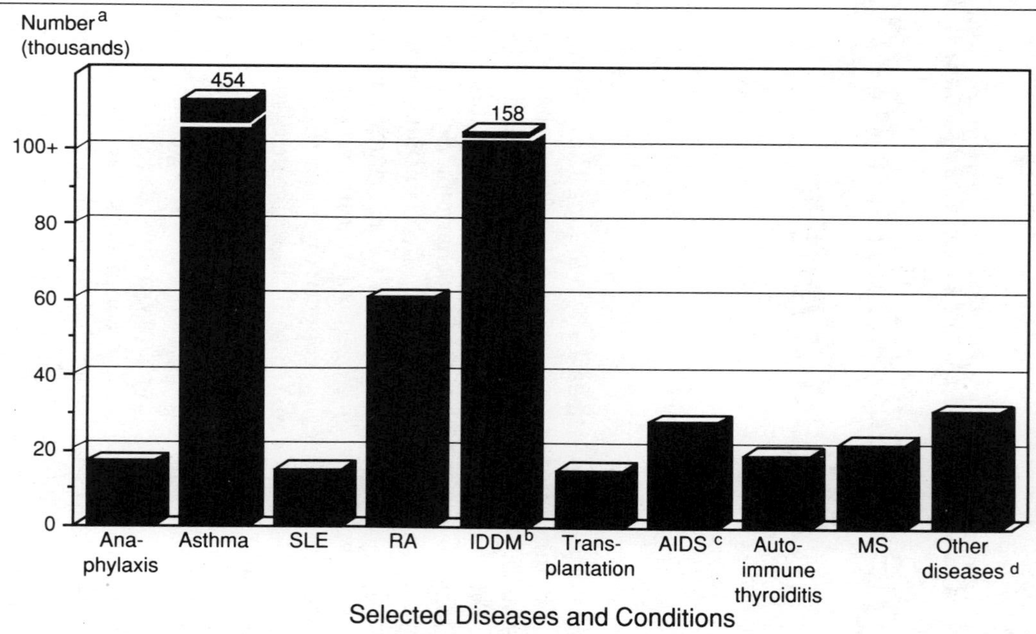

[a] *Based on 1987 Hospital Discharge Survey data, first listed diagnosis (10).*
[b] *Insulin-dependent (type I) diabetes mellitus; see text.*
[c] *AIDS hospitalization based on 1985 estimate (11).*
[d] *Selected other diseases, including urticaria from allergies, hemolytic anemia, myasthenia gravis, contact dermatitis and other eczema, and "other diseases of the immune system."*

46

Table 4.1. *Immunologic diseases, by organ site*

Allergic diseases
  Allergies—insect, food, drug, environmental
Immunologic diseases involving the respiratory system
  Allergic rhinitis/hay fever
  Chronic sinusitis
  Asthma
  Hypersensitivity pneumonitis
Collagen vascular diseases
  Vasculitis syndromes, including Wegener's granulomatosis
  Systemic lupus erythematosus
  Cutaneous lupus
  Scleroderma
  Eosinophilic fascitis
  Panniculitis
  Dermatomyositis/polymyositis
Immune endocrinopathies
  Autoimmune-mediated thyroiditis
  Autoimmune-mediated diabetes mellitus (type I)
  Autoimmune-mediated primary adrenal insufficiency

Immunologic diseases involving the hematopoietic system
  Immunodeficiency diseases
  Acquired immunodeficiency syndrome
  Autoimmune hemolytic anemia
  Idiopathic thrombocytopenic purpura
  Plasma cell disorders
  Amyloidosis
Immunologic diseases involving the nervous system
  Multiple sclerosis
  Guillain-Barré syndrome
  Myasthenia gravis
Immunologic diseases involving the connective tissue
  Rheumatoid arthritis
  Ankylosing spondylitis
  Sjögren's syndrome
Immunologic diseases involving other organ systems
  Eczema/allergic dermatitis
  Immune complex diseases
  Immunologically mediated renal diseases

of immunologic conditions; for example, figure 4.1 summarizes U.S. Hospital Discharge Survey information for several immunologic diseases. However, many of the population-based surveys are not designed to provide comprehensive information on every disease. Therefore, our understanding of the socioeconomic impact of many immunologic diseases is based on fragmented information that has been obtained from smaller, community-based studies. Although substantial information may be gained from this type of review, many critical data on the impact of immunologic diseases are currently unavailable.

Impact of Selected Allergic Conditions

The conditions that are often referred to as allergic diseases represent one of the largest causes of illness and disability in this country. The diseases range in severity from allergic rhinitis, with its clinical expression of moderate nasal discomfort, to asthma or anaphylaxis, where death may be sudden and unexpected. The exact number of persons in the United States who are affected by allergic diseases is uncertain; however, a composite of related information suggests the impact of these conditions. Table 4.2 lists the estimated number of people in the United States who are affected by selected allergic conditions.

Data from NHANES II (the second National Health and Nutrition Examination Survey) provide an estimate that more than 40 million Americans—1 out of every 5—are reactive to at least one of eight selected antigens that are known to contribute to allergic illness (1). Immunotherapy—in this context, defined as the use of allergy shots—is a common drug intervention that is used frequently in ambulatory care for allergic diseases. More than five million allergy shots are prescribed annually for children with asthma and allergic rhinitis (2).

Allergic Rhinitis. Allergic rhinitis, often referred to as hay fever, is a common disorder that affects an estimated 19.6 million individuals in the United States (3). This disorder is the principal reason for more than 8.4 million office visits to ambulatory care physicians. Approximately two-thirds of such visits are by individuals with chronic allergic rhinitis (4).

Ninety percent of the office visits for allergic rhinitis result in medication therapy, which accounts for more than 10.5 million prescriptions annually. Antihistamines constitute the class of drugs prescribed most frequently for this condition (62 percent of all therapy) (5). However, antihistamines are often purchased without prescription,

Allergic Condition	Estimated Number Affected[a]
Allergic rhinitis	19.6 million persons (3)
Chronic sinusitis	32.5 million persons (3)
Contact dermatitis and eczema	5.8 million annual office visits (3)
Allergy immunotherapy	5.4 million administrations to children annually (2)
Skin rashes and allergic skin reactions	12 million annual office visits (4)
Asthma	9 to 12 million persons with active disease (3, 8)
Anaphylaxis and allergic reactions	1 to 2 million episodes annually (6)

[a]*Numbers in parentheses refer to reference list on page 75.*

Table 4.2. *Impact of selected allergic conditions on the U.S. population. ([a]Numbers in parenthesis refer to reference list at the end of this chapter.)*

and therefore the estimated number of prescriptions issued annually for allergic rhinitis is probably a gross underestimate of the total drugs used for this condition (5).

Chronic sinusitis. Chronic sinusitis is the most prevalent allergic disease, with 32.5 million persons reporting this condition (3). Contact dermatitis and other eczemas represent a group of allergic conditions that account for 5.8 million office visits to physicians annually. Concern about skin rashes and allergic skin reactions produces 12 million office visits each year (4).

Anaphylaxis. Anaphylaxis is one of the most dramatic expressions of an allergic disorder—a severe allergic reaction that can lead to the sudden death of an apparently healthy person. An estimated 1 to 2 million people experience severe allergic reactions to insect stings each year (6), and anaphylactic reactions to penicillin are responsible for an estimated 1 to 7.5 deaths per million population (7).

Anaphylactic reactions can occur also from exposure to many other antigens, so the full impact of this condition on the U.S. population is unknown.

Economic Impact of Allergies. Much remains to be learned about the effects of allergic diseases on the U.S. population. In general these conditions are an infrequent cause of hospitalization and mortality; therefore, the national surveillance systems, such as hospitalization and mortality surveys, provide limited insight with respect to the importance of allergic diseases. Furthermore, the economic costs of most of these common illnesses have not been determined. Nevertheless, allergic diseases unquestionably constitute one of the Nation's most common and expensive health problems.

Asthma

Like other allergic diseases, asthma usually is expressed clinically as a chronic illness and is often associated with significant disability. However, unlike other allergic diseases, asthma frequently causes severe morbidity and occasionally causes death. The estimated number of individuals affected with asthma varies according to epidemiologic definition. The information most often used is derived from NHANES II or the National Health Interview Survey (NHIS). On the basis of these two surveys based on 1987 Census data, it is estimated that between 9 million and 12 million persons in the United States have asthma (3,8). There are no national data sources to estimate the incidence of this disease.

Asthma is associated with significant disability. It is responsible for more than 18 million restricted activity days annually, confining individuals to bed for more than 6 million days each year (9). In 1985, asthma was responsible for 6.5 million visits to private physicians and accounted for nearly 1 percent of all office visits to ambulatory care physicians (4). These visits generated 11.5 million prescriptions for drug therapy (5). Additional ambulatory services for asthmatic patients included nearly 5 million visits to hospital outpatient clinics and more than 1.5 million emergency room visits (9).

The clinical expression of asthma can lead to severe morbidity and occasional mortality. In 1987, asthma was the first-listed diagnosis for more than 450,000 hospitalizations (10). Rates for asthma hospitalization in the United States increased 9 percent between 1982 and 1986. Furthermore, in 1981, there were 4,360 deaths from asthma reported in the United States. (Data from 1987 mortality, underlying cause of death, U.S. Vital Records, National Center for Health Statistics.) Although asthma deaths are still infrequent, mortality rates have increased 66 percent since 1980. Non-Whites are almost three times as likely as Whites to die from asthma (8,12,13).

Unlike the case with most other allergic diseases, detailed information has been compiled on the economic impact of asthma in the United States.

Economic Impact of Immunologic Disease: Asthma as a Case Study

With few exceptions, documented information concerning the economic costs of [immunologic diseases] is scarce. Because the most extensive available data are about asthma, this condition is considered in detail here to provide insight regarding the economic costs of immunologic diseases. The estimated costs of asthma can be separated into two broad categories: direct costs and indirect costs. The direct costs for asthma are measured as medical care expenditures. These costs include an estimated $1.3 billion in hospital charges for inpatient, outpatient, and emergency room visits; over $270 million in physician charges for inpatient and private office visits; and $900 million for prescription medications. No available data support estimates of other associated expenditures, such as diagnostic services, nonprescription medications, home health care, or long-term care. The total estimated direct medical expenditures for asthma in 1985 approached $2.5 billion.

The indirect costs associated with asthma include the loss of income from disability and mortality. Loss-of-income figures are derived from both days away from work, absenteeism caused by the need to care for a sick child, and the imputed value of foregone housekeeping. These costs amount to $1.4 billion. An additional indirect cost of illness is based on the reduction of lifetime earnings because of death, $676 million. For asthma, these indirect costs exceed $2 billion annually. Therefore, as summarized in table 4.4, the total estimated annual costs associated with asthma exceed $4.5 billion (1985 dollars). (Based on analysis by Weis, Gergen, and Hodgson—unpublished report.)

The figures in table 4.3 provide a gross estimate of the total economic costs of asthma within the United States. However, they do not give any insight into the economic impact of the disease on affected individuals and their families. A recent study examined the costs associated with the management of childhood asthma, and the results indicate that an average family with a moderately severely asthmatic child will spend 6.4 percent of its yearly income on asthma-related expenses (24).

	Direct medical expenditures ($ millions)
Hospital charges inpatient, outpatient, and emergency room	$1,295
Physician charges inpatient and private office	271
Medications	905
Diagnostic services	n/a
	Indirect costs ($ millions)
Disability through work and school loss	1,417 [a]
Mortality	676
Total estimated costs	$ 4,564

[a] *See text.*

[8] *Based on analysis by Weiss, Gergen, and Hodgson (unpublished report).*

Table 4.3. *Economic Impact of Asthma, estimated direct and indirect costs, 1995.*

Allergic Diseases and Asthma in Children and Young Adults

Immunologic diseases affect persons of all ages and most often are clinically expressed as conditions of chronic morbidity and disability rather than conditions associated with significant mortality. Another important aspect of these diseases is their unique impact on children and young adults. One way to view the impact of immunologic diseases in this younger population is through health care utilization. Table 4.4, for example, shows that in 1980 to 1981, immunologic diseases accounted for 10.5 million, or nearly 1 out of 10, office visits to U.S. pediatricians (2).

Allergic conditions are the immunologic disorders that occur most frequently in childhood. In the United States, there are more than 3 million asthmatic children who are 3 to 11 years old (8), and nearly 40 percent of all physician office visits for asthma are by patients in this age group (2). In addition, more than 5.4 million allergy injections are delivered annually to children by pediatricians (4). In fact, allergy injections are the single most common drug therapy mentioned for pediatrician office visits of all children more than 6 years of age (2).

Asthma is more prevalent among Black children who are 6 to 11 years old than among White children of the same age (rates of 9.4 and 6.2 percent, respectively) (26). In addition, asthma hospitalization and mortality rates are both higher for Blacks than for Whites, and for Blacks the rates are disproportionately increasing (8, 12, 13, 27). Recent evidence suggests that U.S. asthma mortality rates are highest among urban minorities (13, 28). The levels of morbidity and disability related to asthma within other minority populations are not well known; however, the costs of asthma appear to affect minorities disproportionately because these groups tend to be poor. As previously noted, the average family with a moderately severely asthmatic child will spend 6.4 percent of its yearly income on asthma-related costs; for low-income families, however, these costs amount to nearly 12 percent of yearly income (24).

Conclusions and Recommendations

Immunologic conditions represent a broad spectrum of diseases that affect many organ systems. When viewed collectively, these diseases affect nearly 10 percent of the U.S. population. Although only a few immunologic conditions are fatal, most of these illnesses are clinically expressed through years of relentless morbidity and disability. Thus, the economic costs of immunologic diseases differ from those of other diseases. For example, a large proportion of costs for diseases such as cancer and heart disease are related to loss of expected years of life. However, as table 4.4 [on the next page] illustrates, the economic costs of immunologic diseases such as asthma consist primarily of direct medical expenditures and disability. Therefore, the socioeconomic impact of these diseases can be quantified best by measuring the use of ambulatory care and disability such as school days or work days lost.

	Percentage of All Office Visits	Number of Visits (in thousands)
Asthma	2.7	3,415
Allergic rhinitis	2.5	3,162
Allergy immunotherapy	0.9	1,112
Allergies, unclassified	0.8	1,057
Contact dermatitis and eczema	1.3	1,723
Insulin-dependent diabetes mellitus	n/a	n/a
Other immunologic diseases	n/a	n/a
Total	8.2	10,469

SOURCE: **NCHS, Patterns of Ambulatory Care in Pediatrics: The National Ambulatory Medical Care Survey.** *U.S., January 1980-December 1981.*

Table 4.4. *Office visits by children to physicians for selected immunologic diseases.*

References

1. Gergen, P.J.; Turkeltaub, P.C.; Kovar, M.G. The prevalence of allergic skin test reactivity to eight common aero-allergens in the U.S. population: results for the Second National Health and Nutrition Examination Survey. *Journal of Allergy and Clinical Immunology* 80(5): 679-99, 1987.

2. National Center for Health Statistics; Cypress, B.K. Patterns of Ambulatory Care in Pediatrics: The National Ambulatory Medical Care Survey, United States, January 1980-December 1981. *Vital and Health Statistics*, series 13, no. 75. DHHS Pub. no. (PHS)84-1736. Washington, D.C.: U.S. Government Printing Office, Oct. 1983.

3. National Center for Health Statistics; Moss, A.J., Parsons, V.L. Current Estimates from the National Health Interview Survey, United States, 1985. *Vital and Health Statistics*, series 10, no. 160. DHHS Pub. no. (PHS)86-1588. Washington, D.C.: U.S. GPO. Oct. 1986.

4. National Center for Health Statistics; Nelson, C., McLemore, T. The National Ambulatory Medical Care Survey, United States, 1975-81 and 1985 Trends. *Vital and Health Statistics*, series 13, no. 93. DHHS Pub. no. (PHS)88-1754. Washington, D.C.: U.S. GPO, Oct. 1988.

5. National Center for Health Statistics; Cypress, B.K. Medication Therapy in Office Visits for Selected Diagnoses: The National Ambulatory Medical Care Survey, United States, 1980. *Vital and Health Statistics*, series 13, no. 71. DHHS Pub. no. (PHS)83-1732. Washington, D.C.: U.S. GPO, Oct. 1983.

6. Reisman, R. Insect sting allergy in children. In: *Current Therapy in Allergy, Immunology and Rheumatology*, edited by L.M. Lichtenstein and A.S. Fauci. Toronto: B.C. Decker, Inc., 1988.

7. Idsoe, O.; Gruthe, T.; Wilcox, R.R.; deWeck, A.L. Nature and extent of penicillin side-reactions with particular reference to fatalities from anaphylactic shock. *Bulletin of the World Health Organization* 38: 159-63, 1968.

8. Evans, R., et al. National trends in the morbidity and mortality of asthma in the U.S. *Chest* 91(6):65s-74s, 1987.

9. National Health Interview Survey, NCHS, 1983-1987 combined (unpublished data).

10. National Center for Health Statistics; Graves, E.J. Detailed Diagnoses and Procedures, National Hospital Discharge Survey: 1987. *Vital and Health Statistics*, series 13, no. 100. DHHS Pub. no. (PHS)89-1761. Washington, D.C.: U.S. GPO, Oct. 1989.

11. Graves, E.J.; Molen, M. Hospitalization for AIDS, United
     States, 1984-1985. *American Journal of Public Health* 77: 729-
     30, 1987.

12. Sly, R.M. Mortality from asthma, 1979-1984. *Journal of Al-
     lergy and Clinical Immunology* 82: 705-17, 1988.

13. Weiss, K.B.; Wagener, D.K. Changing patterns of U.S. asthma
     mortality: identifying target populations at high risk. *Journal
     of the American Medical Association* (in press): 1990.

14. Lawrence, R.C., et al. Estimates of the prevalence of selected
     arthritic and musculoskeletal diseases in the United States.
     Journal of Rheumatology 16: 427-441, 1989.

15. Felts, W.; Yelin, E. The economic impact of rheumatic diseases
     in the United States. *Journal of Rheumatology* 16: 867-84,
     1989.

16. Yelin, E.; Shearn, M.; Epstein W. Health outcomes for a
     chronic disease in prepaid group practice and fee for service
     settings. *Medical Care* 24: 236-247, 1986.

17. Krolewski, A.S.; Rarram, J.H.; Rand L.I.;, Kahn, C.R.
     Epidemiologic approach to the etiology of type I diabetes
     mellitus and its complications. *New England Journal of Medi-
     cine* 317(22): 1390-1398, 1987.

18. Will, J.C.; Connell, F.A. The preventability of premature mor-
     tality: an investigation of early diabetes deaths. *American
     Journal of Public Health* 78(7): 831-836, 1988.

19. Baum, H.M.; Rothschild B.B. The incidence and prevalence of
     reported multiple sclerosis. *Annals of Neurology* 10: 420-428,
     1981.

20. United Network for Organ Sharing. *Organ Procurement and
     Transplantation Network Annual Status Report to the Health
     Resources and Services Administration: January 1, 1988, to
     December 31. 1988.* Report date: April 21, 1989.

21. USRDS Annual Data Report, 1989.

22. HIV/AIDS surveillance, USPHS, CDC, Division HIV/AIDS, issued October 1989.

23. Winkenwerder, W.; Kessler, A.R; Stolec, R.M. Federal spending for illness caused by the human immunodeficiency virus. *New England Journal of Medicine* 320(24): 1598-1603, 1989.

24. Marion, R.J; Creer, T.L.; Reynolds, R.V.C. Direct and indirect costs associated with the management of childhood asthma. *Annals of Allergy* 54: 31-34, 1985.

25. U.S. DHHS. *Report of the Secretary's Task Force on Black and Minority Health, Volume 1: Executive Summary*. Washington, D.C.: U.S. GPO, 1987.

26. Gergen, P.J., Mullally, D.I.; Evans R. National survey of prevalence of asthma among children in the United States, 1967, to 1980. *Pediatrics* 81: 1-7, 1988.

27. Gergen, P.J., Weiss, K.B. Changing patterns of asthma hospitalization among U.S. children 0-17 years of age, 1979-1987. *Journal of the American Medical Association* 1990 (in press).

28. Weiss, K.B., Wagener, D.K. Geographic variations in the U.S. asthma mortality: Small-area analyses of excess mortality 1981-1985. *American Journal of Epidemiology* 1990 (in press).

29. National Kidney and Urologic Disease Advisory Board. 1990 "Long-Range Plan: Window on the 21st Century" (final draft), November 10, 1989.

30. Division of Health Promotion and Disease Prevention, Institute of Medicine. *New Vaccine Development: Establishing Priorities. Vol. I, Diseases of Importance in the United States*. Washington, D.C.: National Academy Press, 1985.

31. Rice, D.P.; Hodgson, T.A.; Kopstein, A.N. The economic costs of illness: a replication and update. *Health Care Financing Review* 7: 61-80, 1985.

Part Two

Types of Allergic Reactions

Chapter 5

Allergic Rhinitis

Definition, Description, and Importance

Rhinitis, a word derived from *rhin* (nose) and *itis* (inflammation), is an inflammation of the membrane lining the nose. It may result from a number of things: infections, hormones, medications, or an allergic reaction. When inflammation of the nose results from an allergic reaction, the condition is called allergic rhinitis. Evidence suggests that a person's susceptibility to allergic rhinitis is genetically determined.

Years ago allergic rhinitis was misnamed "hay fever," and the phrase has been used since. At that time, hay was falsely believed to cause the disorder, and fever was a term loosely applied to many ailments. Hay fever is not accompanied by a fever, in spite of its name. But, in addition to nasal symptoms, it is not unusual for patients with this problem to experience fatigue, irritability, loss of appetite, weakness, malaise, and even depression.

Allergic rhinitis sufferers know well the symptoms of an attack: a watery nasal discharge, violent sneezing, runny eyes, and an itchy nose, throat, and roof of the mouth. Many experience morning episodes of rapid sneezing, generally 10 to 50 sneezes in a row, that can leave them exhausted. In some, normal sinus drainage is blocked or the eustachian tubes—which connect the back of the throat to the ears—are affected. This may cause hearing problems.

Extracted from NIH Publication No. 80-388.

A 1973 survey estimated that 23.4 million Americans suffered from allergic rhinitis, asthma, or both. In 1975, hay fever sufferers lost more than 3.5 million work days, which cost them more than $154 million in lost wages.

Allergic rhinitis may be seasonal—the traditional hay fever—or year-round. The seasonal form is generally due to pollens from trees, grasses, or weeds. Symptoms appear only during the time of year when the pollens to which the patient is allergic are present. A child with year-round allergic rhinitis can sometimes be recognized by his "allergic salute." This constant upward rubbing of his itchy obstructed nose results, after at least two years, in a permanent crease across the lower part of the nose, another tell-tale sign of a rhinitis sufferer.

Year-round, or perennial, allergic rhinitis results from allergens present all the time. These are usually dust, mold, household contactants, and animal dander.

Chronic rhinitis, however, is not always due to an allergy. The ailment, for example, can be brought about by hormonal conditions such as those during pregnancy. A form called *"rhinitis medicamentosa"* can result from the prolonged use of decongestant nose drops and sprays; certain oral medications, such as the cardiovascular drugs reserpine and propranolol, can also lead to nasal problems. Anatomical abnormalities of the nose, including a deviated septum and nasal polyps, also may lead to chronic rhinitis.

The cause of 60 to 70 percent of chronic rhinitis cases, however, remains undetermined. Physicians have commonly employed a variety of terms—intrinsic rhinitis, vasomotor rhinitis, emotional rhinitis, and stress rhinitis, among others—as diagnoses in those cases where the cause cannot be found. It may be that one mechanism—such as a recently discovered and poorly understood imbalance in the nose's nervous system—may explain all these cases. More likely, however, several different mechanisms cause the same symptoms, just as there can be many causes for a headache. One scientist has microscopically examined small tissue specimens from the noses of rhinitis patients and feels there are 8 to 12 different conditions represented. More work is needed to sort out the diverse mechanisms involved in chronic rhinitis.

Nasal Physiology

The study of the basic processes underlying the workings of the nose is known as nasal physiology. An understanding of nasal physiology is important to understanding rhinitis. Nasal discharge (runny nose) and nasal congestion (stuffy nose) can actually arise from normal responses to the environment. Therefore, knowing what causes these symptoms normally may help us understand what causes the extremely severe or prolonged presence of these symptoms in rhinitis patients.

First, one must look at what the nose does. Aside from serving as a passageway for air to the lungs and its role in the sense of smell, the nose has several major functions. It adjusts the temperature and water vapor content of inhaled air, removes foreign particles and water-soluble gases, maintains clean, moist nasal airway surfaces, and initiates immune processes to protect the body from inhaled foreign materials.

The remarkable effectiveness of these first three functions results from the rich blood supply provided to the nose's mucous membranes and the fluid secretions that line the surfaces of these membranes. Since the air we inhale is subject to frequent changes in temperature and humidity, it is necessary that the nasal blood supply and secretory system be able to adjust rapidly.

This flexibility in adjustment is, in turn, dependent upon the nerve supply to the blood vessels of the nose. Two parts of the nervous system are involved: the **sympathetic (adrenergic) nervous system** and the **parasympathetic (cholinergic) nervous system.** A delicate balance of the two systems is required for the nose to fulfill its function, and yet remain normal.

For example, the nose of a person walking in dry winter air would normally react with a parasympathetic nasal response that increases nasal blood flow and production of mucus; this is necessary to warm and humidify the air being inhaled. Upon entering a warm, moist, indoor atmosphere, the nose must quickly react with a sympathetic response to dry the nose, or the person will continue to experience congestion and mucus secretion, no longer appropriate for the air inhaled.

Thus, any alteration in the timing or degree of these responses can result in disease of the nose. To understand nonspecific types of rhinitis, much more work is needed to determine the role of the blood and nervous systems, and their normal and abnormal responses to various stimuli, including atmospheric conditions and emotional stress.

Airborne Allergens

Science has learned a lot about airborne allergens since their role in allergic rhinitis was first recognized a century ago. But many basic and practical questions remain unanswered. Researchers do know that the solid particles implicated in hay fever are small, usually below 50 microns in size (the width of an average human hair is about 62 microns).

Allergists generally divide allergens into two groups. One comes from outdoor sources in nature and is difficult or impossible to control. The second, more easily controlled, is found in the home or the work place. This division, however, is somewhat artificial and the two groups have overlapping characteristics.

Naturally Occurring Allergens

The naturally occurring allergens primarily include pollens and fungus spores.

Pollens: Pollens, which appear annually, come from trees, such as elms, maples, ashes, oaks, walnuts, hickories, sycamores, and mulberries; grasses, including Bermuda, timothy, and orchard grasses; and weeds, notably the ubiquitous ragweed and, in the Great Plains and Great Basin areas, Russian thistles, sages, and amaranths. Trees generally produce pollen in the spring, grasses in the early summer, and most ragweed species in late summer.

Molds: Molds, which are a type of fungus, release airborne spores. The best recognized are dark-colored microfungi from soil and leaf surfaces. Exposure to dry soil or composting plant materials and such activities as cutting grass, harvesting field crops, or merely walking through tall vegetation may cause rhinitis in mold-sensitive persons. Spores of slime molds, soil algae, and insect debris may also produce an allergic reaction.

Allergens at Work and Home

Allergens in the home or work environment commonly produce a chronic rhinitis without any seasonal increase in severity.

House dust: House dust is the most frequently implicated allergen in the home. Its composition is complex and varies from locale to locale. But vegetable fibers, human skin cells, and tiny insects known as mites dominate most samples. Animal danders and animal products found in the home may also produce rhinitis.

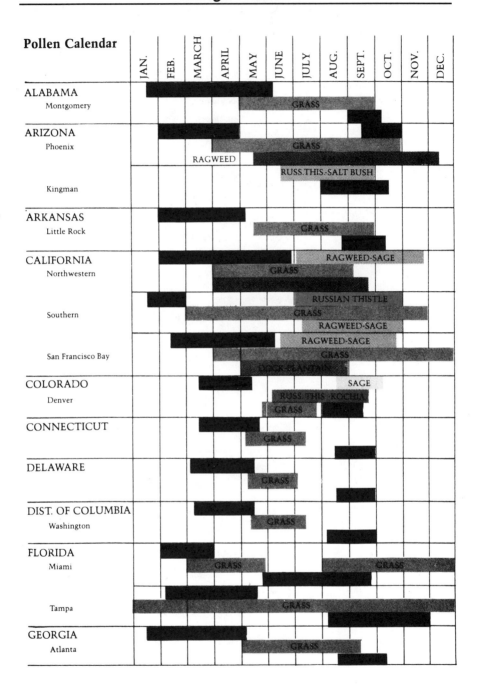

Figure 5.1. Pollen Calendar by State

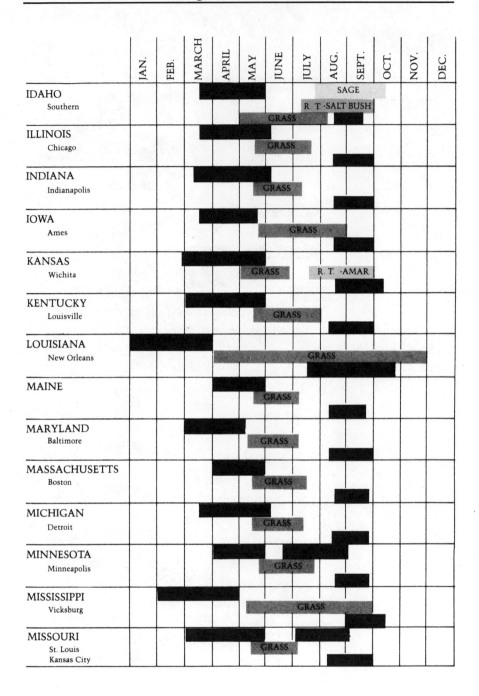

Figure 5.1. *Pollen Calendar by State*

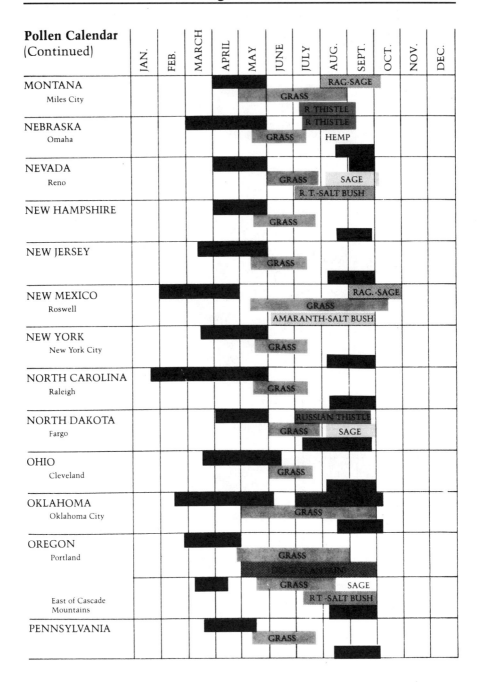

Figure 5.1. Pollen Calendar by State

67

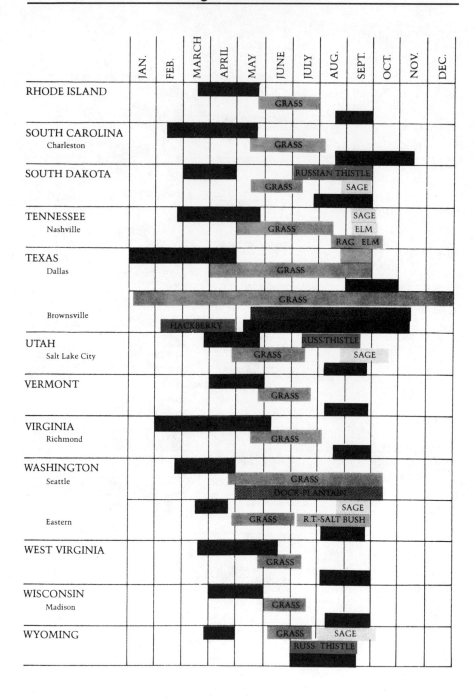

Figure 5.1. *Pollen Calendar by State*

Other Allergens: Other allergens include silk, certain seeds (cottonseed, flaxseed, and castorbeans), and bacterial enzymes, such as those used in some laundry detergents.

Smoke and Fumes: Severe rhinitis may follow exposure to smoke, mists, and fumes from commercial and industrial activities, but these agents seem to function largely as irritants rather than allergens. What remains unknown is whether people with rhinitis are more prone than others to suffer ill effects from such pollutants. *Editor's note: Numerous recent epidemiologic studies have linked second-hand tobacco smoke to cancer and respiratory disease, including asthma and Sudden Infant Death Syndrome. See Omnigraphics' Respiratory Diseases and Disorders Sourcebook.*

Airborne allergens are wide-spread and only limited portions of the continental United States are relatively free even from ragweed pollens. Therefore, relocating to cure one's allergy is usually not the answer and certainly should not be considered without expert medical advice.

However, exposure to many airborne allergens can be reduced. Measures to eliminate dust from the home may be effective, but difficult to follow. Central air conditioning, which allows closed windows, reduces the levels of outdoor allergens found inside homes.

Valuable insights into the role of airborne allergens in allergic rhinitis have been gained by matching clinical observations with measurements of allergens in the air. One study, for example, showed that a pollen count of as little as 20 [grains per cubic meter of air (a little over a cubic yard in volume)] could cause symptoms in grass allergic patients.

Immunologic Response

It is difficult to study an allergic reaction going on inside the body. Therefore, to learn more about these reactions, scientists have tried to duplicate the natural processes by using cells in artificial environments outside the body (i.e., in test tubes). Under these experimental conditions, several interesting findings have been made which may explain what is going on in the nose to cause the swelling, itching, and mucus production during an allergic reaction.

Once a sensitized (made allergic) mast cell encounters an allergen—such as a pollen—the cell releases certain chemicals called mediators.

Figure 5.2. *Air Pollution Sources in the Home*

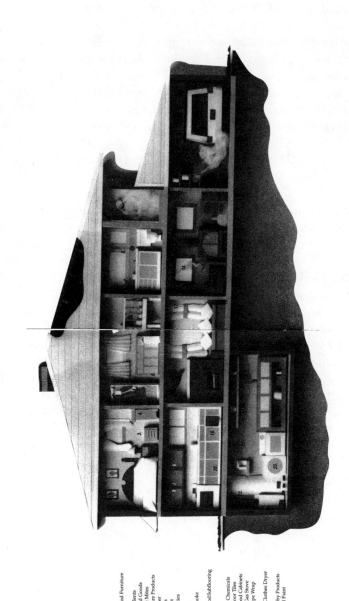

1. Moisture
2. Pressed Wood Furniture
3. Humidifier
4. Moth Repellents
5. Dry-Cleaned Goods
6. House Dust Mites
7. Personal Care Products
8. Air Freshener
9. Stored Fuels
10. Car Exhaust
11. Paint Supplies
12. Paneling
13. Woodstove
14. Tobacco Smoke
15. Carpets
16. Pressed Wood Subflooring
17. Drapes
18. Fireplace
19. Household Chemicals
20. Asbestos Floor Tiles
21. Pressed Wood Cabinets
22. Unvented Gas Stove
23. Asbestos Pipe Wrap
24. Radon
25. Unvented Clothes Dryer
26. Pesticides
27. Stored Hobby Products
28. Lead-Based Paint

These mediators affect surrounding tissues and cause swelling and itching. At least one of these chemicals has a familiar name: histamine. Drugs called antihistamines are already known to combat the effects of allergic reactions. More knowledge about these and other as yet undiscovered mediators and their exact roles in the nose, if any, may lead to the development of more effective medications.

Course, Prognosis, and Complications

Allergic rhinitis can start at any age; it has been newly diagnosed in the elderly and detected in infants as young as 6 months of age. Usually, however, it starts before the age of 40, the peak age of onset being 12 to 15 years.

The disease may range in severity from a petty annoyance during the peak of the pollen season to a condition that makes work or study impossible. Symptoms, in any individual, may vary markedly from year to year, according to geographic location, the amount of inhaled allergens, weather conditions, and a variation in a patient's resistance due to drug or injection therapy. Symptoms may be aggravated beyond the point of tolerance by emotional conflicts. Thus, no one can reliably predict the course and prognosis of an individual patient. Allergic rhinitis sometimes clears spontaneously; but untreated, it usually persists for years, gradually increasing and reaching a plateau.

Sinusitis and nasal polyps are seen occasionally in allergy patients. Some rhinitis sufferers also have, or have had, during infancy and childhood, atopic dermatitis (eczema). It is interesting that some people with positive skin tests do not develop symptoms when they come in contact with the substances that cause their positive tests. Therefore, factors other than the development of IgE which is responsible for positive skin tests must be important in causing hay fever. One study, however, did find that about one-third of symptom-free people who showed positive skin tests had developed symptoms when they were re-evaluated seven years later. This finding may account for people who "suddenly" develop rhinitis when they are older or from contact with a pet that has been in the home for years.

Many allergic rhinitis patients, or their parents, worry about the possibility of later developing asthma. However, in most patients with both allergic rhinitis and asthma, the asthma develops first, or the two ailments appear together. While it is true that children with allergic rhinitis have a greater tendency to develop asthma-like symptoms after exercise, recent investigations suggest the development of asthma is much less a danger than previously thought. A related question concerns the use of immunotherapy in rhinitis patients to prevent asthma.

Diagnostic Procedures

The diagnosis of allergic rhinitis is made presently on the basis of a detailed patient history and, usually, skin tests. These tests involve either injecting a small, diluted amount of each suspected allergen under the skin or applying each substance to a scratch or puncture on the patient's arms or back. In approximately 15 minutes, if the patient has specific IgE antibodies to any allergen, a small raised area surrounded by redness will appear at the allergen's test site. This is called a wheal and flare reaction.

With the development of new methods to identify and measure IgE antibodies, there is increasing interest in perfecting a blood test or some other laboratory test to replace traditional skin testing. Such a test would eliminate the multiple sessions of prick or intradermal injections, thus being particularly helpful for diagnosing children and patients with severe rashes. In addition, this type of test would eliminate patients' reactions to skin-test allergens.

Perfection has not been attained, but two blood tests are in some use. One is called the **radioallergosorbent test (RAST),** and the other is called the **histamine-release test.** The RAST determines how much of a specific kind of IgE antibody is in the patient's blood by measuring its reaction with a disc coated with a pollen or other suspected allergen. The histamine-release test is based on the principle that certain blood cells of an allergic patient will release the mediator, histamine, when these cells are mixed with an allergen that triggers the patient's allergic response. Therefore, measuring the amount of histamine release will give some idea of how allergic the patient is.

Unfortunately, these tests have certain drawbacks. Because they use blood specimens, neither test entirely reflects what is happening in the body's tissues. Testing blood under laboratory conditions is an artificial situation in which many factors may influence the results. There is, for example, a potential interference by antibodies of other classes. Another problem is the difficulty in knowing the condition of the antigen on the disc used in the RAST.

Neither test is as sensitive as skin testing in detecting allergies. Indeed, some patients whose RAST or histamine-release tests show no sign of allergy do have positive skin reactions and the symptoms of allergic rhinitis. However, either of these assays may be of value in cases where skin testing cannot or should not be performed. They are also useful research tools and they, or other tests, may one day be developed to a point where they surpass skin testing.

Drug Treatments

Until the early 1940s, and the general introduction of antihistamines, few drugs existed to relieve the symptoms of allergic and nonspecific rhinitis. Since then, a wide selection of drugs has come into use. These medications have greatly reduced the need for immunotherapy. The development of more effective drugs should reduce further the need for these costly and time-consuming injection treatments.

Allergic rhinitis medications work in one of three ways:

1.   to inhibit histamine;
2.   to block the release of chemical mediators by the mast cells; or
3.   to counteract the effects of the mediators once they are released.

Drugs that inhibit histamine remain the most popular for treating allergic rhinitis. Antihistamines are more effective when given prophylactically or at the first sign of an attack, however, than they are after symptoms develop. They are more effective against nasal discharge than against nasal congestion, and they frequently do little to relieve the itching and watery eyes of hay fever.

There are wide variations in the way patients react to antihistamines, which accounts, in part, for the large number of these preparations on the market. As with most medications, rhinitis drugs may cause undesirable side effects. Antihistamines may produce sleepiness, dry mouth, or blurred vision. In general, the more effective the antihistamine, the greater its chances of producing drowsiness.

One drug that blocks release of chemical mediators has been in use for several years to prevent asthmatic attacks. More recently, it has been tested in the nose and eye against allergies.

Drugs that counteract the effects of the chemical mediators include those that mimic the sympathetic (adrenergic) nervous system (**sympathomimetics** or **adrenergic agents**), drugs that counteract the parasympathetic (cholinergic) nervous system (**anticholinergic agents**), and **anti-inflammatory drugs.**

Sympathomimetics contract the muscles of the blood vessels and are helpful in relieving nasal congestion and itchy eyes. Prolonged use of nasal sprays or drops containing these drugs may produce a "rebound effect" (*rhinitis medicamentosa*). In this, symptoms are at first relieved, but then grow worse, leading to further self-medication. A vicious cycle occurs: as symptoms grow worse, the patient continues to overuse the drug in search of relief. The problem can be corrected by discontinuing the medication. Side effects of the sympathomimetics include rapid heart rate and high blood pressure.

Anticholinergic agents were once popular medications for rhinitis, but are seldom used today because of their side effects of dry mouth and enlargement of the pupils of the eyes.

When traditional drugs fail or their side effects are intolerable, powerful anti-inflammatory agents called **corticosteriods** are highly useful in some patients. The most popular nasal steroid now available in the United States is dexamethasone delivered in an inhaler. While there are no significant side effects from its proper use, it partially suppresses the adrenal system. This ends when use of the drug is discontinued. Research is being conducted on two other steroids which have shown comparably good effects in both seasonal and year-round allergic rhinitis, without the side effect of adrenal suppression.

Long-term use of oral or injected steroids in rhinitis poses a danger of serious side effects. But short-term use of these drugs is often an effective and justified treatment for severe allergic rhinitis. One or two weeks of oral prednisone or a single injection of triamcinolone may produce striking relief.

Drug therapy for allergic rhinitis has expanded in the last 40 years to include an array of medications which evolved as a result of basic research by physiologists, pharmacologists, and immunologists. The current thrust of research in this area lies in developing more effective steroids, nasal sprays, better antihistamines with fewer undesirable side effects, and new drugs based upon the results of basic research.

Immunotherapy

Immunotherapy, developed in the early part of the 20th century, is a standard treatment for allergic rhinitis. In recent decades, the development of new drugs has drastically reduced the need for it. Nonetheless, a large number of people benefit from these "allergy shots."

Immunotherapy was put into widespread use before physicians learned how it worked, how well it worked, and in which cases it was most effective. However, a number of well-conducted studies have now been completed. Over all, they show immunotherapy produces significant effects in rhinitis caused by grass pollen, ragweed pollen, and house dust.

But there has not been uniform agreement in all instances. For example, no significant effect is seen in house dust immunotherapy when relatively low doses or brief courses of treatment are used. Indeed, studies indicate that low-dose immunotherapy is ineffective with all allergens evaluated to date.

One long-advocated use of immunotherapy, in addition to treating symptoms, is for preventing the subsequent development of asthma in allergic rhinitis patients. In the past, this risk has been put as high as 35 percent, or more. It is likely, however, that this is a gross overestimate. A study of one entire community indicated a risk of about 7 percent. The NIAID task force recommended that long-term studies be done to confirm the exact risk of these patients developing asthma and to determine the value of immunotherapy in preventing it. Since drugs and avoidance measures are successful in most allergic patients, the extent to which immunotherapy should be used is controversial. Many experts believe that only a small percentage of patients need this therapy, and that this will decrease as alternative treatments are perfected. Nonetheless, given the enormous prevalence of allergic rhinitis, the absolute number of potential immunotherapy patients appears substantial. Attempts to improve allergy extracts include methods to make them more slowly absorbed so as to decrease the likelihood of an adverse reaction and attain a good response with fewer injections.

Chapter 6

Asthma:
A Severe Allergic Reaction

Bronchial Asthma

People with asthma suffer from a disease that makes it hard for them to breathe at times. For some people, it is a minor problem, but for others it can be life threatening. Bronchial asthma is characterized by a reversible obstruction—a temporary blockage—of the bronchial airways, the tubes through which you breathe. The obstruction is caused by inflammation and mucus in the airways, contraction of the muscles that surround the airways, and airway swelling.

If You Have Asthma, You're Not Alone

Along with its sister allergic diseases, bronchial asthma is among the most common chronic diseases suffered by Americans. Approximately 15 to 16 million Americans suffer from bronchial asthma; between 30 and 35 million have other allergic diseases. In other words, these are very common diseases.

Asthma is often thought to be a benign disease, but about 4,000 Americans die from asthma each year. The group at greatest risk is older asthmatics, above the age of 50; 10 per 100,000 older Americans die each year from asthma. Among the middle-age groups, 1.5 per

---

National Office of Communications, National Institute of Allergy and Infectious Diseases, March 1990, Based on a lecture presented by Michael A. Kaliner, M.D. "What You Need to Know About Asthma."

100,000 people die from asthma each year; but below the age of 9, 2 children per 100,000 die per year from asthma.

Asthma is the number one cause of school absenteeism, and the number one cause of pediatric admissions to the hospital. Overall, for adults as well as for children, it is the number six cause of admissions to all hospitals. There are 10 million office visits per year to physicians' offices for asthma. If you take into account office visits for asthma and allergies, the number becomes 30 million. One out of every nine office visits to physicians in the United States is due to asthma or allergic diseases.

Over-the-counter expenses for drugs to treat asthma exceed $2.3 billion dollars. Including prescription drugs, the expense is greater than $3 billion. Including the expense of office visits and hospitalizations, it's a staggering $4 to $5 billion.

What's Going On?

Asthma is not a problem with breathing in but a problem with breathing out. During normal inhalation, air moves smoothly from the mouth, through the trachea, bronchi, and bronchioles into the alveoli. If you're an asthmatic, you can do the same: you lower the diaphragm, you swing the ribs out, and that makes the lungs bigger. If there is an airway obstruction, the airway opens up and air can slide around the obstruction. However, breathing out is passive. Ordinarily, to breathe out all you do is stop breathing in, and you automatically breathe out. But if you're asthmatic, you can't do that. The minute you relax your ribs and let your diaphragm slide up, the obstructed airways block the airflow and air can't get out. You have a lot of dead air trapped in your lungs, and you end up breathing at the top of your lungs.

The four components that cause asthmatics to have trouble in breathing are secretion of excess mucus, swelling in the airway, inflammation in the airway (white blood cells invade the walls of the airways), and muscle spasm.

If you don't have asthma and want to get a sense of how an asthmatic feels, try this: breathe in. Now, don't let the air out. Hold that deep breath and breathe in and out using only the top of your lungs. You're going to find yourself getting tired. It's uncomfortable to breathe up here, and that's what an asthmatic does. You can relax now, but that exercise gives you an idea of what it would be like to have that trapped air.

Why You Wheeze

Ordinarily, the open airway through which you breathe is empty. The airway itself is lined with ciliated cells, cells topped with little hairs that move mucus. Beneath, there is a very thin basement membrane, an area known as the *lamina propria*, that is fairly devoid of cells. Next there is a thin muscle layer. Around that are submucous glands that secrete about 10 milliliters of mucus a day, about the amount in a tablespoon.

When an asthmatic's airway is full, it contains not only excessive, very sticky mucus but also a lot of other debris, including two kinds of white blood cells-eosinophils and neutrophils. Also, some of the cells that should be lining the airway lift off and resettle in clumps in the airway. Because the cells lift off, the airway itself becomes denuded; it does not have the normal cells that cover and protect it. The airway becomes hyperirritable; like scraped skin, it's sore. When an asthmatic coughs, or breathes in cigarette smoke or irritating fumes, he or she will begin to wheeze—a whistling sound—because the airways are hyperirritable and have constricted.

The basement membrane becomes very thick because of the deposition of additional materials. The area beneath the basement membrane, which has very few cells in the normal condition, grows full of inflammatory cells such as eosinophils and neutrophils. The blood vessels become dilated and full of white blood cells. The muscle layer thickens and muscle contraction occurs. The mucous glands become enlarged and actively secrete mucus that fills up the airway.

What Causes Asthma?

The causes of asthma include allergy, infections, industrial chemical exposures, complications from drugs and chemicals, exercise, vasculitis (inflammatory diseases of the blood vessels), and what are called idiopathic causes.

Allergy

Allergy is the number one cause of asthma. About 90 percent of the people under 10 who have asthma have allergies. If you are younger than 30 and have asthma, there is a 70 percent chance that you are allergic. About half the people over 30 who have asthma have allergies.

How An Allergic Reaction Works

Every tissue in the body has "mast" cells, a name derived from the German "mastung," which means well-fed. Mast cells are most heavily concentrated in the mucous membranes (the skin that lines the nose and the airways), where there are about 10,000 mast cells per cubic millimeter. On the surface of mast cells are many IgE antibodies. Antibodies are proteins made by the body, and ordinarily they protect against invaders like bacteria and viruses. In allergy, a special kind of antibody known as IgE is made by plasma cells and is directed against ordinarily harmless materials like pollen, dust, or food. When mast cells that are sensitized by having IgE antibodies on their surface encounter that antigen or foreign substance, they then trigger the release of histamine and other chemicals from inside the mast cells, and this causes the allergic reaction. You don't exhibit an allergic reaction until you have been exposed to the antigen for a period of time. So, for instance, if you think you are safe because you bought a cat last month and you're not sneezing yet, just wait; you still may have an allergic reaction.

Ragweed is a common plant that can illustrate how this works. Ragweed produces about a billion pollen grains per year, per plant. Ragweed pollen is very light and carried far and wide by wind. When inhaled by an allergic person, the pollen will encounter plasma cells that respond to the pollen by making IgE antibodies. The IgE then coats the surface of the mast cells.

After 2 or 3 years (or seasons) of breathing in an allergen like ragweed pollen, the next time that allergic person breathes in that pollen, instead of simply causing IgE to be produced, the mast cells, now sensitized with IgE, release histamine and other chemicals. These substances released from the mast cells interact with the airways and produce the changes that cause asthma. The same allergy mechanism applies to ragweed, grass, dust, mold, animal allergens, and a variety of other allergens that are inhaled. This can also occur in an asthmatic who is allergic to certain foods. In addition, there are mechanisms in the body that trigger the release of these same chemicals from the mast cells not in response to inhaled allergens or to foods, but to exercise. Asthma that is related to exercise is called exercise-induced asthma, and it does not necessarily involve IgE antibodies at all.

Not everybody is allergic and if you're not, your antibody-producing cells won't make IgE antibodies in response to pollen or other allergens. Allergies are hereditary; if you are a parent with allergies, the likelihood is that one in three or one in four of your children will have allergies. If both parents are allergic, all offspring are likely to be allergic, too.

When is allergy likely to be a contributing factor to asthma?

- when a blood relative—mother, father, sister, brother, aunt, uncle, or child has allergies;
- when the asthma begins at a young age;
- when the asthma symptoms occur or worsen seasonally, such as in fall and spring;
- if other allergic symptoms also occur, such as rhinitis (runny nose), hay fever, or eczema;
- if tests show that the blood and sputum contain an increased number of eosinophils.

Infections

Infections can also cause asthma. Bronchiolitis is a viral respiratory infection that occurs in children younger than two. It is usually caused by one of two viruses—respiratory syncytial virus or parainfluenza virus. A child may get a fairly bad cold and then develop respiratory distress. The child may cough and wheeze and even have croup. About 50 percent of these children, if they have an allergic parent, will go on to develop asthma. Generally, this asthma is fairly mild and is substantially improved before age ten. Nonetheless, it's a very common cause of childhood asthma. Sporadic asthma can occur when people have an upper respiratory tract infection. Many adults only develop asthma as a consequence of a cold, often a cold that leads to bronchitis.

Chemical Causes

Industrial and occupational exposure can lead to asthma. Inhaled substances can act as allergens or as irritants that do not result in IgE production. The most common cause of occupation-related asthma is the inhalation of substances like toluene di-isocyanates, trimellitic anhydrides, and enzymes. Anyone who inhales chemical fumes can develop bronchial irritation or can become allergic to the chemical. It is estimated that as many as 15 percent of asthmatics develop asthma in response to industrial exposure.

A very common cause of asthma is nonsteroidal anti-inflammatory drugs such as aspirin. Aspirin is a very potent drug. The way it takes away pain is to stop the formation of agents known as prostaglandins. There is a whole class of drugs, chemically distinct from aspirin, that acts the same way. About 5 to 10 percent of asthmatics will have asthma triggered by aspirin or other aspirin-like compounds—that includes phenylbutazone, indomethacin, ibuprofen, and other non-steroidal anti-inflammatory drugs.

Patients with aspirin allergy tend to have chronic sinus infections, and often will have nasal polyposis—growths inside the nose. Aspirin-initiated asthma can be a very severe form of asthma. It can be prevented by avoiding aspirin and, in part, by aggressive treatment of the sinuses.

It was once thought that yellow dyes, the F, D, and C No. 5, known as tartrazine yellow, triggered asthma, and, for a while, physicians discouraged patients with aspirin sensitivity from eating foods containing yellow dye. It turned out not to be a real problem. It was also thought at one time that benzoate preservatives could trigger asthma. There is no convincing evidence that this is true.

One group of chemical additives that has in fact been found to trigger asthma attacks in susceptible people is sulfites.

In ancient times, the Romans began adding sulfites to wines as preservatives, and sulfites have been added to wine ever since. People who have asthma or allergies triggered by wine may be sulfite sensitive.

Most people have heard about asthma attacks occurring after someone eats at a salad bar or restaurant. Sulfiting agents (sulfuric acid derivatives) are added to many perishable foods to keep them from turning color. Generally, any fresh food that would turn brown upon standing could have sulfites added to it to prevent that browning. About 5 percent of asthmatics who ingest high concentrations of sulfites will develop a severe asthma attack.

The Food and Drug Administration requires labeling of sulfite-containing foods and prohibits salad-bar restaurants from adding sulfites to their fresh foods. However, other processed foods that are available at salad bars, for example, still may contain sulfites.

- Foods with the Highest Concentration of Sulfites (ppm)

  Pizza Dough 11-20
  Instant Tea 5-6

Wine Vinegar 75
Fresh Shrimp 4-36
Grapes 15
Dried Fruits (Apples, Raisins) 275
Grape Juice 85
Lemon Juice 800
Canned Vegetables 5-30
Instant Potatoes 35-90
Corn Syrup 30
Fruit Topping 60
Molasses 125
Beer 10
Wine 150

Beta blockers (beta adrenergic antagonists) have, since their first day of introduction, been recognized to cause asthma. Beta adrenergic antagonists are used for many purposes, including the treatment of migraine headache, glaucoma, rapid heart rate, high blood pressure, tremors, and many other conditions.

If you have asthma and have been advised to take a beta adrenergic blocking agent, tell your doctor that you have asthma and ask if an alternative drug can be prescribed. There is no question that Beta Blockers will make mild asthma more severe and dramatically complicate the treatment of asthma.

Exercise

Exercise is a potent stimulator of asthma. When you exercise, you hyperventilate by taking rapid, shallow breaths. Just as evaporating water cools the skin, hyperventilation cools the airways. A reflex reaction to this cooling of the airways causes asthma.

Exercise is as important for people with asthma as it is for everyone else. Fortunately, there are effective medications that prevent most exercise-induced asthma. Swimming doesn't cause much of a problem in people with asthma, biking causes somewhat more; and running is the worst type of exercise for asthma sufferers. Swimming is best because you are inhaling very moist air, thereby slowing down the cooling of the airway. If you want to exercise without taking medication, you can wear a surgical mask, enabling you to re-breathe humidified air and avoid asthma symptoms. A proper warm-up period also reduces exercise-induced asthma.

Vasculitis

A rare cause of asthma is a type of vasculitis (inflammation of the blood vessels) known as the Churg-Strauss syndrome. In this disease, which occurs equally among males and females, allergic asthma suddenly and for no apparent reason gets much more severe. It is often diagnosed by an abnormal x-ray, which will show a white patch, indicating infiltration of inflammatory cells into the lungs.

Idiopathic Causes

Often physicians can't determine what is triggering someone's asthma, and they call it idiopathic, which is the medical term for "I'm not sure of the cause." This undefined type of asthma occurs most often in older individuals who have some bronchitis, a lot of excess mucus secretion, and perhaps sinus infection. For lack of a better definition, this is called idiopathic asthma, and it accounts for about 25 percent of the individuals above the age of 30.

Triggers of Asthma

Conditions that trigger asthma symptoms include sinusitis, gastroesophageal reflux, pregnancy, intense emotions, and hyperthyroidism.

Sinusitis

Some asthmatics only have asthma symptoms in relationship to a cold and sinus infection. You'll recognize sinusitis because you will feel mucus dripping down the back of your throat. Often you will have headaches in the sites where the sinuses are, and you may run a fever. Sinusitis commonly causes asthma to worsen. The asthma and the sinusitis should be treated at the same time.

Gastroesophageal Reflux

Gastroesophageal reflux means the backup of acid from the stomach up into the esophagus, or swallowing tube. In this case, asthma generally occurs at night, because when you are lying in bed, acid can leak out of your stomach and into your esophagus, thereby irritating the lining of the esophagus, setting up a reflex reaction in the chest, and triggering night-time asthma.

Pregnancy

Asthma complicates pregnancy about 1 percent of the time; about 1 woman in 100 develops asthma because of her pregnancy. But many asthmatics get pregnant. About half of people with asthma are women. And when those women become pregnant, one-third of them get better, one-third of them get worse, and one-third of them don't change.

In the one-third who get worse, the asthmatic symptoms that occur during the first pregnancy are generally the same in the second, third, and fourth pregnancies.

Fortunately, the asthma medications now in use do not have any bad effects on the unborn baby. Asthmatic patients go on to have normal pregnancies, normal deliveries, and normal children.

Emotions

Intense emotions can trigger asthma. That doesn't mean that asthma is all in your head, it means that psychological stress can cause an asthmatic attack the same way that sinus inflammation and gastroesophageal reflux can.

Hyperthyroidism

Hyperthyroidism, which means over-activity of the thyroid gland, often causes an increase in asthmatic symptoms. It is one of the possibilities doctors consider when an asthmatic who has been stable suddenly gets much worse.

Diagnosis

When a person with asthma symptoms comes into the doctor's office, the doctor usually gives the patient pulmonary function tests, which, for example, measure tidal volume. That is the amount of air you breathe in and out with a regular breath; it's usually about 500 milliliters. The doctor will then ask the patient to take a maximum inhalation and a maximum exhalation. By measuring the maximum expiratory level and the maximum inspiratory respiratory level, the doctor will calculate total lung capacity.

In a healthy person, about 75 to 85 percent of the air comes out within 1 second of a maximum exhalation (blowing out as hard as possible). By 3 seconds, the lungs have been essentially emptied. Asthmatics can't breathe in as much, because they have all that air trapped in the back of their lungs. Even at 6 and 7 seconds, they are still blowing out air. At that point, the normal person would have already been ready to breathe in again. But a person with asthma can't move air out.

Treatment

There are two major ways to treat asthma: by avoiding substances or events that trigger asthma, and by using various medications.

Avoidance

Pets. If an asthma sufferer is allergic, the best treatment is avoidance of the irritating substance. You should avoid cats, for example, if you are allergic to them. The source of allergen from both cats and dogs is saliva. Cats preen themselves, and it's the dried saliva left on their skin that becomes aerosolized and acts as such a potent allergen. Dogs hardly ever clean themselves, so generally a dog turns out to be a much less important source of allergen than is a cat.

People who are allergic to cats should not live with cats. People who are allergic to dogs should not have dogs. But many animal lovers are very attached to their pets. If you must have a dog or cat indoors, at least don't let your pet in the bedroom. Give yourself 8 hours away from inhaling the allergen, if you can. Even birds should be avoided indoors, since feathers are a potent allergen. Feather pillows are another major source of allergy.

Pollen. If you have to be outdoors, recognize that airborne pollen levels are highest in the early morning on bright, sunny, windy days. Use air conditioning in your car during pollen season whenever possible.

Dust. A major source of allergens in dust is the dust mite. This microscopic bug lives mostly during the summer. During the winter, house dust contains parts of dead dust mites and their feces, which are actually the major source of dust allergens.

Dust mites live in wall-to-wall carpeting, in the springs and mattresses of beds, and any place dust collects. You can cover the springs and mattresses with allergy-proof encasements. You can keep table tops free from knick-knacks. Shades are preferable to venetian blinds or curtains. Hardwood floors, or linoleum floors, and washable throw rugs are preferable to wall-to-wall carpeting. Closets are particularly laden with dust, so, if possible, use a clothes closet outside of the bedroom.

Air-filtering Devices. Air conditioning is extremely effective at clearing air particles, so during the pollen season, if you have air conditioning throughout the house, you will be less likely to suffer from allergy-induced asthma.

Electrostatic air precipitators are now safe and effective, although expensive. Older models produced ozone, which, even in very low concentrations cause asthmatic symptoms to get worse, since ozone is an irritant to mucosal membranes—the skin that lines the nose and the bronchi. But room air filters (the most effective ones are known as HEPA filters, high-efficiency particulate activating filters) are less expensive, are very efficient in removing air particles and don't produce ozone. Before buying a filter, rent one for your bedroom and see if it makes a difference.

If you have a choice, hot-water heat or radiator heat is better than forced hot-air heat. Forced hot-air heat distributes dust and mold throughout the house every time it circulates the air; radiators don't do that.

Medications

Cromolyn Sodium. There is a preventive drug for allergies. It is known as cromolyn sodium. It is used in an inhaled form for asthma, in an eye-drop form for allergic eye diseases, and in a nasal spray for allergic rhinitis. What this drug does is prevent the mast cell from secreting the chemicals that cause allergies.

Unfortunately, cromolyn sodium does not work for everybody, but for those persons in whom it works, it works well. For anyone with allergic asthma, this drug is worth a try. It is also excellent for preventing exercise-induced asthma.

Bronchodilators. More commonly used than cromolyn sodium are bronchodilators. Bronchodilators relax the smooth muscles that line the airways, thereby opening those airways, if the muscle is contracted. There are three classes of bronchodilators: anticholinergics, methylxanthines, and beta adrenergic agonists.

- **Anticholinergic Drugs.** Known as atropine or atropine-like drugs, stop the action of acetylcholine, which triggers the muscles to contract. They relax the muscle by blocking its contraction. These are medium-potency drugs, certainly less potent than beta adrenergic agonists. Their duration of action is shorter. They are very important for the treatment of patients who produce excess mucus, and will be very important in the treatment of patients who have chronic pulmonary disease, but they are less important for treating asthma. However, clinical practice, particularly in some children and adults, has shown them to be very effective.

- **Methylxanthines** have been around for quite a long time but have only become popular in the last 15 to 20 years. That's because we now have ways of monitoring methylxanthine blood levels, and we now have pills that can be taken once or twice a day. Therefore, methylxanthines are the major drug used in the United States for the treatment of asthma. The most commonly known methylxanthine is theophylline. People who can't tolerate theophylline can usually take another compound called oxtriphylline. By the way, caffeine, found in coffee and tea, is a derivatve of methylxanthines. Caffeine is a very mild bronchodilator so it wouldn't be effective to treat asthma with coffee or tea.

  Theophylline acts by stopping some of the enzymatic actions in smooth muscle cells and thereby relaxing them. This is a very potent, very popular form of therapy, and there are no long-term complications from its use.

- **Beta Adrenergic Agonists.** The last class of bronchodilators is beta adrenergic agonists. These are drugs related to the chemical adrenaline. When you are frightened, your heart starts beating more rapidly, your airways dilate, and the pupils of your eyes dilate, due to adrenaline. Because adrenaline causes the airways to dilate, scientists were able to modify it into a very specific agent that works only in the lungs, causing them to open without affecting the rest of the body. One of the most impressive things that's happened in the past 15 years in the treatment of asthma has been the creation of inhaled bronchodilators. We can now deposit bronchodilators, like these beta adrenergic drugs, directly into the airways and have the site of action only on the airways. They work very quickly, within minutes, and their effects last up to 6 to 8 hours. So these are the mainstays of therapy. Bronchodilators like methylxanthines and beta adrenergic agonists are the two drugs most prominently used in the treatment of asthma.

Corticosteroids. These are clearly the most effective drugs for the treatment of asthma. However it is important to know how to use them, when to use them, who should use them, how long to use them, and when to stop them. They work by reducing swelling, reducing mucus secretions, stopping inflammation, reducing mast cell number and secretion, and even stopping the production of the IgE antibody.

On the other hand, corticosteroids are powerful drugs with serious side effects: they cause osteoporosis, a thinning of the bones; they cause weight gain; they lead to peptic ulcers; they can cause diabetes and increased infections; in children, they can stop growth.

Should we use them? Knowing how to use them properly minimizes the negative effects. Also over the past 5 to 10 years, inhaled steroids have been introduced; these have been pharmacologically engineered to work only in the lungs and have no systemic action. They work on asthma but don't create side effects. That's been the major breakthrough in the treatment of asthma in the past 10 years. While we once hesitated to use corticosteroids because of their side effects, we now use inhaled corticosteroids on many, if not most, asthmatics because of their safety and effectiveness.

Immunotherapy. Also known as allergy shots, immunotherapy is appropriate in people whose asthma has clear-cut allergic causes that are not adequately controlled with medication and avoidance of triggers. When immunotherapy works, it reduces not only the need for other treatments but also the disease itself.

Peak Flow Meters

In addition to avoidance of triggers and careful use of medications, the use of a peak flow meter can contribute to effective asthma management, particularly in children. This simple device helps patients monitor their own breathing. It measures the peak expiratory flow rate, which means the ability to breathe out quickly. A normal peak flow rate is first determined when an asthmatic child is feeling well, by blowing into the meter as hard and fast as possible several times. This measurement indicates how open the large airways are. The highest reading is recorded.

Peak flow monitoring is usually done several times a day or when the child feels ill. If the rate drops significantly, it may indicate that additional medication is needed to prevent asthma symptoms. Taking medication before severe symptoms are noticeable may prevent a full-blown asthma attack.

Some Myths About Asthma

Though very common, asthma is not very well understood by most people. Misconceptions about its causes and treatment abound. Here are a few of these misconceptions:

"There's no sense treating my child. He's going to outgrow his asthma."

This is both true and false. About 50 percent of the asthmatic children whose asthma develops between the ages of 2 and 10 will not have asthma in their teenage years; they'll have a spontaneous reduction in their asthma. But often the asthma recurs when those people reach their thirties. So it goes away, but it doesn't go away permanently. Lung function tests of former childhood asthmatics show that they still have abnormal airways disease.

Should you wait to treat them? No. Asthma is a serious disease. It impairs the capacity of your child to exercise, it impairs your child's self-image, and it shouldn't be ignored. There are effective ways to treat asthma, and there is no reason to let a child suffer, waiting to get better. Have your child seen by a specialist in asthma and allergies, and have him or her treated adequately.

"Asthma is all in your head." Or, "Parents can cause asthma."

Asthma is not "all in your head," and parents can't cause it. Psychological stress is one of the things that triggers asthma, but that doesn't mean that asthmatics are crazy or that parents are responsible. Emotional stress can make asthma worse, but you shouldn't feel guilty that your child has asthma. Your child has asthma because of other conditions over which you had no control. Psychological stress can trigger asthma symptoms, but it does not cause the disease.

"Asthmatics shouldn't exercise."

Asthmatics should go out and exercise just like their friends. Eight percent of the athletes who represented the United States in the 1988 Olympics had exercise-induced asthma. They were able to perform in the Olympics because of proper medications to prevent asthmatic attacks caused by exercise.

"Allergic mothers shouldn't breast-feed."

In fact, by breast-feeding, you reduce the opportunities for your child to become allergic to foreign proteins. Although breast milk is a distillate of proteins that you've eaten, your breast-fed child has a reduced exposure to non-human proteins. When a baby is born, its gastrointestinal tract is immature and it absorbs proteins that are much larger than proteins absorbed by adults. Adults break those down to very simple amino acids. By absorbing proteins that are macromolecules, the infant's body recognizes these as foreign antigens and makes antibodies to them. That's one reason children have such a high incidence of food allergy. Mothers who are themselves allergic, and therefore are more likely to have an allergic child, should breast-feed for at least 6 months to a year, if at all possible.

"Recurring asthmatic attacks lead to emphysema."

Patients can have asthma all their lives and when they die, their lungs don't show any more damage than those of a non-asthmatic. There are two exceptions to this. There is a rare disease known as alpha-1-antitrypsin deficiency, which is a congenital enzyme deficiency that can present as asthma and leads to a very early and very destructive form of emphysema. The second is an unusual condition called allergic bronchopulmonary aspergillosis, which is an infection in the airways that leads to destruction of the airways. Other than those two very unusual causes of asthma, asthma does not lead to emphysema. Asthma is a fully reversible disease in its uncomplicated state. If you have asthma, don't worry about emphysema, but don't ignore the asthma; you still need to be treated.

"Smoking does not affect asthma."

Asthmatics should not smoke. Inhaling someone else's smoke is also harmful to an asthmatic because smoke further irritates the airways. Parents should be very concerned. Recent studies suggest that children of smoking parents are at greatly increased risk of developing asthma.

"Certain foods can cause asthma."

Clearly, foods can cause allergies, but they are rarely a cause of asthma. Except in the case of sulfites, foods should not be restricted for asthmatics.

"Over-the-counter drugs are all an asthmatic needs."

If over-the-counter drugs were as potent as prescription drugs, they would not be sold without a prescription. Over-the-counter drugs are used much more than prescription drugs for asthmatics because they are easier to get to and they don't necessarily involve the expense of an office visit, but you sacrifice potency and specificity in the treatment. The drugs that are available over-the-counter are mild, non-specific agents that are mild bronchodilators, far less potent and far less effective than the drugs you can get by prescription. If you or your child has asthma, you should see a specialist, an allergist, or a pulmonologist who understands asthma and its treatment. As stated earlier, the two major advances in asthma treatment in the past 20 years, inhaled steroids and beta adrenergic agonists, are both prescription-only drugs.

Research

At many research institutions around the country, including the National Institute of Allergy and Infectious Diseases, scientists are working to better understand the mechanisms involved in asthma, to develop new and improved treatments for asthma, and to find better means of preventing asthma symptoms. We have come a long way in our search to improve the quality of life for people with asthma and certainly hope that we will make even more progress in the decade ahead.

For Further Information

American Academy of Allergy & Immunology
611 East Wells Street
Milwaukee, WI 53202
1-800-822-ASMA

American College of Allergy & Immunology
800 E. NW Highway, Suite 1080
Palatine, IL 60067
1-800-842-7777

American Lung Association
1740 Broadway
New York, NY 10019

Asthma & Allergy Foundation of America
1717 Massachusetts Avenue, NW, Suite 305
Washington, DC 20036
1-800-7-ASTHMA

Mothers of Asthmatics
10875 Main Street, Suite 210
Fairfax, VA 22030
(703) 385-4403

Based on a lecture presented by Michael A. Kaliner, M.D. Chief, Allergic Diseases Section Laboratory of Clinical Investigation, National Institute of Allergy and Infectious Diseases, National Institutes of Health.

Chapter 7

Sinusitis: A Painful Response to Allergies and Infections

sinusitis/si-na-sit-as/n: inflammation of a sinus.

This simple definition gives little indication of the misery and pain caused by sinusitis, nor of the millions of dollars Americans spend each year for medications that promise relief of their symptoms.

Sinuses are hollow air spaces, of which there are many in the human body. But when people say, "I'm having a sinus attack," they usually refer to one or more of four groups of cavities known as paranasal sinuses. These are located within the skull or bones of the head surrounding the nose.

The Sinuses Are Obsolete Troublemakers

It's amazing how many parts of the human body don't seem to have any useful purpose. No one knows for certain why these air pockets in the skull exist. It has been suggested that, at one time in human development, they aided the sense of smell—a distinct advantage for those of our ancestors who depended on their noses to sense danger or seek food.

Other theories suggest that the sinuses may have evolved to play a role in vocalization, or that they produce protective mucus for the nasal cavity, equalize pressure changes in the nose during breathing,

FDA Consumer, Dec. 1984-Jan. 1985 and NIH Publication No. 77-540.

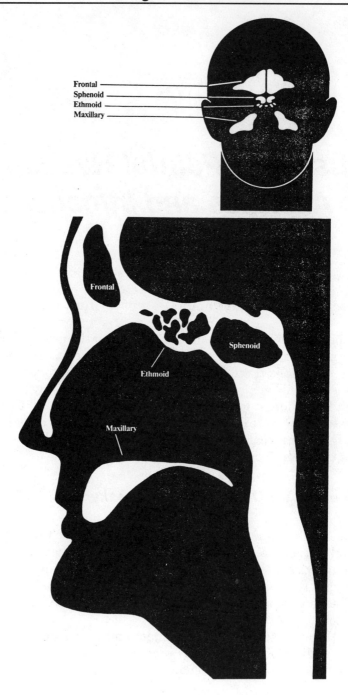

Figure 7.1. The sinuses

or even serve to make us a little more lightheaded. For many people who suffer bouts of sinusitis, these air spaces have only one purpose—to cause misery.

The sinuses are hollow spaces in certain bones of the skull. They usually come in pairs, one on each side of the head, and are individually identified by their location. The frontal sinuses are just over the eyes; the maxillary sinuses, largest of the lot, are in the maxillary (the upper jaw bone); and the ethmoid sinuses are located in the ethmoid bone, situated just back of the eyes. The ethmoid sinuses are the only multi-compartmentalized or honeycomb type of sinus. Deep in the head, at the back of the nasal cavity, are the sphenoid sinuses, located in the sphenoid bone.

Although they are paired, the sinuses are not necessarily symmetrical. The frontal sinuses, in particular, come in different sizes and shapes in different people and can also vary in the same person. Some people may have no frontal sinuses at all. The frontal sinuses are the only ones that cannot be seen on X-rays of newborns. Girls develop sinuses earlier than boys; men have larger sinuses than women.

Each sinus has an opening into the nose for the free exchange of air and mucus and each is joined with the nasal passages by a continuous mucous membrane lining. Therefore, anything that causes a swelling in the nose, be it a viral or bacterial infection or an allergic reaction, can similarly affect the sinuses. Air trapped within an obstructed sinus, along with pus or other secretions, may cause pressure on the sinus wall. The result is the intense pain of a sinus attack. When air is prevented from entering a paranasal sinus by a swollen membrane at the opening, a vacuum can be created with a similar end result of pain.

The symptoms of acute sinusitis are very much like those of a bad cold. The patient has a runny nose (the discharge may be pus-filled), headache and discomfort. What distinguishes the sinus infection is localized pain plus tenderness and disturbances of taste and smell.

The Sinus Pain Signal

Sinusitis carries its own localized pain signals, depending upon the particular sinus affected. If the maxillary sinuses are involved, the pain is felt in the cheek on the affected side. Sometimes this pain radiates to the ear on that side, to the opposite side of the face, or to the forehead. There also may be toothache, tenderness over the sinus area, and slight swelling of the lower eyelid. Putting the heel down hard while walking can jar the head and cause pain in the involved sinus.

Pain in the frontal sinus area in the forehead is relentless and severe and can be aggravated if the patient bends forward or if the head is jarred. Often the pain starts before or just after rising in the morning and persists for a few hours until it diminishes in the early afternoon. It is not unusual for a patient to have nearly incapacitating pain in the morning, yet feel perfectly well in the afternoon. It is believed that relief comes as a result of changes in pressure related to posture.

There is no facial swelling with frontal sinus infection, except for an occasional slight swelling of the upper eyelid. Tenderness over the affected area can be felt when pressure is applied.

Infection of the ethmoid sinuses causes pain behind and between the eyes and a frontal headache that is often described as "splitting." The upper and lower eyelids may be swollen.

Sphenoid sinusitis is often hard to diagnose, since the pain is not conveniently localized. It can occur behind the eyes, in the forehead, in the back of the head, or in an odd site such as over the canine teeth. The headache of sphenoid sinusitis is throbbing and can come and go with a change of position. It is usually worse in the morning. There may be malaise—a vague feeling of discomfort—and a variety of nasal problems, such as obstruction, runny nose or postnasal drip.

The pain of chronic, or persistent, sinusitis is dull and lingering in contrast to the sharp pain of acute sinus disease. Headache may be a feature of chronic maxillary sinusitis. Chronic disease involving the ethmoid sinuses tends to be associated with nasal polyps—outgrowths of the mucous membrane inside the nose.

Chronic disease in the frontal sinuses can take one of two forms. One is a recurring but minor sinusitis characterized by mild tenderness and persistent headache with intermittent drainage in the nose. The second form is a mucocele, a cyst in the respiratory lining that continues to secrete mucus painlessly, expanding the sinus and the thin surrounding bone. These cysts can break through the wall of the eye socket, resulting in swelling of the upper eyelid and displacement of the eyeball.

Sinusitis can be diagnosed by the patient's symptoms, feeling of swollen or tender areas, X-ray examination, and transillumination. This last procedure, which takes place in a dark room, involves a hooded light being placed in the patient's mouth. With the patient's eyes open, if the sinuses are normal, the doctor should be able to see a contraction of the pupils and a crescent of light corresponding to the position of the lower eyelids. With the eyes closed the patient should have a sense of light in the eyes. If not, the sinuses are probably affected. Transillumination is useful only in diagnosing frontal and maxillary sinusitis.

Viral, Bacterial and Fungal Infections

Any virus that enters the body through the nasal passages can set off a chain reaction resulting in the misery of a sinus attack. For example, the common cold, influenza, and measles all cause congestion in the nose.

When this swelling involves the adjacent mucous membranes of the sinuses, air and mucus are trapped and, unless the sinuses are open enough to permit drainage, an attack of acute sinusitis occurs.

Many types of viruses cause the "common cold." Eighty-nine distinct types of rhinoviruses already classified are believed to cause a majority of the common cold symptoms that appear in September and October. Another family of viruses, the coronaviruses, is also known to cause many of the colds adults suffer in midwinter, from December through February.

But only one-third to one-half of the colds that occur can be traced to a specific virus; in the other colds studied, the infectious agent has not yet been isolated. Some of the 32 types of adenoviruses (so named because they were originally found in the adenoids) cause acute respiratory illness, especially in young children who live in institutions or boarding schools and in military recruits in training camps.

Bacterial organisms also can contribute to sinus infections. Staphylococcal and streptococcal infections in infants usually begin with symptoms in the upper respiratory tract. *Hemophilus influenzae,* a bacterial organism, attacks the nose and throat and can settle in the maxillary sinuses; if untreated, this condition may persist for months in a chronic form. The organism also can cause a very acute infection of the ethmoid sinuses.

Many apparently healthy people harbor certain bacteria in their upper respiratory tract with no apparent ill effects until the body's defenses are weakened or drainage from the sinuses is impeded by a cold or other viral infection. Then the bacteria that may have been lurking harmlessly in the nose, throat, or sinus area move in to create a secondary infection in the same location.

Still another form of respiratory tract disease that can involve the sinuses is caused by the family of fungi known as *Mucoraceae.* Although these organisms are abundant in the environment, scarcity of the infection in healthy individuals indicates that there is a natural resistance to them. The fungi are found most often in patients with uncontrolled diabetes, those with such blood ailments as leukemia, or individuals who have been treated for a considerable period of time with steroids. Because more such patients live longer than was previously the case, incidence of *Mucoraceae* disease is increasing.

Sinusitis in Allergic Patients

The combination of allergic and infectious sinusitis has long been considered the most difficult form of sinus disease to treat. The patient with uncontrolled nasal allergies frequently experiences a high degree of congestion, swelling, excess secretions, and discomfort in the sinus areas.

An allergic individual is one who is highly sensitive to certain substances with which he comes in contact. These substances are known as allergens. Inhaled allergens, such as dust, molds, animal hairs, or the pollens of trees, grasses, and weeds, often set off the allergic reaction that, in turn, contributes to a sinusitis attack. As body cells react against these foreign substances, chemical compounds, such as histamine, are liberated at the mucosal surface. This, in turn, produces swelling and blockage of the nasal passages and sinuses.

Drugs, too, can set off a nasal reaction with accompanying sinusitis. For example, intolerance to aspirin has frequently been noted as an associated condition in patients with bronchial asthma, nasal polyps, and sinusitis.

Conversely, sinusitis caused by bacterial infections often seems to be associated with asthmatic attacks. One study, conducted at Scripps Clinic and Research Foundation in California, indicated that of 160 asthmatic patients examined, nearly 50 percent without demonstrable allergies were found to have bacterial infections of the sinuses.

Prevention of Sinusitis

Although all sinus disorders cannot be prevented any more than all colds or bacterial infections can be avoided, certain measures can be taken to reduce the number and severity of the attacks and possibly to prevent the condition from becoming chronic.

Appropriate amounts of rest, a well-balanced diet, and exercise can help the body function at its most efficient level and maintain a general resistance to infections.

Many sinusitis victims find partial relief from their symptoms when humidifiers are installed in the home, particularly when the room air is heated by a dry forced-air system.

Air conditioners help to provide an even temperature and electrostatic filters attached to heating and air conditioning equipment are valuable in removing dust and pollen from the air.

Cigarette smoke and other air pollutants should be avoided by a person susceptible to sinus disorders, particularly one who is also allergic. Allergic inflammation in the nose predisposes a patient to a strong reaction to all irritants. Since alcohol causes a swelling of the nasal-sinus membranes, its ingestion should be curtailed.

Sinusitis-prone individuals may be uncomfortable in swimming pools treated with chlorine, since this substance is irritating to the lining of the nose and sinuses. Divers often experience congestion and infection when water is forced into the sinuses from the nasal passages.

Air travel, too, poses a problem for the individual suffering from acute upper respiratory disease, chronic sinusitis, or allergic rhinitis. A bubble of air trapped within the body expands as air pressure in a plane is reduced. This expansion causes pressure on surrounding tissues and can result in a blockage of the sinuses or eustachian tubes. The result may be discomfort in the sinus or middle ear during the plane's ascent or descent. Use of decongestant nose drops or inhalers before flight are recommended to avert this difficulty.

If a person suspects that his sinus inflammation may be related to an allergic reaction to dust, mold, food, or pollen—or any of the hundreds of allergens that can trigger a respiratory reaction—he would be wise to seek his physician's referral to an allergist. Such a specialist can perform certain tests to determine the substances to which a patient is allergic and recommend various steps to reduce or limit the allergic manifestations.

It may be necessary to prescribe medications or to eliminate certain foods or medications from the diet. In severe conditions, in which the patient does not respond to routine medical therapy, a series of desensitization injection treatments may be attempted. Materials for injection are made up of dilute solutions of the causative allergens and, when administered in increasingly larger doses over a period of time, help the body develop immunity to the offending substance, thus lessening sensitivity.

Treatment of Sinusitis

A stuffy nose, though a symptom of sinusitis, occurs in other conditions and many people confuse simple nasal congestion with sinusitis. However, by physical examination and X-rays, a physician can make a precise diagnosis and prescribe a course of treatment that will clear up the source of infection and relieve the symptoms.

Treatment of sinusitis is aimed at re-establishing drainage of the nasal passages, controlling or eliminating the source of the inflammation, and relieving the pain. To accomplish this, the physician may prescribe medication to reduce the congestion, antibiotics to control a bacterial infection, and painkillers to relieve the discomfort.

A sinus infection cannot be cured by home remedies, but the discomfort that accompanies such an inflammation often can be lessened by inhaling steam from a vaporizer or tea kettle. A hot water bottle, hot, wet compresses, or an electric heating pad applied over the inflamed area also can prove comforting.

Stuffy noses can be unstuffed with nonprescription nasal decongestants, usually in the form of drops and sprays. Such products do their job by constricting the tiny blood vessels in the nasal lining, thus shrinking the mucous membranes and promoting drainage. While relief is prompt and dramatic, nasal drops and sprays also pose a threat. Overuse of these products can lead to a phenomenon known as "rebound congestion" in which the mucous membranes become even more congested and swollen than before the spray was used.

An advisory panel of experts reviewing ingredients in nonprescription drugs for FDA said that ephedrine, naphazoline hydrochloride, oxymetazoline, phenylephrine and xylometazoline are safe and effective ingredients for use in nasal decongestants.

Sinus sufferers who use nasal decongestants—sprays, drops or pills—should read the label carefully and follow the directions to the letter.

Severe cases of sinusitis may require special procedures by a physician. One technique requires the patient to lie on his back with his head over the edge of the examining table. A decongestant fluid is placed in the nose, and air is suctioned out of the nose so that the decongestant fluid can shrink the sinus membranes sufficiently to permit drainage. Or, a thin tube can be inserted into the sinuses for washing out entrapped pus and mucus.

Only rarely are more serious surgical operations required. In children, problems often are eliminated by removal of adenoids obstructing nasal-sinus passages. Adults who have had allergic and infectious conditions over the years sometimes develop polyps—small growths on the mucous membrane lining of the sinuses—which interfere with proper drainage. Removal of these polyps and, where necessary, repair of a deviated septum (the bony partition separating the two nasal passages) to insure an open airway often provides considerable improvement.

Research on Related Problems

Sinusitis has been described as both a very complex and very common disease entity. Since a number of infectious or allergic processes can cause sinusitis, it has been reasoned that control or prevention of the underlying cause is the best approach toward eliminating sinusitis symptoms.

One of the medical research arms of the Federal government primarily concerned with the study of allergic disorders as well as viral, bacterial, and fungal infections is the National Institute of Allergy and Infectious Diseases (NIAID) of the National Institutes of Health. An intensified research effort by NIAID began in 1971 with the establishment of a network of Asthma and Allergic Disease Centers throughout the United States. These Centers conduct laboratory experiments and carry out research studies on a variety of allergic disorders.

The common cold often precedes sinus infection. Study of the viruses which have been implicated as common cold agents has been a major research effort of the National Institute of Allergy and Infectious Diseases. The World Health Organization has designated NIAID as an International Reference Center for Respiratory Diseases other than Influenza. Many grantee investigators across the country are engaged in an effort to develop methods to control agents of upper respiratory tract infections.

Scientists at NIAID and elsewhere at one time thought it might be possible to develop a vaccine to prevent a person from being infected by a cold virus. Early in the study of colds it was suggested that a "cocktail" vaccine be developed against the main rhinoviruses, but this idea has not proved feasible. The great number of rhinoviruses and the absence of any one major cold-causing virus have made the possibility of successful vaccination extremely unlikely.

While research continues on the cold viruses, NIAID scientists and their collaborators at medical centers throughout the United States are seeking other approaches to control of the common cold. A promising area of research relates to stimulation of antiviral activity in infected body cells, that is, the production of substances that can halt the ability of a virus to take over the cell's genetic material and reproduce itself. One such antiviral substance being intensively studied is interferon, produced by the body's natural defense system. Several years ago a group of NIAID-supported investigators reported the successful testing of interferon as a preventive of the common cold. However, the scientists cautioned that interferon is still too costly and difficult to recover from cells and is far from being a practical remedy for colds.

In Summary

It would be difficult to persuade a person suffering an acute sinusitis attack or the chronic sinusitis sufferer that his discomfort could point the way to improved health. But this is actually the case. The presence of sinusitis is an indication that an allergic or infectious process is undermining the individual's well being. By consulting a physician who can make the diagnosis and prescribe the proper course of treatment, whether that be allergy therapy or antibiotic medication, the sinusitis sufferer has the opportunity to forestall more serious conditions that may cause irreversible damage.

Chapter 8

Dermatologic Allergies

Introduction

Allergic skin diseases are common and, at times, devastating health problems that have great socioeconomic consequences. In the past 15 years, we have learned a good deal about these disorders, especially those that involve the immune system.

This chapter discusses six skin diseases: atopic dermatitis (eczema), allergic contact dermatitis, urticaria (hives), vesiculobullous (blistering) diseases, vasculitis (inflamed blood vessels), and lupus erythematosus (a skin inflammation associated with other organ involvement). Improved understanding of the immune system has led to a greater understanding of these diseases. And, in turn, the study of each of these ailments has added to our understanding of the immune system. However, further progress in treating these disorders requires a more detailed understanding of their causes and further investigation of their immunologic bases.

Atopic Dermatitis (Eczema)

Atopic dermatitis is a chronic, itching, superficial inflammation of the skin occurring in nearly 7 per 1,000 persons in the United States. This common disease can sometimes have drastic economic, social, and psychological repercussions. About 90 percent of all cases appear between the second month of life and age five.

Excerpted from NIH Publication No. 80-388.

Itching is the major symptom of eczema. Other symptoms include a redness of the skin, swelling, and "weeping" blisters. In its chronic state, the patient's skin thickens, darkens, cracks, and scales. Symptoms most often appear on the neck and face and in the bends of the knees and elbows. Most people rarely need hospitalization for eczema. However, occasionally admissions are necessary to treat severe cases and to control serious infections. No one can predict what course an individual case will take, but many children outgrow eczema. Some heal in infancy, and with most, improvement is common around puberty. However, children with a family history of eczema and those who develop asthma and hay fever are more likely to continue to have eczema as adults.

Eczema can affect occupational opportunities. The results of three studies showed: from 20 to 57 percent of eczema patients were hindered by their disease in their work activities; the disease hindered 30 to 45 percent in selecting a career; and 3 to 20 percent changed jobs at least once because of this disorder.

All evidence indicates that a tendency to develop eczema is inherited and involves more than one gene. The development of the disease depends on factors both inside and outside the body but the cause of eczema is still uncertain.

Eczema is associated with allergic diseases. Most patients also have or go on to develop hay fever or asthma or have a family history of these diseases. Moreover, eczema patients usually have positive skin tests for allergens, and studies show elevated IgE antibodies in 43 to 80 percent of these patients. However, this disease has not been shown to result from an allergic response. Twenty to 57 percent of these patients do not have elevated IgE levels. Also, the ailment can occur in people who are unable to produce IgE antibodies. Furthermore, routine allergy therapy shown to be effective in hay fever has little or no effect on eczema. An important exception to this rule is the possible manifestation of food allergies as eczema, particularly among infants.

Advances in immunology and cell biology have opened new avenues of research in eczema. Recent studies suggest that defects in the body's cell-mediated immunity may be associated with eczema. They include: the finding of an increased incidence of unusually severe skin infections among eczema patients; changes in the functioning of the immune system's white cells associated with the disease; and an association of eczema with certain immune-deficiency disorders.

A number of physiologic features are associated with eczema. Changes in blood vessels, for example, result in a pale, raised welt—called white dermographism—when the skin is scratched or stroked.

Intramuscular injections of histamine produce a greater increase in skin temperature and histamine level in eczema patients than in normal people. Significant variations in several other body chemicals are reported in eczema patients. Whether these changes are a cause or an effect of the disease remains unresolved.

In addition to its unpleasant symptoms, eczema carries a risk of additional complications and problems, including the development of other skin disorders. As mentioned, patients have a high susceptibility to several types of skin infections. Also, severe eczema has associated with it an increased incidence of cataracts.

The major emphasis in treating eczema is the relief of symptoms. Antihistamines suppress itching; and, thus, reduce the scratching that can lead to infection. Moisturizing agents help prevent the drying and cracking of skin. Corticosteroids applied to the skin are the mainstay of therapy. When necessary, antibiotics may be given to treat infections. Some dermatologists recommend that eczema patients avoid soap, which dries the skin, and use a non-alkaline cleanser or grease-free lotion instead. In the most difficult cases, corticosteroids, such as prednisone, may be given orally to combat acute symptoms. Changes in climate—to the mountains, the seaside, or warm, dry areas—usually help only temporarily.

Psychological and physical factors interact in eczema and often create a vicious cycle. Attempts to relate specific psychic disturbances or personalities to eczema have failed. But physicians find that providing psychological support may help patients cope with their disease.

The benefit of immunotherapy in eczema remains unproven. In a recent study, 13 of 16 patients treated with immunotherapy over 2 years showed improvement, as compared to only 4 of 10 patients treated with a placebo. However, other studies have found no benefit in immunotherapy, and several suggest immunotherapy makes eczema worse.

In some cases, physicians may try avoidance, instructing the patient to avoid foods, animal danders, or other possible allergens that a careful medical history suggests may be implicated in the eczema. Avoidance seldom works in eczema, with the exception of elimination of certain foods from infant diets.

Allergic Contact Dermatitis

A type of rash called contact dermatitis can result from an allergic reaction. Symptoms include a red rash, swelling, and intense itching. Blisters may develop and break open, forming a crust. In severe cases, the rash and blisters may spread all over the body.

A variety of substances that touch the skin may cause the disease. These include poison ivy, poison oak, drugs, antibiotics, cosmetics, certain metals such as nickel and chromates, and a number of environmental, industrial, and synthetic chemicals.

Allergic contact dermatitis, or ACD, may develop at any age. Its precise prevalence is unknown, but the disorder probably affects several percent of the U. S. population. The disease may be acute or may become chronic. It is less common than irritant dermatitis, but more serious, since relapses commonly occur and job changes may be necessary.

Symptoms may appear 7 to 10 days after the first exposure to an allergen. More often, the allergic reaction doesn't develop for many years, and may require many repeated low-level exposures. Once the sensitivity does develop, however, contact with the triggering allergen will produce symptoms within 24 to 48 hours. An attack builds in severity from 1 to 7 days. Even without treatment, healing often occurs in 1 or 2 weeks, although it may take a month or longer.

Often ACD's rash will occur in new areas of the body, appearing to "spread." People mistakenly blame fluid oozing from the rash's blisters; but the blister fluid does not carry the rash to other parts of the body, nor can someone else catch the disease from this fluid. The extension of the rash is caused by renewed contact with whatever triggered the initial outbreak. The substance that causes poison ivy is oily. It can contaminate and remain on clothing, or even on the fur of a pet. Thus, a person may come in contact with it several days in a row without actually touching the plant again. As a result, new areas of skin become involved and the victims believe the original rash is spreading.

A common myth is that bathing will spread the blister fluid, and thus the disease. On the contrary, exposed skin should be cleansed thoroughly and clothes washed to get rid of the allergen that triggered and can continue to trigger the ACD. Certain substances, film developers, rubber chemicals, zirconium, mercury, and beryllium, for example, cause symptoms other than the classic red rash and blisters. In some cases, ACD may look like hives.

The disease is a type IV (cell-mediated) allergic reaction. It begins when an allergen binds to the skin and, in susceptible individuals, is recognized as foreign. The immune system responds by producing a variety of white cells, primarily T lymphocytes, to attack the foreign allergen. This response produces the skin inflammation that we call allergic contact dermatitis.

Detailed questioning about the work and leisure activities often pinpoints the cause of ACD. Careful skin examinations are important for identifying possible causes, and because ACD can be mistaken for other skin disorders. Patch tests are the best means of helping to confirm the disease's specific causes. These tests consist of applying suspected allergens to the skin, covering them, and waiting for two days to see if a reaction occurs.

Acute ACD is easily treated with drugs. If the offending allergen can be avoided, the problem will not recur. However, if the allergen cannot be identified or avoided, allergic contact dermatitis may become chronic. In that event, the patient must be treated for chronic dermatitis, while the search for his or her allergen continues.

Urticaria/Angioedema

Urticaria (more commonly called hives) is characterized by red, swollen, intensely itchy blotches on the surface of the skin. If the swelling occurs deeper in the layers of the skin, or in the tissue below the skin, it is called angioedema. The two may appear together, or separately, in any location; however, angioedema most often occurs on the hands, feet, and face. These swellings arise suddenly, rarely persist longer than a day or two, and may recur indefinitely.

Urticaria is a common and bothersome skin disorder that responds poorly to skin medications. More than one-fifth of the population has suffered an eruption at some time in their lives. Urticaria has many causes, both immunologic and non-immunologic. In a very small number of cases, hives may be a symptom of a more serious underlying disease. However, in chronic cases, a vast majority (greater than 70 percent) are of unknown cause. Some cases apparently result from an allergic response, such as to certain drugs and foods. Seasonal hives in people suffering from asthma, hay fever, or eczema also presumably result from an IgE-mediated allergic reaction. Why some people should react with hives to allergens that usually cause respiratory symptoms remains unknown.

Hives sometimes follow the use of aspirin, or foods colored by tartrazine, a yellow food dye (yellow #5). These cases do not involve immunologic reactions, but may stem from an interference with an enzyme called prostaglandin synthetase.

Another mechanism is involved in **hereditary angioedema,** a potentially fatal inherited disease that produces episodic swelling of the face and extremities. In addition, swelling may occur in the tongue, throat, or larynx, shutting off air to the lungs. This disease is associated with a deficiency of a blood protein that is part of the complement system.

An associated disorder is dermographism, a hive that appears when the skin is briskly stroked with a firm object and which may be an allergic reaction involving IgE but without a defined antigen. Swellings that arise after constant pressure on the skin applied by such things as elastic in socks, tight wrist bands, and brassiere straps are termed pressure urticaria. Cold-induced urticaria is a disorder brought on by cold temperatures and is IgE-mediated in at least some cases; rarely, it may lead to shock and death. Solar urticaria follows exposure to the sun or a sun lamp. Another type of hives (cholinergic urticaria) occurs after an increase in body temperature following such activities as exercising or bathing in warm water.

Recurrent episodes of hives, if there is no underlying illness, are best treated with antihistamines. The effectiveness of this treatment varies, and often different types of antihistamines must be tried before one is found that relieves itching and swelling, and prevents further outbreaks.

When the type of disorder can be identified, specific drugs give the best results. For example, acquired cold-induced urticaria frequently may be controlled with the antihistamine cyproheptadine, and cholinergic urticaria may be improved with the antihistamine hydroxyzine. Life-threatening hereditary angioedema can now be treated effectively with hormones. Antihistamine treatment is not always successful in hives. Corticosteroids may help some of these patients, but long-term therapy with these drugs carries the risk of adverse side effects.

Vesiculobullous Diseases

Blistering can be a symptom of any of the several vesiculobullous diseases. The past decade has seen major advances in our understanding of this phenomenon and of three uncommon but debilitating diseases: **pemphigus vulgaris, bullous pemphigoid,** and **dermatitis herpetiformis.** Greater knowledge about these disorders has come from a better understanding of the immune system. The immunological basis for each of the three diseases is probably quite different.

As a result of basic and clinical research, the outlook for people afflicted by these blistering disorders is far better than it was 10 years ago. New diagnostic techniques allow physicians to diagnose the diseases earlier and with greater certainty. New therapies have reduced disability and death.

Pemphigus Vulgaris. This rare, chronic disease has now been documented in all races and ethnic groups. Thin, flaccid blisters form on normal appearing skin. The disease usually begins in the mouth, and involves the mucous membranes. Ruptured blisters heal slowly, if at all. The exact mechanisms causing this disease are unknown. However, some studies suggest involvement of immune complexes with local activation of complement. Other studies indicate that "pemphigus antibody" in the absence of complement can induce blister formation.

Before drugs were found to combat the disease, about half its victims died in the first year or two after onset. Recent studies report death rates of 9 to 24 percent, and several research teams now report remissions of longer than 2 years in patients. The disease can be controlled with high doses of corticosteroids. More recently, a combination of corticosteroids and immunosuppressive drugs has proven effective.

Bullous Pemphigoid. This disorder occurs mostly in the middle-aged and elderly. Firm blisters with reddened bases form, mostly on the neck, groin, and armpits. Recently physicians have found the disease may occur as isolated blisters on only one part of the body, especially the lower legs. As in pemphigus vulgaris, studies of this blistering disease suggest a role of local complement activation. In addition, most of these patients have been found to have an antibody directed against a layer of skin known as the **basement membrane.**

Bullous pemphigoid is disabling, but rarely fatal. The disease responds well to corticosteroids, alone or in combination with immunosuppressive drugs. Treatment usually lasts 4 to 6 months; thereafter, many patients go into prolonged remission.

Dermatitis Herpetiformis. Chronic, debilitating, but not fatal, this disease may occur at any age. Firm blisters with reddened bases form in small groups, most often on the buttocks, lower back, shoulders, elbows and knees. These cause intense itching.

IgA antibodies appear to play a role in the disease, and immune complexes have been detected in many patients. The complement system also appears involved. A significant number of patients suffer bowel disorders, but the relationship between the gut and skin diseases is unknown.

Several drugs provide prompt relief; symptoms may abate in as little as three hours after treatment. A gluten-free diet corrects gastrointestinal problems associated with dermatitis herpetiformis in many patients and in a few, gluten avoidance helps their skin disorder.

Cutaneous Necrotizing Angiitis

This is a chronic form of vasculitis, or inflammation of the blood vessels. Small, solid elevations, dusky red to purplish, appear on the skin and do not blanch when pressed. Hives (mostly in women), nodules, blisters, ulcers, tissue death, and a mottling of the skin are less common symptoms.

The disease produces itching or burning, and, occasionally, pain. Patients may also suffer fever or malaise. Symptoms may recur over weeks or years, leaving a temporary darkening of the skin or even scars. The disorder can cause ulceration and prolonged disability.

Cutaneous necrotizing angiitis may be more than a skin disorder, it may reflect a serious systemic disease. Infections or drugs may cause the disease in some cases but many other cases develop for unknown reasons. Evidence suggests the disorder results from a type III allergic reaction involving immune complexes, and that the complement system plays a major role. Recent findings indicate that chemicals released by mast cells may also be involved.

Several drugs, including certain antihistamines, can alleviate symptoms, but they do nothing to combat the disease. In some patients, corticosteroids and immunosuppressive drugs have proved beneficial in treating the disorder. When another disease is associated with cutaneous necrotizing angiitis, treating that ailment often improves the skin.

Lupus Erythematosus of the Skin

This inflammation of the skin takes three forms. Discoid lupus forms round or oval red spots an inch or more in width, which may leave skin discoloration or scarring upon healing. A second form is often found in patients with early systemic lupus erythematosus, or SLE, a serious disorder of the connective tissue. This type involves a sensitivity to sunlight. It consists of red, swollen spots on parts of the body exposed to light, such as the cheeks, bridge of the nose, and arms. These may heal without scarring. A third type, a "butterfly rash," is often seen in patients with SLE. This red eruption on the face usually lasts only a few days and normally passes without scarring or permanent skin changes.

Evidence of numerous immunologic activities can be found in patients with lupus erythematosus of the skin. Studies to date, however, suggest that the skin reaction is due to a cell-mediated immune response, rather than to the work of antibodies. When the skin disorder accompanies SLE, it is a reflection of the underlying, more serious disease. Thus, studying the skin disorder should shed new light on SLE.

Chapter 9

Allergic Drug Reactions

The Problem

For thousands of years, people have been treating their illnesses with various drugs. At first these were natural substances such as herbs and the juices or saps from plants that were eaten or applied to the skin. Doctors still use some of these natural products—for example, quinine obtained from the bark of the cinchona tree and digitalis prepared from the dried leaf of the foxglove plant. Today, however, most drugs available to the doctor are man-made chemicals designed to combat specific diseases or sets of symptoms.

As more drugs become available and are used, the number of adverse reactions to them increases. The World Health Organization's definition of an "adverse drug reaction" is any response to a drug that is harmful and not intended and that occurs at doses given to individuals for prevention, diagnosis, or treatment of disease.

One of the major public health problems today is drug-induced illness. Between 3 and 5 percent of medical hospital admissions are due to adverse drug effects, and 10 to 20 percent of patients hospitalized for other reasons have an adverse response to a drug prescribed while they are hospitalized. The Department of Health and Human Services has estimated that the annual cost of treating adverse drug reactions in U.S. hospitals is approximately $3 billion. Thus, in addition to the individual suffering and even death in rare cases, adverse drug reactions

NIH Publication No. 80-388 and 82-703.

have become a costly problem indeed. Some of these adverse reactions to drugs are recognized as allergies.

Useful drugs have specific actions which correct abnormalities associated with disease states. Aspirin relieves pain and reduces fever; penicillin kills bacteria that cause a number of diseases; digitalis increases cardiac contraction and helps control several heart ailments. Since drugs work by inducing changes in the body's complex balance, no drug is totally safe for every person. Even the safest will produce adverse reactions in a few patients. This problem of drug reactions is a growing concern, both among doctors and patients.

The U. S. Food and Drug Administration's laws place great emphasis on safety during the initial evaluation of new drugs. However, once a drug is approved for general use, the exact frequency of undesirable side effects is not always closely followed. Thus, estimates of drug reactions, allergic and otherwise, rest on a group of specific studies, rather than national statistics.

Hospitalized patients, who generally receive more than one drug during their stay, are the people most carefully monitored for side effects. About 30 percent of them develop some drug reaction during their hospitalization. Most of these are not allergic reactions, but many of the more serious ones are. Statistics gathered by the Boston Collaborative Drug Surveillance Program show that 6 percent of the drug reactions in hospital patients result from an allergic response. Other studies attribute 2.7 to 34.4 percent of all drug reactions to an allergic response. Overall, the risk of suffering some type of allergic drug reaction in the hospital appears to be between 1 and 4 percent.

As part of the Boston study, allergic drug reactions were studied in 45,122 patients. The percentage of patients suffering allergic reactions to 40 specific drugs ranges from 0 percent of 3,828 people taking digoxin (a heart drug) and of 1,819 taking aminophylline (an asthma drug) to 5.2 percent of 2,344 patients receiving the antibiotic ampicillin (all of the ampicillin reactions may not have been allergic). Rash, fever, and itching were the most common reactions, but more serious ones occurred, including anaphylaxis. Aspirin had one of the lowest allergic reaction rates, 0.1 percent of 1,615 patients. Other clinical trials suggest allergic reactions to aspirin may run as high as 3 percent.

The Boston Collaborative Study produced the most comprehensive data available on allergic drug reactions. But because it applies only to hospitalized patients and because of its emphasis on certain symptoms while excluding others, the study undoubtedly underestimates

Drug	Total number of patients treated	Percentage of allergic reactions
Digoxin	4683	0
Aminophylline	1876	0
Furosemide	3497	0.3
Ferrous sulfate	1636	0
Heparin sodium	1553	0.8
Warfarin sodium	1035	0
Propoxyphene	2976	0.3
Flurazepam HCl	1862	0.1
Barbiturates	4658	0.5
Regular insulin	1101	0
Acetaminophen	2827	0
Aspirin	1942	0
Milk of magnesia	4933	0
Phenytoin	905	0.1
Methyldopa	809	0
Chlorthiazide	707	0.3
Glutethimide	221	0.5
Indomethacin	229	0.5
Chlorpromazine	622	0
Procainamide HCl	381	0
Allopurinol	1015	0
Potassum iodide	525	0
Ampicillin	2988	5.2
Cephalosporins	1308	1.3
Clindamycin	104	0
Erythromycins	481	0.2
Gentamycin	607	1.6
Nitrofurantoin	219	0.9
Penicillin G	3286	1.6
Chloramphenicol	292	0.7
Isoniazid	675	0.3
Kanamycin	257	0
Streptomycin	351	0
Tetracyclines	1182	0

Table 9.1. *Frequency of allergic skin reactions to selected drugs*

the overall importance of drug allergy as a health problem. It is estimated, for example, that between 0.3 and 0.5 percent of allergic drug reactions are severe enough to require hospitalization. These reactions include life-threatening anaphylaxis, serum sickness, and lung, kidney, and skin complications.

Deaths from allergic drug reactions, however, appear rare. The Boston collaborative program found the risk of anaphylactic death in the hospital was 0.6 per 1,000 patients. Another study found one allergic drug death among 7,423 hospital admissions. A Swedish study reported that 2.7 percent of patients who suffered drug-caused anaphylaxis died, and 0.22 percent of all allergic skin reactions caused by drugs resulted in death.

Types of Allergic Drug Reactions

Our knowledge about allergic drug reactions is limited, but growing. A number of reactions are proven; others are suspect. Not all allergic drug reactions are due to the drug itself. Occasionally, the immune system responds to traces of impurities or additives in a medicine or to a drug's metabolites, the substances that result from the chemical breakdown of the drug in the body. Some drugs generally produce a single type of reaction; others can trigger a number of effects. An allergic reaction to penicillin may manifest itself in any one of at least seven forms, including anaphylaxis, fever, and severe contact dermatitis. Certain parts of the body seem more susceptible to allergic drug reactions, particularly the skin, lungs, liver, kidneys, blood, and blood vessels.

Because drugs may affect several organs in the body, it is sometimes hard to decide whether a patient's symptoms result from the illness itself or from an allergic reaction to a drug. For example, a rash may appear during or after some streptococcal infections. Yet a rash may also be a symptom of an allergy to penicillin, an antibiotic used to treat the same streptococcal infections.

The symptoms that will appear in those who develop allergic reactions to drugs are impossible to predict ahead of time. A drug allergy may affect a single organ and a localized area of the body or it may affect many organs and many sites at the same time. Reactions on the skin are obvious and common. Reactions in other parts of the body may be difficult to detect; these are probably more frequent than people may think. The most common allergic responses of various parts of the body are reviewed here.

118

Allergic drug reactions include:

Anaphylaxis. This is an extreme allergic reaction that produces potentially fatal shock. Often severe anaphylactic shock is preceded by the sudden onset of violent itching, especially on the soles of the feet and palms of the hands, and by reddening of the skin as if it were sunburned, particularly around the ears. Hives may occur, and the face may become distorted with swelling. The patient may feel faint and anxious. The blood pressure becomes dangerously low. Breathing may suddenly become extremely difficult and the patient may suffer cough, extensive itching, a rapid pulse rate, and a bluing of the skin caused by a lack of oxygen. Unconsciousness, convulsions, shock, or vomiting may occur. Abrupt anaphylaxis most often occurs after an injection of a medication. Severe anaphylaxis may also occur after taking a drug by mouth, but usually there is a longer time between the onset here than there is when the drug is injected. Penicillin is the most common cause of drug-induced anaphylaxis; but a number of other drugs may cause the reaction, including opiates, hormones, vitamins, streptomycin, and tetracycline.

Serum Sickness. This disease—characterized by fever, rash, hives, swollen lymph glands, and painful joints—occurs in humans after repeated injections of rather large quantities of foreign antigens (animal serum). Many drugs, however, cause an allergic reaction similar to serum sickness. These include penicillin, the sulfonamides, thiouracil (used in hyperthyroidism and some heart disorders), and phenytoin (a drug used to control epilepsy).

Symptoms of serum sickness generally appear 2 to 3 weeks after the last dose of the triggering drug. They disappear after the drug or its metabolites are cleared completely from the body. Most of the symptoms are thought to be mediated by IgG, and possibly IgM, drug complexes. However, it is probable that the hives in this reaction result from IgE antibody or immune complex triggered histamine release.

Angioedema or giant hives. Angioedema or giant hives is the sudden appearance of massive swollen areas of the skin, mucous membranes, and occasionally, internal organs. Angioedema in the throat causes the airway to become blocked and makes breathing difficult. Such cases may be life-threatening and need emergency medical treatment. The symptoms of swelling in areas other than the throat may be unpleasant but are not usually life-threatening.

119

Drug Fever. This usually occurs 7 to 10 days after onset of drug treatment. Discontinuing the drug promptly relieves the fever, but if the medication is given again, the fever will return. Penicillin, streptomycin, barbiturates, and phenytoin are among the most common causes of this reaction.

Skin Reactions. An estimated 15 percent of all visits to dermatologists involve adverse reactions to drugs. Many of these are allergic reactions. One of the more common forms of the allergic skin responses is hives; the drug that causes this condition most often is penicillin. Other conditions that may be drug-induced include eruptions of blisters and solid elevations of the skin. Another type of reaction that can result from many drugs is exfoliative dermatitis, a severe skin disorder in which the entire skin becomes red and scaly and peels off. Chills and fever are common.

Contact dermatitis, which produces swelling, reddening, itching, or eruptions on the skin at the site of contact with a drug, often develops in nurses or druggists who handle drugs. Patients may also develop contact dermatitis from medications applied directly to the skin. Allergic reactions may be provoked by soap and antibiotic creams as well as by local anesthetics used to numb pain. Examples are procaine (Novocain), which dulls the pain of dental work, and many over-the-counter sprays containing benzocaine that are applied to the skin to numb the pain of sunburn, minor cuts, and insect bites.

Symptoms of contact dermatitis may appear within several hours or as long as 48 hours after the medicine is applied to the skin. If the person stops using the offending drug promptly, the reaction usually will end in a few days.

Another type of drug allergy that affects the skin is a "photosensitivity" reaction. Reddening and eruptions appear on areas of the skin exposed to sunlight after a person has taken a sensitizing drug by mouth or injection or has applied it to the skin. For example, some people who venture out into the sun after taking griseofulvin (an anti fungal agent), sulfa drugs and tetracyclines (antibiotics), chlordiazepoxide (a sedative), or thiazides (diuretics) may get a rash that looks like a sunburn.

Lung Involvement. A number of allergic-drug reactions may occur in the lung. Anaphylaxis is one. Inflammations of various types are others. One acute inflammation, accompanied by rash and fever, follows treatment with nitrofurantoin (used against urinary tract infections) and sulfasalazine (used in ulcerative colitis). This usually ends with no permanent damage after the drug is stopped, but some cases of fibrous damage to the lungs have been reported. Another lung inflammation, hypersensitivity pneumonia, may occur in people inhaling pituitary preparations as treatment for a metabolic disorder called diabetes insipidus. A form of pneumonia may follow the use of sulfonamides or penicillin. Certain drugs may cause a sudden onset of bronchial asthma; other drugs such as para-aminosalicylic acid (used to treat TB), sulfa drugs, and penicillin may induce pneumonia. Still others such as hydralazine (used to lower blood pressure) produce symptoms that mimic a disease known as lupus by causing inflammation of the membrane (pleura) that lines the lung. Other allergic responses in the lungs, including swelling and the formation of fibers in the air sacs, may occur as the result of certain drugs. Usually damage to the lungs is not permanent, and after treatment is stopped the lung function becomes normal.

Other Proven Reactions. Allergic drug reactions may manifest themselves as forms of liver or kidney diseases. A number of medications may cause widespread inflammation of the blood vessels in the skin and internal organs. Allergic drug reactions may also cause several serious and potentially life-threatening diseases of the body's blood cells, including a rare anemia, a decrease in the number of blood platelets, and the destruction of white cells involved in immunity. Less serious changes in lymph cells can occur that may be mistaken for Hodgkin's disease.

Pseudoallergic Reactions. Some drug-induced reactions resemble an allergic response in many respects, but laboratory tests have failed to find evidence of the immune system's involvement. The most common symptoms in these cases are hives and/or angioedema, rashes, bronchospasm, spasms of the larynx, and shock. Some drugs known to induce these reactions are aspirin, tartrazine (yellow food dye #5), dyes used in some x-ray studies, and ampicillin.

Approximately one million Americans have pseudoallergic reactions to aspirin, and many of them have allergy-related problems. Among people with chronic hives, 23 percent suffer adverse reactions to this drug, usually in the form of an increase in the severity of their condition. Of all asthmatics, 3.8 percent react to aspirin, usually developing acute bronchospasm. Almost 1 percent of normal individuals and 1.4 percent of hay fever patients have aspirin intolerance.

Type of population	%
Chronic Urticaria	23.2
Asthma	3.8
Rhinitis	1.4
Normal	0.9

Table 9.2. *Frequency of aspirin intolerance in various conditions*

Acetidine	Charger	Persistin
Alka-Seltzer	Coricidin	Say-Sayne
Anacin	Dristan	Stanback
Anahist	Ecotrin	Theracin
APC	Empirin Compound	Triaminicin
Aspergum	Excedrin	Trigesic
BC	Inhiston	Vanquish
Bromo-quinine	Measurin	
Bromo-Seltzer	Midol	
Bufferin	Pepto-Bismol	

Table 9.3. *Some over-the-counter drugs that contain aspirin*

Many preparations that can be bought without a prescription contain aspirin. In addition to most headache drugs, these include pain-killers, allergy medications and cold remedies. People with pseudoallergic reactions to aspirin are also at risk of developing similar reactions to other drugs. For example, an estimated 15 percent of Americans with aspirin intolerance also react adversely to tartrazine and thus must avoid foods and drugs containing this dye. Other drugs associated with aspirin intolerance include indomethacin (used in arthritis), sodium benzoate (a food preservative and antifungal agent), mefenamic acid (an anti-inflammatory drug), phenylbutazone (used in rheumatism), and ibuprofen (an anti-inflammatory agent).

Contrast dyes injected to provide clearer pictures in some x-ray studies may cause hives, bronchospasms, laryngospasm, shock, and even death. One review of 10,000 consecutive contrast-media injections found 1.7 percent of the patients experienced pseudoallergic reactions. Another study reported that fatal reactions occur in 1 out of 50,000 patients.

Ampicillin, a frequently prescribed antibiotic, can cause a non-allergic skin rash that may be mistaken for allergic dermatitis. The rash occurs in about 9 percent of people treated with ampicillin, and in perhaps half of the infectious mononucleosis patients who take the drug.

Which Drugs Are the Major Culprits?

Antibiotics

The numbers of antibiotics available today that may cause allergic reactions are too numerous to record here. This section deals with only a few.

Penicillin. Penicillin is probably the most common cause of drug allergy, with some type of allergic response occurring in one of every 50 persons who take this antibiotic. About 76 percent of these responses are skin reactions (hives, rashes, contact dermatitis) and about 22 percent are systemic (serum sickness, drug fever, vasculitis, angioedema, wheezing); only 2 percent of the reactions to penicillin involve anaphylactic shock.

Neomycin. Neomycin, an antibiotic that may be an ingredient of eye drops, often causes allergic contact conjunctivitis (pink eye). As an ingredient of ointments, neomycin may produce symptoms similar to allergic contact dermatitis.

Streptomycin. Allergic responses to streptomycin may range from mild reactions of the skin to drug fever and even to anaphylactic shock.

Chloramphenicol. Chloramphenicol, used in the treatment of Rocky Mountain spotted fever, typhoid fever, and certain types of meningitis, may affect the production of blood cells. An especially severe reaction to this antibiotic is aplastic anemia, a blood disorder in which the body's bone marrow fails to produce enough blood cells.

Sulfonamides. The new sulfonamides (sulfa drugs) now on the market produce fewer allergic reactions than did the sulfa compounds produced many years ago. However, the long-acting sulfa drugs may cause allergic responses such as hives, angioedema, skin rashes, fever, blood disorders, hepatitis, inflammation of the lungs and blood vessels, or a form of pneumonia. Included in this category of long-acting sulfas are those used as diuretics (drugs to counter fluid retention) as well as antibiotics.

Insulin. Allergic reactions to insulin are common. The symptoms range from pain and swelling at the site of injection to hives all over the body and severe reactions such as shock.

Insulin is prepared from both pork and beef pancreas, and because it is an animal protein, it can cause allergic reactions. The main factors that appear to be related to insulin allergy are the type of insulin used when treatment is begun and the genetic makeup of the patient. Most patients with insulin allergy have only delayed local reactions at the injection site; these last just a short time, and the patients are able to continue treatment without further problems. (Whether these are truly allergic responses is questionable.)

Although most insulin reactions are due to the hormone itself or to the animal protein, other reactions are due to incidental components. For example, some of the allergic skin reactions to insulin are now thought to be caused by zinc, which is used in commercial preparations of insulin. Zinc-free insulin, which is now available, has not produced any allergic responses in zinc-sensitive people.

Other drugs. Some of the common drugs that may also cause allergic reactions include anti-tuberculosis medications and other antibiotics not discussed above, anticonvulsants, barbiturates, local anesthetics, heavy metals, organ extracts, vaccines, tranquilizers and sleeping pills, laxatives, and drugs used to treat hyperthyroidism and heart disorders.

Which Drugs Reactions Are Non-allergic?

More than half of the adverse drug reactions reported by doctors are not allergic by definition. Such reactions may be classified as overdosage, idiosyncrasy, side effects, paradoxical response, or drug interactions. All drugs, even over-the-counter ones, can cause these responses. Great variations occur in the symptoms, their frequency, and their severity among different patients.

Symptoms of overdosage may obviously result from too large an amount of medication taken. For example, an overdose of aspirin may cause a "ringing" in the ears. Yet overdosage may also be caused by the unexpected accumulation of a drug in a patient whose impaired or inadequate body function is unable to break it down or excrete it at a normal rate.

Many abnormal or unexpected reactions to drugs are termed "idiosyncratic." Examples include an unexpected response to an ordinary dose of a drug (e.g., reduced production of blood cells with use of the antibiotic chloramphenicol); a toxic response to a low dose of a drug (e.g., "ringing" in the ears with use of quinine, sometimes prescribed to relieve muscle cramps); or an unusual resistance to a large dose of a drug. Some idiosyncratic reactions are now known to have a genetic basis.

Side effects of drugs—undesirable yet unavoidable actions of medications and not related to the desired effect—are frequently encountered. Sleepiness after taking antihistamines and diarrhea that sometimes accompanies use of antibiotics are common examples. Patients may sometimes find it necessary to tolerate annoying yet harmless side effects of a medication in order to experience its curing effects.

Paradoxical responses are ones that vary from the reactions usually expected after a drug is administered and result in the opposite effect. One example is a case of the "jitters" after taking a sedative.

The interaction of one or more drugs being taken by a patient at the same time may also cause adverse reactions. These interactions occur when one drug alters the body's ability to use another drug or when a combination of two or more drugs modifies the effects of each drug. The interaction of two common drugs, alcohol and tranquilizers, can cause reactions that range from drowsiness to death.

Thus it is probable that a person may experience an adverse reaction to a drug without being allergic to it. The symptoms of non-allergic and allergic reactions to medication are sometimes very similar.

The Allergic Mechanism

Animal studies provide considerable information about how antibodies form and react with chemicals in drugs. This information has given immunologists new insights into human drug allergies. The immune system's response is complex and depends upon the drug's chemical characteristics, how it is given, and a number of factors within the body.

Drug Characteristics. The size of the molecules that make up a drug and their structural complexity influence the immune system. The larger and more complex the molecules, the more likely they are

125

to cause an allergic reaction. Proteins and carbohydrates are particularly potent at producing an immune response. The repeated use of foreign enzymes for therapy always carries the risk of a serious allergic reaction. Reactions to foreign hormones are less frequent, but these may create autoimmune problems when they occur. The key to whether a small molecule provokes an allergic reaction depends upon the molecular bonds it forms with larger molecules. If these bonds are stable, even a small molecule can generate an immune response. Most drugs used clinically, however, do not form stable bonds.

In some drugs, minor contaminants or metabolites appear to be responsible for the allergic reaction. Purified penicillin salts rarely provoke an immune response, for example. But penicillin contaminants will, and penicillin itself breaks down into several compounds that are strong allergens.

The phenomenon of **cross-reactivity** also plays a significant role in drug allergy. Once the body is sensitized (made allergic) to an antigen, it produces antibodies to that antigen. Sometimes, however, specific antibodies will react with a different compound, one whose chemical structure is quite similar to the antigen that originally stimulated the formation of the antibodies. This is called antigenic cross-reactivity, and it can cause allergic reactions to drugs a person has never previously taken.

The Body's Response. How a drug is administered influences its potential for an immune response. For example, some drugs will readily cause an allergic reaction if applied to the skin, yet almost never produce a response if taken by mouth. Certain drugs carry a risk of serious, even fatal, anaphylaxis when injected. A number of drugs (e.g., antihistamines) applied directly to the skin may sensitize, but they will have less allergic effect when given by injection or by mouth.

Some people appear more susceptible to allergic drug reactions. Several animal studies suggest this may be related to how well certain scavenger cells (macrophages) function. How genetically determined factors influence human drug reactions remains unknown. But the question is of considerable importance and, according to NIAID's task force, should be vigorously studied.

In general, a person's gender makes little difference in allergic drug reactions. Age, however, appears important. Evidence suggests at least some allergic drug reactions are less common in infants and the aged. This may be because the immune system is immature in babies and tends to be less reactive in the elderly. It is unclear whether a person who is allergic to one drug is predisposed to allergic reactions to a new drug. Certainly, one should avoid further exposure to drugs having the same chemical makeup as the drug that first provoked the allergic response. Exposure to the sun sometimes increases the chance of an allergic reaction to certain drugs applied to the skin and even to some taken by mouth. When the intestines, kidneys, or liver are damaged and malfunction, the risk of allergy is greater because of the resulting inability of these organs to metabolize and excrete drugs.

The breakdown products of a drug that are formed as the body uses the drug occasionally may be the culprits rather than the drug itself in causing the reaction. In some cases, the body's allergic response is caused not by the drug or its breakdown products but by other chemicals added to the drug to preserve it (e.g., benzoic acid, methylparabens) or to improve its flavor or odor (e.g., terpenes).

Environmental Factors. The environment within the body may also influence the immune system. Tissue injury, for example, may increase the likelihood of an allergic response to antibiotics. Exposure to the sun appears to increase allergic reactions to certain drugs applied to the skin, and even to several taken orally. Damage to the intestine, kidney, or liver—which can alter the metabolism of drugs or their excretion—enhances the risk of allergy.

Diagnosis, Prevention, and Treatment

Practicing physicians frequently confront three questions of great importance regarding allergic drug reactions:

- Was a given drug reaction caused by an allergic response?

- If a drug reaction was allergic, which of several drugs taken by the patient caused the response?

- If a patient has experienced an allergic reaction to a drug in the past, what is the current risk of an allergic reaction if the drug is given again?

Currently, physicians must rely more on clinical judgment than tests to answer these questions. Useful diagnostic tests generally do not exist to tell a doctor whether a drug reaction was allergic, what caused it, or if a patient will suffer an allergic response to a drug the physician wants to prescribe.

A number of tests detect a human immune response against drugs and simple chemicals. Unfortunately, these rarely prove a certain drug caused or can cause an allergic reaction. Many people will show an immune response to a drug in these tests. But when they take the drug, no symptoms of an allergic reaction occur. Others show no response to the test, but develop allergic reactions. A useful test must not only show immune activity to a drug, it must show that this immune response produces undesirable effects in the person receiving the drug.

The diagnosis of drug allergy is usually made on the basis of the patient's medical history. Often the patient is the one who first notices the symptoms. Skin rashes, hives, swelling, fever, cough, and asthma may be signs of an allergic reaction to a drug and should be reported to the doctor, even if the reaction is slight. The doctor relies strongly on information that the patient supplies about the drug taken: when, how much, the length of time before symptoms appear, and what other medicine is being taken at the same time. Too often patients fail to report use of laxatives, nose drops, tonics, cold and cough remedies, antihistamines, vitamins, ointments, birth control pills and creams, douches, suppositories, aspirin and other pain killers, headache remedies, and antacids because they do not consider these compounds to be "drugs."

If the doctor suspects that an allergic reaction to a drug has occurred and if the symptoms generally begin to subside within 24 to 48 hours after the drug has been removed, it is likely that the drug has indeed caused the reaction. Occasionally, however, especially severe symptoms may continue or become worse for a week after a drug is stopped. A long-lasting drug may even cause allergic reactions for weeks or months after a patient has stopped taking it.

Depending on the patient's symptoms and the length of time before they subside, the doctor may again prescribe small amounts of the same medication to confirm the diagnosis. Such a repeat challenge can be very dangerous, especially if the patient has had a previous life-threatening allergic reaction. The doctor's decision to reuse the drug must be based on the need to know whether the patient has a drug allergy, the severity of the allergic reaction, the seriousness of the disease, and the availability of acceptable drug substitutes.

Although skin tests are used to detect allergies to pollens, molds, dust, animal danders, and food substances, most attempts to diagnose sensitivity to a drug by using the drug itself for skin testing are usually unsuccessful. This is because the exact derivative or breakdown product of the drug that acts as the antigen is not known. The patch test, if applied carefully, may help to diagnose contact dermatitis caused by drugs or chemicals. However, useful diagnostic tests generally do not exist to tell whether a drug reaction was allergic, which drug caused it, or whether a patient will suffer an allergic response to a drug that the doctor wants to prescribe.

Thus the diagnosis of drug allergy at present relies heavily on circumstantial evidence—the medical history, present symptoms, and time lapse between use of the drug and appearance of the symptoms. Careful diagnosis is important because it may affect not only the person's current therapy but also medication in the future.

This inadequacy in testing poses a difficult problem for a doctor. Should the physician withhold a drug because of its potential for triggering an allergic response, or because the patient has appeared to react to it in the past? In some cases, the physician may decide to withhold all drugs, because none can be proven innocent of harm.

NIAID's task force recognizes a great need for more sensitive and predictive tests. Indeed, they feel that the need for greater accuracy and precision in diagnosing allergic drug reactions cannot be overstated. Better diagnostic tests would provide a two-fold benefit. First, they would reduce the harmful effects, and even deaths, that result from these allergic responses. Second, they would allow many patients to receive drugs now withheld because physicians can not tell whether the medications will trigger a severe allergic reaction.

Preventing adverse drug reactions, of course, is more desirable than treating them after they occur. Many serious ones can be prevented, because the past often foreshadows the future. That is why physicians question patients about any previous drug reactions and review patients' medical records for mention of previous drug responses. Drugs known to produce frequent adverse reactions are used sparingly, and oral drugs are used more often than injections, which carry a higher risk of reaction.

The first step in treating drug allergy is identification of the offending drug. An unexplained rash, fever, swollen lymph glands, wheezing, or a gastrointestinal upset may signal trouble. Often, withdrawing the drug at this point is all that is needed. Mild symptoms will disappear without treatment in a few days or weeks after a patient stops taking the drug. Severe skin reactions require local or systemic treatment. Local treatment includes soothing baths, lotions, and steroid creams. (However, creams containing methylparabens should be used with caution, for such creams may themselves provoke contact dermatitis.) If secondary bacterial infections develop, antibiotics may be used unless a patient has shown an allergic reaction to a specific antibiotic. For severe systemic reactions, fluids or diuretics may help to eliminate the drug from the body and hasten recovery. Life-threatening anaphylactic reactions require the prompt use of epinephrine (Adrenalin), assurance that the airway passages are open, and administration of oxygen and intravenous fluids. When reactions to a drug are similar to serum sickness, the symptoms usually disappear after the drug clears the body. Sometimes, however, antihistamines are given to control hives and aspirin is used to ease joint pain (if the patient is not sensitive to aspirin). Corticosteroids are used for severe symptoms of the skin and joints and for treatment of blood vessel inflammation and involvement of internal organs as a result of an allergic response.

Patients who are intolerant to insulin during the early stages of treatment of their diabetes usually are able to tolerate it with continued administration. In some cases, however, the allergy persists. The administration of antihistamines or corticosteroids or a change in the animal source and/or purity of the insulin may give relief. When other methods are not successful, severe systemic reactions to insulin can be treated by desensitization. The patient at first receives small doses, which are increased gradually under the supervision of a doctor as tolerance is achieved.

If skin tests show that the patient is actually allergic to the zinc component of the insulin preparation, zinc-free insulin is recommended. Purified human insulins manufactured by new procedures are undergoing clinical trials and are expected to be of great value in the treatment of diabetes and insulin allergy.

When prompt preventive treatment for tetanus is required by patients who have not previously been immunized for tetanus, human hyperimmune tetanus gamma globulin should be used rather than horse tetanus antitoxin. The best preventive treatment, however, is for the patient to maintain the active tetanus immunization with a booster injection once every 10 years.

Substances chemically related to an allergy-causing drug often produce similar adverse reactions. In aspirin-sensitive people, however, drugs that are not chemically related to aspirin (such as tartrazine) may provoke similar reactions. Such reactions are not predictable.

Substitute medications are usually available for persons with sensitivity to a particular drug. Aspirin can be replaced by acetaminophen. Tests can be conducted to find which antibiotic other than penicillin is effective against a bacterial infection.

Occasionally, drug reactions occur in cases where continued use of the drug is vital to life itself. If no alternative drug exists, then physicians must decide whether the patient faces a greater risk from continuing the drug, or from his underlying disease. With certain drugs—including penicillin, insulin, tetracycline, and streptomycin—immunotherapy may work. The drug is given in slowly increasing doses until therapeutic levels are reached. In some patients, the immune system comes to tolerate the drug and no longer generates an allergic response to it.

Subacute bacterial endocarditis, an infection of the inner lining of the heart, is perhaps one of the few infections that calls for immediate treatment with penicillin, even if the patient is allergic to this antibiotic. Such patients are desensitized by being given small doses of penicillin at frequent intervals, with the amount increased gradually until the therapeutic dose is tolerated. Of course, the patient is hospitalized during this treatment and a doctor is constantly in attendance, with all emergency measures available. Unfortunately the desensitization, which allows penicillin to be tolerated, may last only for the duration of the immediate treatment, and the allergy may return after a period of time.

The best way to prevent recurrence of allergic reactions to a drug is to avoid use of the drug. The patient should be aware of hidden sources of the drug, such as ingredients of over-the-counter medications. Treatment with several drugs in combination should be avoided if possible. Patients with asthma and nasal polyps should be very careful in their use of aspirin. The allergic patient should learn both the generic name and the trade name of the offending drug and should inform other doctors who will provide care in the future. A special identification card should be carried, or a *Medic Alert* tag or bracelet should be worn in case of an accident. *Medic Alert* tags and bracelets can be ordered from the Medic Alert Foundation, Box 1009, Turlock, California 95380 or are generally available in local pharamacies.

Chapter 10

Chemical Photosensitivity: Common Products Can Make You Allergic to Sunlight

Since childhood, my brother Blair always developed a dark tan without ever sunburning. Now a college soccer coach in Iowa, he is constantly outside practicing in the sun. Recently, Blair suffered a severe sunburn after only 45 minutes of sun exposure on a cool, partly sunny morning. Consulting his physician, he learned that the commonly prescribed colitis medication Azulfidine (sulfasalazine), which he was using at the time for a colon infection, was the cause of his problems.

Azulfidine is one of the many medications included in the Food and Drug Administration's most recent listing of medications that increase sensitivity to light and can cause a wide variety of health problems known as photosensitivity disorders. In some individuals, these medications can produce adverse effects when the person is exposed to sunlight and other types of ultraviolet (UV) light of an intensity or for a length of time that would not usually give the person problems. Some products are more likely to cause reactions than others. And not everyone who uses the products will be affected.

Photoreactions

Chemicals that produce a photoreaction (reaction with exposure to UV light) are called photoreactive agents or, more commonly, photosensitizers. After exposure to UV radiation either from natural sunlight or an artificial source such as tanning booths or even those "purple-lighted" mosquito zappers, these photosensitizers cause

FDA Consumer, May 1996.

chemical changes that increase a person's sensitivity to light, causing the person to become photosensitized. Medications, food additives, and other products that contain photoreactive agents are called photosensitizing products.

FDA has also reported that photoreactive agents have been found in deodorants, antibacterial soaps, artificial sweeteners, fluorescent brightening agents for cellulose, nylon and wool fibers, naphthalene (mothballs), petroleum products, and in cadmium sulfide, a chemical injected into the skin during tattooing.

Photoreactive agents, such as Azulfidine, can cause both acute and chronic effects. Acute effects, from short-term exposure, include exaggerated sunburn-like skin conditions, eye burn, mild allergic reactions, hives, abnormal reddening of the skin, and eczema-like rashes with itching, swelling, blistering, oozing, and scaling of the skin. Chronic effects from long-term exposure include premature skin aging, stronger allergic reactions, cataracts, blood vessel damage, a weakened immune system, and skin cancer.

Widely used medications containing photoreactive agents include antihistamines, used in cold and allergy medicines; nonsteroidal anti-inflammatory drugs (NSAIDs), used to control pain and inflammation in arthritis; and antibiotics, including the tetracyclines and the sulfonamides, or "sulfa" drugs.

Sometimes this quality can be put to good medical use. For example, two well-known photoreactive chemicals, psoralens and coal-tar dye creams, are used together with UV lamps to treat psoriasis, a chronic skin condition characterized by bright red patches covered with silvery scales.

Pioneering Research

European scientists pioneered photosensitivity disorder research during the 1960s. In 1967, Danish researchers attributed strange skin lesions (any abnormal change on the skin) on women to perfumed soap. In 1967, British researchers discovered that sandalwood oil in sunscreens and facial cosmetics caused photoallergies and later reported that quindoxin, a food additive in animal feed also caused phototoxic erythemal skin patches on British farmers handling the feed.

Shortly thereafter, French scientists demonstrated that bergamot oil in sunscreens caused photosensitivity disorders. German researchers isolated photoreactive agents in colognes, perfumes and oral contraceptives.

In 1972, American scientists linked sunlight-activated aniline compounds (found in drugs, varnishes, perfumes, shoe polish, and vulcanized rubber) to hives and skin conditions such as dermatitis and dandruff.

Scientists were soon publishing laundry lists of photoreactive agents found in these substances as well as those in hair dyes, hair styling creams, and household items such as shoe polish and mothballs. Current research focuses on identifying what photoreactive agents are found in which medicinal products and how to control photosensitivity disorders.

Photosensitizers can cause either photoallergic or phototoxic reactions.

Photoallergies

In photoallergic reactions, which generally occur due to medications applied to the skin, UV light may structurally change the drug, causing the skin to produce antibodies. The result is an allergic reaction. Symptoms can appear within 20 seconds after sun exposure, producing eczema-like skin conditions that can spread to nonexposed parts of the body. But sometimes, photoallergic reactions can be delayed. For example, Yuko Kurumaji reported in the October 1991 issue of *Contact Dermatitis* that photoallergic sensitivity disorders to the topically applied NSAID Suprofen (not approved for use in the United States) took up to three months to develop.

Other regularly used products that can cause photoallergic reactions are cosmetics that contain musk ambrette, sandalwood oil, and bergamot oil; some quinolone antibacterials; and the over-the-counter (OTC) NSAID pain relievers Advil, Nuprin and Motrin (ibuprofen), and Aleve (naproxen sodium).

Phototoxicity

Phototoxic reactions, which do not affect the body's immune system, are more common than photoallergic reactions. These reactions can occur in response to injected, oral or topically applied medications.

In phototoxic reactions, the drug absorbs energy from UV light and releases the energy into the skin, causing skin cell damage or death. The reaction occurs from within a few minutes to up to several hours after UV light exposure. Though sunburn-like symptoms appear only on the parts of the body exposed to UV radiation, resulting skin damage can persist.

For example, Henry Lim, M.D., reported in the March 1990 issue of *Archives of Dermatology* that several patients previously exposed to photoallergens continued to have phototoxic skin eruptions up to 20 years after discontinuing medication use, even though they avoided further exposure to the photoallergens.

Frequently prescribed medications that cause phototoxic reactions include tetracycline antibiotics, NSAIDs, and Cordarone (amiodarone), used to control irregular heartbeats.

Because drug-induced photosensitivity disorder symptoms mimic sunburns, rashes and allergic reactions, many cases go unreported. Also, although research has shown that the numbers of photosensitized individuals may be high, most people do not associate the sun's light with the development of their skin eruptions.

Photophobia

Some medications can cause photophobia. Although literally, photophobia is fear of light, photophobic photosensitivity disorder patients avoid light not because they're afraid of it but because their eyes are painfully sensitive to it.

Some medications that induce photophobia include several drugs prescribed for irregular heartbeat, such as Crystodigin (digitoxin) and Duraquin (quinidine), and several drugs for diabetes, such as Tolinase (tolazamide) and Orinase (tolbutamide).

Who Gets a Reaction?

The degree of photosensitivity varies among individuals. Not everyone who uses medications containing photoreactive agents will have a photoreaction. In fact, a person who has a photoreaction after a single exposure to an agent may not react to the same agent after repeated exposures.

On the other hand, people who are allergic to one chemical may develop photosensitivity to another related chemical to which they would normally not be photosensitive. In such cross-reaction, photosensitivity to one chemical increases a person's tendency for photosensitivity to a second. For example, J.L. deCastro reported in the March 1991 issue of *Contact Dermatitis* that 17 patients allergic to the antiseptic thimerosal, used in some contact lens preparations, developed photosensitivity to the NSAID Feldene (piroxicam), yet none of them had had any previous photoreaction to Feldene.

Although those with fair skin are more susceptible to photosensitizing, it is not uncommon for dark-skinned individuals to have chronic photodermatitis.

People infected with HIV, the virus that causes AIDS, are more susceptible to photosensitive disorders so they need to exercise special care in UV light exposure. In a study published in the May 1994 *Archives of Dermatology*, Amy Pappert, M.D., reported that if apparently healthy patients exhibit certain photodistributed skin problems of unknown origin, the possibility of HIV infection should be considered.

What is termed a "photo-recall" can take place when a non-photoreactive product prompts the repeat of a previous reaction to a photoreactive agent.

Photoreactive products can also aggravate existing skin problems like eczema, herpes, psoriasis and acne, and can inflame scar tissue. They can also precipitate or worsen autoimmune diseases, such as lupus erythematosus and rheumatoid arthritis, in which the body's immune system mistakenly destroys itself.

A Few Common Photosensitizers

These are just a few of the more commonly used drugs that can cause photosensitivity reactions in some people.

Brand Name	Generic Name	Therapeutic Class
Motrin	ibuprofen	NSAID, antiarthritic
Crystodigin	digitoxin	antiarrhythmic
Sinequan	doxepin	antidepressant
Cordarone	amiodarone	antiarrhythmic
Bactrim	trimethoprim	antibiotic
Diabinese	chlorpropamide	antidiabetic (oral)
Feldene	piroxicam	NSAID antiarthritic
Vibramycin	doxycycline	antibiotic
Phenergan	promethazine	antihistamine

Table 10.1.

Do Sunscreens Help?

Does using sunscreen help protect against photosensitivity? The answer is not clear. Sunscreens do lessen the effects of UV radiation, but some contain ingredients that themselves may cause photosensitivity in some people. Also, most sunscreens protect only from short-wave UV light (UVB), whereas most phototoxic compounds are activated by longer wavelengths of UV light (UVA). Sunscreens containing bergamot oil, sandalwood oil, benzophenones, PABA, cinnamates, salicylates, anthranilates, PSBA, mexenone, and oxybenzone can all cause photosensitivity reactions. Titanium dioxide is the least likely sunscreen to cause photosensitivity disorders.

Before going out in the sun, it's a good idea to check with your doctor to see if any of the medications you're taking is likely to cause problems and decide how to best avoid such reactions. Read the labels of OTC drugs and note if they may be photosensitizing.

If you get symptoms after being out in the sun, you may want to consider what drugs and chemicals you are using and contact your doctor immediately for advice.

Tanning Booths Bigger Problem

Tanning booths and the use of indoor tanning products can be more of a problem than natural sunlight, and this is true with photosensitivity reactions as well as in general. FDA enforces policies in which sunlamp product manufacturers must develop an exposure schedule and establish a maximum recommended exposure time (and therefore the maximum timer interval) based on the characteristics of their particular products. This information must appear on the product's warning label and is no way to be considered as a safe limit.

FDA warns that some tanning operators may claim that UVA sunlamps are safer than the sun and UVB lamps. This is not true. In fact, exposure to the UV radiation from sunlamps adds to the total amount of UV radiation you get from the sun during your lifetime, further increasing your risk of cancer.

For further information on the dangers of indoor tanning, write to FDA (HFZ-342), 5600 Fishers Lane, Rockville, MD 20857 and ask for DHHS Publication No. (FDA) 87-8272.

—by Craig D. Reid, Ph.D.

Craig D. Reid, Ph.D., is a writer in New Haven, Conn.

Chapter 11

Occupational/Environmental Asthma and Related Allergic Respiratory Diseases

The Problem

The link between certain occupations and respiratory diseases dates back to the 18th century. It was then that physicians first described attacks of breathlessness among grain sifters and millers. That was also the time when physicians came to recognize the great importance of inquiring about a patient's work when considering his illness.

The problem of occupational illness is now widely recognized. Industries produce or use numerous materials capable of inducing lung ailments in workers, and, sometimes, in people living close to factories. (See list in this chapter.) These ailments include asthma, chronic bronchitis, emphysema, some cancers, fibrosis, granulomatous disease, and hypersensitivity pneumonitis.

Studies in the metal-refining industry, for example, suggest that almost all workers regularly exposed to the complex salts of platinum develop disorders of the upper or lower respiratory tract. In the cotton industry, byssinosis (a lung ailment caused by inhaling cotton dust) has been found in a large percentage of cardroom workers and in a smaller percentage of spinners. Long-term, prospective studies in the polyurethane foaming industry suggest chemicals used there may decrease lung function among exposed workers.

The immune system plays a varying role in occupationally caused respiratory diseases. Immunologic reactions are responsible for the

Extracted from NIH Publication No. 80-388.

139

development of certain types of occupational asthma and all types of hypersensitivity pneumonitis. This chapter focuses primarily on the occupational and environmental factors that influence the development and course of bronchial asthma, and also discusses asbestosis, berylliosis, and silicosis.

Occupational/Environmental Asthma

The proportion of asthma cases caused or influenced by occupational and environmental factors in the United States is unknown. Estimates from several other industrialized nations, however, suggest that about 2 percent of all asthma cases have an occupational origin. In Japan, about 15 percent of the asthma in men is attributed to an industrial cause. By extrapolating either of these figures to the United States, a large number of Americans must suffer from occupational asthma and its social and economic hardships.

Material	Industry
Animal, bird, fish and insect-serum, dander, secretions, excreta, contaminated water	Veterinarians, animal and poultry breeders, laboratory workers, fishermen, sericulture
Castor bean Green coffee bean Papain Pancreatic extracts Organic dusts Molds	Oil and food
Flour	Bakers, farmers, & grain handlers
Enzymes from *Bacillus subtilis*	Detergent
Hog trypsin Ethylenediamine Phthalic anhydride Trimellitic anhydride	Plastics, rubber, and resin
Phenylglycine acid chloride Sulphone chloramides	Pharmaceutical
Complex salts of platinum	Metal refining

Table 11.1. *Industrial materials known to cause allergic problems*

Some data are available on the risk of asthma from specific industrial exposures in the United States. A study of workers exposed to toluene di-isocyanate (TDI), a substance used in making the thermoplastic material, polyurethane, found that 5 percent developed occupational asthma. A recent study suggests that 6 percent of the people breeding or studying animals for scientific purposes develop asthma. Worldwide studies in the detergent industry show that about 2 percent of all exposed employees develop asthma symptoms from inhaling those enzymes used in enzyme-containing detergents. Moreover, susceptible people living near an industrial plant may develop asthma from breathing air contaminated by a specific chemical produced or used there. This, for example, is true of TDI.

There is evidence that chemicals used in homes and offices may provoke asthma. These include hair sprays, perfumes, insecticides, and household cleaning products, especially those packaged in aerosol or spray form.

Aerosols and sprays	Insecticides
Aromatic plants and trees	Lint
Car and diesel engine fumes	Medicinals
Cooking odors	Newspapers
Cosmetics	Paints
Deodorants	Perfumes
Household cleaning products	Tooth pastes and powders

Table 11.2. *Household items that may irritate airways*

Clear definition of the relationship between asthma and general air pollution—the accumulation of injurious manmade or natural substances in the atmosphere so often found in urban areas—remains unsettled. So, too, does the role of weather and climate in asthma. Under certain extreme and unusual climatological conditions, however, pollutants, pollens, and fungal spores may rise to such high levels that they trigger attacks in asthma patients.

The Development of Occupational Asthma

Three separate mechanisms may account for the development of occupational asthma—irritant effects, allergic factors, and pharmacologic factors.

Irritant Effects. The airways of asthmatics respond much more readily to inhaled irritants than do the airways of non-asthmatics. Consequently, concentrations of dusts, vapors, or other irritants that have little or no effect on healthy people may cause bronchoconstriction in asthma patients. The result is airway obstruction and an asthma attack. Irritants are thought to precipitate asthmatic episodes in several ways. One concept is that irritants stimulate special receptors of the vagus nerve. The nerve's response contributes to the bronchoconstriction.

Many industrial materials act as irritants and may induce attacks in people already asthmatic. Moreover, some of these substances—such as TDI and formaldehyde vapor—may act as both irritants and as sensitizing agents in certain people.

Allergic Factors. Many cases of occupational asthma result from IgE-mediated (type I) allergic reactions. In these cases, there may be months or even years between the first contact with the sensitizing industrial material and the development of symptoms. People with existing allergies are more likely to develop occupational asthma than non-allergic individuals.

An allergic response to occupational chemicals has been documented in a number of asthmatics by skin and bronchial-challenge tests. More recently, specific IgE antibodies against certain industrial materials have been found.

Among the materials proven to provoke asthma by an allergic mechanism are: enzymes from the bacterium *B. subtilis* (used in detergents); trimellitic anhydride (used in plastics, rubber, and resin); the complex of salts of platinum; castor beans and green coffee beans; and pancreatic extracts used by some food processors. Possible causes of allergic occupational asthma include salts of nickel, natural resins used in printing, organic phosphorus, soldering fluxes, and cotton dust.

Although TDI causes asthma in some 5 percent of the workers exposed to it, TDI-induced asthma is no more common in allergic individuals than in non-allergic. TDI-induced asthma may be allergic asthma, or it may involve some non-allergic mechanism.

142

Material	Industry
Salts of nickel	Metal plating
Grain (including insect and related grain contaminants)	Farmers, grain elevator operators
Wood dusts	Wood mills, carpenters
Vegetable gums (Acacia, Karaya), natural resins	Printers
Ampicillin Spiramycin Piperazine Amprolium hydrochloride Antibiotic dusts	Pharmaceutical
Diisocyanates (TDI, HDI, MDI)	Polyurethane, printers, adhesives
Pyrolysis products of polyvinyl chlorides Price labels and adhesives Soldering fluxes	Meat wrappers, electrical trade
Organic phosphorus	Farm workers
Cotton Dust	Textile and cotton seed oil
Formalin	Medical, pharmaceutical

Table 11.3. *Industrial materials presumed to cause allergic problems*

Pharmacologic Factors. Certain substances may cause the direct release of cell chemicals capable of constricting bronchial smooth muscle. In test-tube experiments, for example, high concentrations of extracts from cotton, flax, and hemp have been mixed with human lung tissue and incubated. These tissues were not from subjects allergic to the extracts, yet they released histamine. The complex salts of platinum also cause direct histamine release in experimental animals. However, whether these pharmacological reactions play a role in occupational asthma in humans remains unknown.

The cause of respiratory reactions—often called meat cutter's asthma or meat labeler's asthma—that follow the inhalation of fumes from attaching price labels with hot irons to plastic materials remains unknown. More than one type of mechanism may be involved, however.

Diagnosis

A detailed history is vital in diagnosing occupational asthma. Most often, as with other forms of the disease, an immediate attack of wheezing, shortness of breath, and tightness of the chest occurs after the patient inhales some material at work. The symptoms usually clear after leaving the factory and are often absent on weekends and holidays. Frequently, however, the patient has an early morning cough, sometimes with sputum. These symptoms may extend over weekends and short holidays, making the diagnosis more difficult.

The immediate asthma attack is the most common response. However, in some occupational asthmatics, delayed attacks may occur or there may be prolonged or late attacks triggered by a single exposure. The late reactions may involve immune-complex formation, but this remains unclear. The nature of the recurrent nighttime asthma that can follow a single, short exposure to industrial materials is even less clear.

If the physician suspects an occupational cause for asthma, s/he may do tests—both before and after work—which measure the amount of air a patient inhales and exhales. If an IgE-mediated allergic reaction is involved, and if appropriate samples of the suspected material are available, skin testing can provide important answers.

The most specific way of determining what triggers occupational asthma is a lung challenge test. This technique, however, is available only at large medical centers, and then only when specialized test materials and personnel are available. It is usually done by mixing the suspected compound in water. Using certain precautions, the patient inhales first small, then increasing, concentrations of this mixture as a mist. Signs of an asthmatic reaction indicate that the compound can cause symptoms and is a likely source of the patient's problem. At this point, the testing is stopped. This test is sometimes the only way to prove a specific material can cause symptoms of asthma.

However, one research center is experimenting with a special device called a challenge chamber to determine which substances are causing asthma in workers. In this room, a patient is exposed to air containing the suspected compound—either as dust or vapors—in the same concentrations as exist in the working place. Experiments with TDI in this chamber show that the greater the concentration of TDI, the more likely susceptible individuals are to suffer an asthma attack.

Treatment and Prevention

The most effective treatment for occupational asthma is preventing people from further exposure to the materials that cause their disease. This may be accomplished by moving a worker to a job in some other part of the plant. However, minimal amounts of a substance may provoke asthma attacks. Consequently, some workers may have to change occupations completely.

This choice may be unacceptable because of personal or economic reasons. In such cases, physicians may use drugs, such as sodium cromoglycate, which can inhibit asthmatic reactions to a number of inhaled materials. This approach requires regular consultations between patient and physician. Moreover, the long-term effects of using these drugs to counter occupational asthma are not totally known.

Prevention, rather than treatment, is the ultimate goal in occupational asthma. And prevention requires awareness by workers and employers of the possible dangers inherent in various occupations. NIAID's task force believes that workers have a right to know what substances may cause adverse reactions. Furthermore, management and union representatives should educate and encourage workers to report respiratory symptoms. This can alert an industry to the need to reduce exposure at the earliest stages of the problem. The detergent industry's experience demonstrates the value of skin testing as a means of monitoring workers. Evidence gathered there indicates that skin tests become positive before respiratory symptoms appear. Workers exposed to materials known to cause occupational asthma should also be monitored with routine respiratory-function tests.

Work areas should be designed and maintained so exposure to asthma-causing substances is kept at the lowest possible levels. It is important that researchers determine at what concentrations these materials cause reactions in allergy-prone individuals. This may provide a level of exposure below which sensitization and later symptoms will be minimal, at least for IgE-mediated allergic asthma.

The detergent industry has proved the effectiveness of such efforts. After *B. subtilis* enzymes were identified as the cause of occupational asthma among its workers, the industry moved to decrease exposure of employees. The result has been a dramatic drop in sensitization of employees and this form of occupational asthma.

Other Allergic Occupational Respiratory Diseases

In addition to occupational asthma and hypersensitivity pneumonitis, three other occupationally induced lung diseases deserve discussion. These are the inorganic dust diseases of silicosis, asbestosis, and berylliosis. Each involves complex interactions of the immune system with materials used by industry. In each, much remains unknown about the nature of the immune response and its effects on the disease's course.

Silicosis. Sandblaster's silicosis, or grinder's disease, is a severe and rapidly fatal form of lung disease. It results from inhaling dust from stone, sand, or flint that contains silica. Substantial amounts of dusty particles may deposit in the lungs, leading to the formation of damaging nodules and fibrous tissue.

Estimates place the number of workers engaged in abrasive operations in the United States at about 100,000, some 70,000 of whom are exposed to free silica. In southern Louisiana alone, at least 2,000 men blast metal surfaces, and the majority use sand to do their work. The national prevalence of sandblaster's silicosis is unknown, but 140 cases with 37 deaths have been identified at one medical center since 1958.

Many abnormal immune responses occur in people who develop this respiratory disease. Animal experiments show silica can destroy the scavenger cells called macrophages, which help protect the lung. These cells, in turn, release certain enzymes, which cause further macrophage destruction. This chain of events may initiate the development of nodules and fibrous tissue in human lungs. Other immune reactions also occur, and a high incidence of autoimmune diseases is associated with silicosis.

Silicosis, both in its chronic and more rapidly developing forms, results, to a large extent, from physiologic and immunologic events. Understanding its immunologic origin and development has great biomedical and economic significance.

Asbestosis. Here, inhaled asbestos fibers cause a chronic inflammation of the lung. This results, at least in part, because unlike most other foreign matter, these fibers are not eliminated by the immune system.

Asbestosis patients have reduced numbers of lymphocytes, the white cells so vital to immunity. Moreover, certain asbestos fibers can activate the alternative pathway of the complement system, which plays a major role in inflammation. And, as happens in silicosis, some asbestosis sufferers develop antibodies against their own lung tissue. All these factors lead to the development of fibrous material, which replaces the lungs' air sacs and causes breathing difficulties and even death.

Berylliosis. This lung inflammation results from inhaling beryllium fumes or fine beryllium dust. It may be an acute episode, whose severity depends on the amount of beryllium inhaled and the length of exposure, or it may be chronic. The chronic form is more insidious, and patients eventually develop potentially fatal fibrous lung damage.

As with silicosis and asbestosis, berylliosis involves immune events, especially in its chronic form. Beryllium salts stimulate cell-mediated immunity, for example, in both humans and animals. Laboratory experiments suggest beryllium may produce an allergic reaction, and that it is highly toxic to macrophages that protect the air sacs of the lungs.

Farmer's Lung and Related Diseases

Definition, Description, and Importance

Allergic pneumonia, also called **hypersensitivity pneumonitis,** results from inhaling any of a wide variety of substances, such as dusts and molds. Farmer's lung, an example of allergic pneumonia, is caused by antigens inhaled from moldy hay. Unlike problems due to the immediate type of allergy (IgE-mediated), symptoms in this disease are delayed. Four to 10 hours after exposure, a susceptible person suffers cough, fever, chills, and shortness of breath.

Some forms of allergic pneumonia are rare; others appear to be surprisingly common. The disorders often have quite graphic names: mushroom worker's disease, bird fancier's disease, coffee worker's lung, sauna taker's disease, maple bark stripper's disease, and New Guinea lung. They affect both city and country dwellers; and the molds that cause farmer's lung may thrive in air conditioners and humidifiers.

Our knowledge of the incidence of farmer's lung and its related disorders is incomplete. Nonetheless, there seems little doubt that farmer's lung is an important occupational illness, and that the disease may be frequently missed or misdiagnosed because patients and physicians are unaware of the disorder. Many cases of rarer types of hypersensitivity pneumonitis (wheat weevil disease, bagassosis, and furrier's lung, for example) also undoubtedly go unrecognized.

Estimates of the socioeconomic impact of these diseases are difficult to make, since so little is known about their incidence and prevalence. However, if a dairy farmer must give up farming because of farmer's lung disease, the potential for financial hardship is great. Most farmers know no other occupation; most farm wives are ill-equipped to enter the job market.

Disease	*Exposure*
Farmer's lung	Moldy hay and other fodder
Bagassosis	Moldy sugar cane
Mushroom worker's disease	Mushroom compost
Humidifier lung	Contaminated system
Air conditioner lung	Contaminated system
Malt worker's disease	Moldy malt
Sauna taker's disease	Contaminated appliance
Bird fancier's disease	Pigeon, budgerigar, parrot, hen, turkey droppings
Maple bark stripper's disease	Moldy maple logs
Sequoiosis	Moldy redwood sawdust
Wood pulp worker's disease	Moldy logs
Pituitary snuff taker's disease	Desiccated pituitary
Suberosis	Moldy cork dust
Cheesewasher's disease	Cheese mold
Wheat weevil disease	Wheat flour
Furrier's lung	Hair dust
Coffee worker's lung	Coffee dust
New Guinea lung	Thatched roof dust

Table 11.4. *Causes of Hypersensitivity Pneumonitis*

Three Forms

Farmer's lung and the other types of allergic pneumonia appear in three forms. This variation, and the fact that symptoms of the three forms mimic more common ailments, account for many missed diagnoses.

Acute Form. This is usually characterized by chills, fever of 101 to 104 degrees Fahrenheit, dry cough, breathlessness without wheezing, and malaise. Symptoms generally peak within a few hours after onset (8 to 12 hours after exposure), and most disappear after a day. But breathlessness and fatigue may persist, up to several weeks. The severity of an attack depends in part on the amount of mold or dust inhaled, and partly on how the patient's immune system responds.

In some patients, exposure will produce an immediate asthmatic reaction, followed by the typical symptoms of farmer's lung a few hours later. The asthma attack may subside with or without treatment.

Subacute Form. This is a more insidious form of hypersensitivity pneumonitis. It resembles progressive chronic bronchitis, with cough, shortness of breath, easy fatigue and a weight loss. These patients may have decreased oxygen in their blood. Corticosteroid drugs and avoidance of the triggering antigens usually lead to improvement of this condition unless permanent lung damage has occurred.

Chronic Form. Prolonged, sufficiently intense exposure to antigens can gradually cause irreversible lung damage and disabling respiratory problems in exposed individuals. Fibrous material develops in the lungs and interferes with lung functioning. As a result, the body fails to get adequate oxygen, and debilitating breathlessness and fatigue occur. Lung scarring may progress and can be fatal.

Corticosteroids, bronchodilator therapy, and avoidance of triggering molds and dusts normally provide only minimal improvement at this late stage.

The Immune Response

Hypersensitivity pneumonitis is not the typical allergic response seen in hay fever and many asthma patients. Exactly what type of immune response causes it is still debatable, although antigen-antibody reactions and, more recently, cell-mediated immunity have been considered as participants in the production of lung damage.

The late reaction that characterizes an acute attack of farmer's lung and similar disorders suggests a type III allergic reaction, the type mediated by IgG antibodies. And, indeed, certain IgG antibodies are present in about 90 percent of hypersensitivity pneumonitis sufferers.

It may be that farmer's lung and the other disorders result from a combination of type III and type IV (cell-mediated) allergic reactions, but further studies are necessary to determine this. The role of heredity in these diseases is also uncertain and warrants further study.

Physical Changes

Whatever the allergic mechanism, the physical changes caused by hypersensitivity pneumonitis may depend more on the amount of antigen inhaled and the time between exposures than they do on the type of mold or dust. Whether the disease is farmer's lung, mushroom worker's lung, or bird fancier's lung, the type of lung damage seems similar. In addition, clinical symptoms are similar.

After exposure to inhaled antigen, a susceptible person's lungs become inflamed. The alveoli—the lungs' tiny air sacs—thicken and swell. This process can lead to the death of certain cells within the lung.

These inflamed areas become surrounded by nodules of tissue. Parts of the bronchiolar airways may be destroyed, and other airways become narrowed by inflammation, tissue debris, and an influx of scavenger cells that come to clean up the debris.

If a person is only slightly sensitive or if the dose of mold or dust is small and no further exposure occurs, the acute episode may be followed by little or no long-lasting damage. If there is continued exposure to the antigen, the inflammation will continue and damage is likely. Fibrous tissue builds up in the air sacs and airways. Eventually, severe scarring occurs and air sacs are destroyed. The lungs lose their elasticity and remain over-inflated.

Diagnosis, Prognosis, and Complications

These disorders pose difficult diagnostic problems. Because farmer's lung and the other related types of allergic pneumonia are rare and because the symptoms resemble those due to infectious lung diseases, the initial diagnosis is often incorrectly made as viral or bacterial pneumonia. Considering the possibility of hypersensitivity pneumonitis in a given case is often the key to diagnosing it.

Even when the disease is suspected, however, the diagnosis is not easy to verify. A physician can not diagnose the disorder based on a single test or on a specific feature of the ailment. Rather, a combination of typical symptoms, physical findings, x-ray studies, and lung and immunologic tests are needed.

With the exception of farmer's lung, no research group sees more than a small number of people with a specific form of hypersensitivity pneumonitis. Moreover, not all people develop the disease after exposure. Among those who do, some voluntarily avoid further exposure without physician evaluation. For these reasons, exact incidence is uncertain and much remains unknown about the disease's natural history. However, some general information does exist about the course and prognosis of these diseases. A brief exposure, even though intense, will produce an acute reaction in a susceptible individual. This is followed by a return to normal in most acute cases, while continued exposure leads to progressive and irreversible disease.

Two Footnotes

Two forms of hypersensitivity pneumonitis deserve brief comment.

Maple Bark Stripper's Disease. This is an example of a disorder essentially eliminated as a result of understanding its origin. The disease is caused by inhaling the spores of *Cryptostroma corticale*, a mold that grows beneath the bark of maple logs.

In 1962, an epidemic occurred among workers at a Wisconsin paper mill. High concentrations of the mold spores were found in the dust of the mill's wood room. To combat the problem, the company installed new equipment, changed its operating methods to reduce drastically spore levels, and cautioned workers against spending excessive time in high-dust areas. No new cases of disease have occurred at the paper mill since 1964.

Forced-Air System's Lung. A number of recent cases of hypersensitivity pneumonitis have resulted from exposure to a variety of organisms contaminating forced-air systems in homes and work areas. Air conditioners, heating systems, and humidifiers have all been implicated. Thus, diseases similar to farmer's lung can occur in urban office workers, since some organisms can grow in air conditioners and humidifiers, as well as in hay. Forced-air system's lung is thought to occur more frequently than generally recognized, and it may represent a serious health problem.

Major Related Diseases

Several disorders related to hypersensitivity pneumonitis may be associated with special health problems.

Grain Dust Exposure. This is not a single disease state. The spectrum of health problems that grain workers confront as a result of inhaling dust is varied, with respiratory abnormalities similar to chronic bronchitis and asthma the most common.

The number of Americans regularly exposed to grain dust is substantial. The U.S. Bureau of the Census put the number of people living on farms at 8,250,000 in 1976. Perhaps one-quarter of these handle grain. An estimated 100,000 persons work in the Nation's large and small grain elevators; people transporting grain are also exposed to its dust.

Between one-half and three-quarters of the exposed workers develop cough, sputum production, chest discomfort, and wheezing. These symptoms generally disappear shortly after exposure stops. However, in many grain workers, these symptoms become chronic.

A number of workers also experience "grain fever," a combination of fever, chills or both, often accompanied by general malaise, which lasts for several hours. These symptoms may occur upon return to work after a period of absence, or after an intense exposure. Grain handlers also commonly experience acute and chronic eye and nose irritation.

The exact mechanisms by which grain dusts produce these effects remain undetermined. However, comparisons of grain handlers who smoke with those who don't reveal that smokers have a significantly higher incidence of respiratory symptoms and lung-function impairment. Allergy also seems to play a role. Wheezing and abnormal lung function are more common among allergic than non-allergic grain workers. Allergic individuals are more likely to develop an immediate or late asthmatic reaction after inhaling grain dust.

Pulmonary Mycotoxicosis. This rare ailment is an acute reaction similar to farmer's lung. It occurs following the "uncapping" of a silo, a common practice among dairy farmers.

A silo is filled with freshly cut forage and covered. Two or three feet of forage is placed atop the covering. This dries quickly, supporting the growth of huge numbers of fungi and bacteria. In the process of opening the silo, the moldy top layer is usually thrown off by hand. Fungal and bacterial fragments contaminate the air the farmer breathes. Examinations of the lung tissues taken from patients with pulmonary mycotoxicosis reveal innumerable fungal spores deposited in their lungs.

An attack generally comes on promptly with severe itching about the eyes and the back of the nose and mouth. Fever, chills, extreme exhaustion, and breathing problems follow. Symptoms usually disappear several days to 2 weeks after exposure ends, and the farmer has little or no further difficulty.

The exact cause of the disease has not been determined. Specific evidence for an immune reaction has not yet been found.

Allergic Bronchopulmonary Aspergillosis (ABPA). This syndrome, which occurs in some asthma patients, is caused by an allergic reaction to a genus of fungus, aspergillus, growing in the bronchi. A physician should suspect ABPA in any asthma patient who develops recurrent fever, pulmonary infiltrates (shadows seen on the lung x-ray), mucus lodged in the lungs, and brownish sputum. The origin of ABPA is not entirely understood. It appears, however, to involve a combination of type I (IgE-mediated) and type III (IgG-mediated) allergic reactions.

ABPA is fairly common in the United Kingdom, but has been considered rare in the United States. Now, however, more cases are being recognized and a reasonable estimate is that 10,000 cases exist here. The condition can progress to extensive lung scarring. These late destructive changes cannot be completely reversed. Although some patients remain stable for years, in others, the lung disease can lead to slow but progressive damage of the respiratory system.

Oral corticosteroid drugs reverse acute flares. Chronic administration of the steroid, prednisone, may be necessary to prevent ABPA recurrences.

Efforts to Control the Diseases

Theoretically, hypersensitivity pneumonitis could be prevented by eliminating all organic dusts from the environment. Unfortunately, this is impossible. Currently, the best advice to patients with the disease is to avoid the molds and dusts that trigger their ailment.

Everyone inhales organic dusts in varying amounts. Therefore, preventing hypersensitivity pneumonitis will depend eventually upon identifying all sensitizing dusts, the quantities and conditions necessary for the disease to develop, and the factors that predispose certain people to the disorder. NIAID's task force recognizes the necessity of conducting much more research to gain the knowledge required to design effective and feasible prevention programs.

Chapter 12

Pediatric Allergies

Importance and Impact

Asthma and allergic disorders constitute a major health problem among children in the United States. Two to three million youngsters suffer from asthma and 80 percent of these cases are allergy associated. More than six million are afflicted with hay fever (allergic rhinitis), and about two million have allergy-associated eczema (atopic dermatitis). Food allergies, too, are a significant problem, particularly in infants and young children, although the incidence is difficult to estimate. All together, well in excess of six million children in the United States suffer from at least one allergic disease, and many suffer from more than one.

Asthma and chronic allergic diseases are responsible for millions of lost school days, thus adversely affecting the education of these children. About one out of every five children visiting a pediatrician has either a minor or a major allergic disorder. And asthma is a leading cause of hospitalization among young children. The impact of these ailments on the emotional, intellectual, and physical development of children, and their families and society, is great.

Profound physiological changes during the fetal, neonatal, and adolescent periods of life affect the development and expression of allergic diseases. At these critical times, and indeed throughout childhood, the study of pediatric allergies provides unique opportunities

Extracted from NIH Publication No.80-388.

to gain new understandings of the immunological, biochemical, anatomical, environmental, and psychosocial aspects of allergy. Children are not merely small adults; they respond differently from adults to diagnostic tests and treatments. NIAID's task force believes that better understanding of the evolution and effects of pediatric allergies will benefit millions through improved diagnosis, treatment, and prevention.

Common Childhood Allergies

- Allergic rhinitis (hay fever)
- Atopic dermatitis (eczema)
- Infantile asthma
- Gastrointestinal disorders due to food allergies
- Serous otitis media

Genetic Factors

As early as 1190, Maimonides, the famed rabbi and physician, recognized that asthma tended to run in families. But it wasn't until early in the 20th century that the first extensive study of heredity in asthma occurred. It found that 48 percent of the allergy patients surveyed had an immediate family history of allergies, but only 12 percent of the non-allergic people studied had such a family history. That suggested asthma followed a simple Mendelian recessive inheritance pattern. But later studies have shown the genetic pattern of allergy is more complex. Most geneticists now regard allergies as polygenic, meaning that more than one gene is involved. While the tendency to become allergic may be inherited, it is quite possible for a child to suffer allergies, even though neither of his parents do. It is also possible a person will live his life allergy-free when both parents are allergic.

Recent studies involving children in several countries suggest parasitic infestations may have been one evolutionary force responsible for the development of allergies. Allergies develop in susceptible people when IgE antibodies react with allergens, such as pollen or dust. The new theory argues that this IgE response originally developed to protect people against parasites. If parasites are no longer present, then people direct their IgE production against basically harmless things like pollens. Studies have found that people from regions of the world where parasites are common tend to have higher IgE levels than people from areas where parasites are less of a problem. Also, in the

West African nation of Gambia, researchers found that IgE levels were significantly higher in rural children, as compared to children living in urban areas where parasite control and nutrition are better. Yet asthma was almost unknown in the rural communities, while quite common in urban school children.

Developmental Aspects

Preventing allergic diseases depends in large part on gaining a better understanding of how developmental changes in the body affect the onset and expression of the disorders. A major question is when and how allergy-prone youngsters are sensitized to allergens. Are some babies born allergic? Or do allergies develop only after birth?

Studies have shown that the immune system develops relatively early in gestation. The fetus is capable of forming IgE antibodies at 22 weeks, yet such low quantities are usually made that they are often undetectable at birth. IgE does not normally cross the placenta. Therefore, it is unlikely a newborn infant can be passively sensitized with IgE antibodies from its mother. Nonetheless, there are reports of newborns who react to skin tests for pollens or foods to which they have never been exposed since birth. Strong evidence suggests that specific IgE antibodies are present in the sera of some umbilical cords.

Thus, the intriguing possibility exists that a fetus can be sensitized to allergens ingested or inhaled by the mother. This untested notion suggests that allergens enter the mother's bloodstream, cross the placenta, and sensitize the susceptible fetus.

Evidence indicates that mothers can pass antigens to their infants by breast feeding. For example, studies of babies who were fed exclusively by nursing have shown that many have IgE antibodies to cow's milk, and, indeed, are allergic to it. The implication is that infants are sensitized by cow's-milk antigens present in their mother's milk. Reports suggest that infants also may develop allergies to other foods through breast feeding, making this a subject worthy of more systematic study, according to NIAID's task force.

They also recommended that, based on recent findings, the practice of feeding cow's milk substitutes to children genetically at risk of developing allergies needs to be reevaluated. In 1953, research destined to have a major impact on the feeding of infants was reported. Scientists found that significant allergy symptoms developed within the first year of life in more than half of the at-risk children studied who were fed cow's-milk formula from birth. But only 14 percent of the children at risk who did not drink cow's milk developed symptoms. This finding was confirmed in a 13-year follow-up study.

These studies stimulated a new industry: the production of canned soybean formula as a substitute for cow's milk. However, the task force feels that important limitations of the investigations supporting this concept, along with new findings, make a restudy mandatory. A 1973 survey of over 400 children found no difference in the incidence of allergy in infants fed cow's milk, soy formula, or mother's milk. Moreover, recent work suggests soy formula may act to increase the allergic response, if allergies develop.

The immune system can be affected by antigens absorbed intact into the blood from the intestine. This process seems more common in children than adults. Obviously, the allergic response can be significantly affected by developmental changes in the processes that alter the absorption, digestion, or metabolism of foods.

Other critical developmental changes may affect the severity of allergic symptoms. One example, important in asthma, is the reaction of infants' airways, compared to those of older children and adults. Any narrowing of the small airways will create a proportionally greater increase in airflow resistance in infants, and thus produce greater disease.

Environmental Factors

Environmental factors may cause or trigger allergic diseases. Controlling these factors appears most beneficial to infants and young children, for doing so might prevent the development of some allergies altogether. There is evidence to support this idea in certain food studies. Eliminating or reducing the exposure of at-risk children to infectious viruses, certain household antigens, and airborne irritants may also help.

Asthmatic children often experience their first attack while suffering a respiratory infection. Several viruses, among them respiratory syncytial virus, influenza type A, and adenovirus, are associated with the onset of asthma. A possible explanation for this was developed recently. Investigators found that bronchial smooth muscle increased its response to histamine 100-fold in volunteers infected with a weakened live virus. This work suggests that viruses damage the airways' protective lining, exposing receptors that respond easily to histamine, and perhaps to other more powerful bronchoconstrictors released by mast cells.

Dust and other household allergens are probably the most important airborne antigens affecting infants and children. They are common triggers for allergic rhinitis and allergic asthma. House dust is comprised of many things, but in many geographic locations the major allergen in it is the dust mite. Cockroach remains and rodent hairs are two other components of some house dust. Studies find that children from low socioeconomic backgrounds are more likely to react to dust than children from high socioeconomic backgrounds. This finding may reflect greater infestation by roaches and rodents in their homes. Such a finding suggests that living in a non-infested home may reduce the risk of allergies.

Evidence suggests that parents' smoking may increase the risk of respiratory ailments in their children. But whether breathing in cigarette, cigar, or pipe smoke increases a child's risk of developing allergies remains uncertain. One study did find that tobacco smoke aggravated asthma in half the asthmatic children studied, and in 67 percent of those whose parents smoked.

There are several well-documented cases of acute asthma associated with smoking and the presence of positive skin tests to tobacco. This association has been noted in both smokers and nonsmokers.

Marijuana or hashish smoking can result in acute symptoms of bronchitis, asthma, pharyngitis (sore throat), and rhinitis. Preliminary evidence now suggests that long-term, chronic marijuana smoking may predispose some people to bronchitis and emphysema. The substantial use of marijuana by adolescents emphasizes the need for greater research on these problems, according to NIAID's task force.

Specific Childhood Allergies

Several allergic diseases occur rather frequently among children. The most common are allergic diseases of the upper respiratory tract. Any severe allergy can adversely affect a child's emotional, intellectual, and physical well-being.

Allergic Rhinitis. This ailment, commonly called hay fever, afflicts more than five million children and adolescents. Up to age 10, the disease is more common in boys; after age 10 and through adolescence, new cases appear more often in girls. (Allergic rhinitis is discussed in detail in an earlier chapter.) Symptoms include a stuffy, runny nose, sneezing, and watery eyes. Complications may include dental disorders (maxillary overbite and maldevelopment of the dental arches), sinus and eustachian tube problems, hearing loss and serous otitis media.

Serous Otitis Media. This inflammation of the middle ear is a common ailment in infants and children with allergic rhinitis. A sterile fluid with varying consistency accumulates in the middle ear. A child may feel pain, a bubbling or pressure in the ear, and hear popping sounds. Temporary hearing loss may occur, and occasionally some permanent damage is done to hearing.

Such fluid accumulation can result from several other causes, including abnormalities in the middle ear itself, abnormalities in the structure or the functioning of the eustachian tube, or non-allergy-related nasal abnormalities.

Serous otitis media appears to result from a series of immunological disorders of the middle ear that follow infectious or allergic diseases. Further indication that an allergic reaction may play a role in this condition is the presence of an increased number of mast cells in the middle ears of patients with chronic serous otitis media.

Atopic Dermatitis. This type of eczema generally develops early in life and is associated with a hereditary tendency to hay fever and asthma. An acute attack brings redness of the skin, swelling, and blisters that discharge fluid. In the chronic state, the skin thickens, darkens, cracks, and scales. The neck, face, and bends of the knees and elbows are the most often affected. Symptoms may be mild or severe, and they tend to occur at different body sites at different ages.

Atopic dermatitis is common in allergic children. A major U.S. study found this condition to be present in 4.3 percent of 1,753 children followed from birth to age 7; and the eczema occurred in fully one-third of those children who developed allergies. The ailment commonly appears after the second month of life. Sixty percent of the cases appear before age 1, and 90 percent by age 5. Most children outgrow eczema, with improvement usually occurring at puberty. But it is impossible to predict which cases will clear, and which will continue into adulthood. Atopic dermatitis is a common disease in children, affecting primarily the neck, face, and bends of the knees and elbows. The main symptom is itching, along with redness, swelling, and weeping blisters; in a chronic condition, the skin darkens, thickens, cracks, and scales. The exact cause is unknown, but food allergens have been implicated particularly in infants. Most children outgrow the disease, improvement usually occurring at puberty.

The impact of atopic dermatitis on a child's emotional, social, and intellectual development can be great. One study found the disease prevented or interfered with the schooling of 35 percent of the patients.

The disease's exact cause remains uncertain. Eczema patients may have abnormal sweating, which may contribute to their inability to maintain soft and pliable skin.

The role of allergens in the development of atopic dermatitis is controversial. Considerable evidence implicates certain foods as triggers, particularly in infants. Inhaled pollens, molds, and dust appear inconsequential in the disease, although contact with animal dander may provoke eczema in some individuals.

Infantile Asthma. Of the 67 million children under age 17 in the United States, more than 8 million experience asthma at some time in their childhood, and 2.1 million suffer chronic asthma. Nearly three-quarters of these chronic asthma patients are 12 years of age or younger. Since there is no objective test to diagnose asthma in infants, the true incidence, prevalence, and impact of the disease in this group remains unknown.

Although the death rate from asthma in this age group is low, the suffering caused by this disease is high. The effects of the disease on family life, school performance, and on the development of a child's independence and self-image are also great.

About four out of five young asthmatics have an allergy involved in their disease. Of these, a relatively small proportion of infants with asthma possess a hypersensitivity to certain foods, including milk, wheat, eggs, and corn. In a few of these infants, milk may cause a rare syndrome in which their lungs concentrate iron, an anemia develops in which the red blood cells are reduced in size and hemoglobin content, and gastrointestinal problems occur. The substitution of a non-milk formula in their diets solves the problem. Although both IgE and IgG antibodies to milk have been found in children with this syndrome, their role in the disorder has yet to be established.

Gastrointestinal Disorders. Food allergies can affect the gastrointestinal tract. In one severe disorder called allergic gastroenteropathy, for example, an allergic reaction to food produces diarrhea, abdominal pain, and, often, nausea and vomiting. Unfortunately, simple elimination diets fail to ease these symptoms, and usually patients require corticosteroids for relief. Recent trials with oral doses of sodium cromolyn indicate it can reduce or eliminate the need for steroid therapy, which carries a high risk of adverse side effects.

Several other disorders have been blamed on an intolerance to certain foods or food additives. Hyperactivity and learning disabilities in a large number of children have been attributed to preservatives, food dyes, and other additives. Although this idea has gained adherents and support from some parents' groups, no well-controlled study has confirmed it. Similarly, tension-fatigue syndrome has been linked to eating certain foods. NIAID's task force recommends that well-controlled studies be conducted to establish the validity of these theories before significant political and social actions are taken.

Cystic Fibrosis

Cystic fibrosis is not an allergic disorder, but a disease that involves a general malfunctioning of the exocrine glands which produce saliva, mucus, and sweat. Mucus clogging and infection of the lungs result in breathing difficulties in these children. Some children with cystic fibrosis also suffer asthma and allergic diseases.

Conventional wisdom suggests that asthma might adversely affect the course of cystic fibrosis and other chronic inflammatory diseases of the bronchi. NIAID's task force recognizes the need to survey cystic fibrosis patients to learn the incidence of asthma and allergic diseases among them as well as to know how each of these allergic disorders affects morbidity and mortality in cystic fibrosis.

Chapter 13

Allergic Emergencies

Anaphylaxis

Anaphylaxis (literally meaning without protection) is a very serious manifestation of the allergic response. It is an IgE-mediated reaction that results when mast cells suddenly release chemical mediators that overwhelm the body.

The onset of anaphylaxis is usually sudden. Symptoms develop within minutes after exposure to some triggering allergen; and death, when it occurs, generally follows within less than two hours. The first evidence of anaphylaxis may be swelling and redness of the skin, often accompanied by hives. The victim may experience a feeling of great anxiety. Vomiting, abdominal cramps, and diarrhea are other frequent symptoms. Life-threatening breathing difficulties may develop due to swelling of the larynx or severe bronchospasm; a drastic drop in blood pressure can send a person into potentially fatal shock; in many severe cases, irregular heart beats develop.

Prevention remains the best treatment for anaphylaxis. Physicians carefully question patients about any history of allergies and drug reactions. However, anaphylaxis may occur without warning. In all cases, rapid treatment is essential.

The three therapies which control anaphylaxis are epinephrine, oxygen, and fluids by vein. Antihistamines and corticosteroids are also used. These drugs do not reverse anaphylaxis, but some evidence indicates they may prevent a later worsening of the reaction.

Extracted from NIH Publication No. 80-388.

Why some people react with anaphylaxis remains unknown. It is not even certain that a genetic tendency to IgE-mediated asthma or other allergic diseases predisposes people to anaphylaxis.

There is another response that is often confused with anaphylaxis. It is called the **anaphylactoid reaction,** and its symptoms are essentially the same as those of anaphylaxis. However, antibodies play no role in the anaphylactoid response.

Drug-Induced Anaphylactic Reactions

A lifesaving drug may, on occasion, cause a life-threatening anaphylactic reaction. Such a reaction may occur without any previous indication that the patient is allergic. But often people suffer a milder adverse response to a drug before they experience a potentially fatal allergic reaction. That is why physicians ask patients if they are allergic to any medications, especially penicillin.

Penicillin. Penicillin-induced anaphylaxis is an immediate allergic reaction that begins 2 to 30 minutes after the patient takes the first dose in a new series of treatments with the antibiotic.

About 1 person in 50 who receives penicillin has some sort of allergic reaction to it; about 1 person in 2,500 suffers anaphylaxis; and about 1 person in 100,000 dies. Anaphylactic deaths from penicillin are estimated to be 400 to 800 annually in the United States. Allergic reactions occur with both oral doses and injections. The incidence of anaphylaxis resulting from semisynthetic penicillins is unknown. However, evidence suggests that it is about the same as penicillin, at least for such widely used semisynthetics as ampicillin.

Clinical studies indicate that penicillin-induced anaphylaxis is IgE-mediated. In one study, for example, all the patients who suffered an immediate allergic reaction to the antibiotic had IgE antibodies against penicillin. In another study, three-quarters of the patients found to have IgE antibodies to penicillin developed hives or rashes when later given the drug.

Other Drugs. A number of other drugs may induce anaphylactic reactions. In the Boston Collaborative Drug Surveillance Program, for instance, 12 anaphylactic reactions involving 9 drugs occurred among 32,812 consecutive ward patients. Many drugs have been reported as causing anaphylaxis. However, it is often difficult to determine if the drug reaction is antibody-mediated or the result of some non-immunologic mechanism.

Reactions to Vaccines

Adverse reactions to vaccines may range from mild to fatal, and may be immunologic or non-immunologic. Some are impossible to classify. But the most life-threatening reactions, again, are the IgE-mediated anaphylactic responses and unclassified anaphylactoid reactions.

Tetanus and diphtheria. Tetanus and diphtheria vaccines have been widely used for years. Life-threatening anaphylactic or serum-sickness reactions occur in about 1 in every 1,000,000 inoculations. The danger of a tetanus reaction appears to increase with the frequency of immunization. Therefore, physicians now recommend booster shots be given only every 10 years, and in the event of an injury, no vaccine be injected if the patient has been inoculated within the previous 5 years.

Since diphtheria vaccine is usually given in combination with tetanus or whooping cough vaccines, the incidence of allergic reactions to it alone is uncertain.

Whooping cough, typhoid, paratyphoid, cholera, plague, and tuberculosis. The commonly used bacterial vaccines protect against whooping cough, typhoid, paratyphoid, cholera, plague, and tuberculosis. Mild reactions to each are common; but serious immunologic reactions to each occur only rarely. Children over the age of 6 should not be vaccinated against whooping cough, because of the danger of an adverse reaction.

Viral vaccines. Viral vaccines, too, induce reactions that range from mild to fatal. Local swelling and fever are common; fortunately, hives, serum-sickness, central nervous system disorders, and anaphylactic reactions are far less common. Viruses used in vaccines are grown in a variety of cell cultures including: chick and duck embryo cells; calf lymph; and monkey, rabbit, and dog kidney cells. Reactions to components from these cell cultures—which are incorporated into the vaccine during its production—account for many of the problems.

Rubella, mumps, rabies and yellow fever. Severe allergic reactions to the current rubella (German measles), mumps, rabies, and yellow fever vaccines are extremely rare. Serious problems with influenza vaccines are uncommon; but, rarely, cases of **Guillain-Barré**

syndrome—a paralysis of the nervous system of apparently autoimmune origin—do occur.

Reactions to Diagnostic and Therapeutic Allergens

A variety of diagnostic and therapeutic allergens can produce serious IgE-mediated allergic reactions. The severity and speed with which these develop depend on the nature of the agent, its concentration, how rapidly it is absorbed, and the sensitivity of the patient. Although it rarely happens, an allergen used in diagnosing allergies can, under certain circumstances, cause anaphylaxis in an extremely allergic person.

Physicians closely question patients before testing them for an allergic response. This often enables a doctor to pinpoint likely allergens, and thus limit the number of skin tests given. It can also alert physicians to the potential for serious adverse responses to the tests.

Immunotherapy, which reduces a person's immune response to a specific allergen, can help many allergy sufferers. But physicians must carefully administer the immunotherapy inoculations to avoid an adverse reaction. Such a reaction may occur for unexplained reasons. Adverse reactions may also occur if the amount of allergen given initially is greater than the patient's tolerance; if the amount of allergen is increased too rapidly in subsequent doses; if the timing between doses is not correct; if doses are not adjusted properly during times when the patient is exposed to natural sources of the allergen (such as pollens in the air); and if the dose is inadvertently injected into the bloodstream.

The most severe reactions to immunotherapy usually occur within the first few minutes after injection. Thus, physicians ask patients to remain for 15 to 30 minutes after their allergy injections as a safety precaution. While reactions may occur beyond this time period, they are usually not serious.

Anaphylactic Reactions to Insect Stings

Insect stings can induce anaphylactic reactions in an estimated 0.4 percent of the population, or more than 850,000 Americans. About 40 deaths a year are attributed to insect stings, but many others probably go unrecognized.

Reactions to insect stings may occur at any age, in people with or without a history of allergies. Indeed, several studies find that some people have no warning that they might be susceptible to a life-threatening reaction to an insect sting until it occurs. Most reactions are reported in people under age 20, and twice as often in males as in females. These statistics, however, probably reflect only the greater exposure of males and young people to insects.

Identifying the insect responsible for an allergic reaction is often difficult. Bees leave their stingers, but other insects do not. Recognizing this limitation on cataloging insect stings, the most commonly identified cause of insect-sting reactions is the yellow jacket, followed by the bee, wasp, and hornet.

Efforts to diagnose and treat insect sting allergy date to the 1930s. Research then suggested the allergens that induced insect sting reactions were present throughout the insects' bodies. Thus, extracts for diagnostic tests and for immunotherapy were made by crushing or grinding the whole insect body. Many knowledgeable allergists believe that this therapy is effective; others question the validity of this approach. The use of pure venoms to diagnose and treat insect sting allergies has been evaluated by both patient responses and laboratory tests. In these research settings, the venoms have been found to be very effective. This form of therapy is now available for general patient use.

Certain ants inject venom that can cause potentially fatal allergic responses. The problem in the United States is most serious in the southeastern and south central parts of the country. Of the many types of ants, the one most frequently implicated in severe allergic reactions is the imported fire ant. The name is derived from the insect's painful sting.

Currently, whole body extract is generally used to protect sensitive people against allergic reactions from fire ant stings. A pure venom treatment is in the experimental stage.

Anaphylactic Reactions to Foods

Surprisingly, everyday foods are a relatively common cause of anaphylaxis. Certain foods—nuts, fish, eggs, and seeds among them—are highly allergenic in some people, and for them, a minimal exposure can provoke severe symptoms. For example, anaphylaxis has occurred in several people who simply smelled cooked fish. Less common are severe reactions to such foods as milk, chocolate, grains (barley, rice, wheat), various fruits including tomatoes, and such vegetables as corn, spinach, potatoes, and soybeans.

Most often allergists diagnose a food sensitivity based primarily on a history of the patient's past experiences. Skin tests may be done and they may help confirm a diagnosis of an anaphylactic sensitivity to food. However, positive skin tests do not establish a food as a cause of anaphylaxis. Once a food allergy is diagnosed, it is vital for the patient to avoid the food. Immunotherapy, either through oral administration or injections, has not proven effective in preventing food-induced anaphylaxis.

Anaphylactoid Reaction to Injected Dyes

The use of dyes injected into the body in the course of certain x-ray studies poses a difficult problem, one that physicians have only partly resolved. In studying patients given dye injections for kidney studies, it was found that fewer than 1 in 1,000 had life-threatening reactions. But among those who react, about 35 percent will react again if they are injected with the dye a second time.

The mechanism of this reaction remains a mystery. Research has failed to identify either antibodies or cell-mediated immunity as the cause. However, it may be that the dyes themselves, rather than any immunologic mechanism, induce mast cells to release the chemical mediators that bring on the severe reaction.

These reactions present a problem because the use of these dyes is a vital part of many sophisticated x-ray studies. In a number of serious illnesses, there is no substitute for the diagnostic procedure, and no substitute for the dye. Nor is there a reliable way to predict who is at risk of suffering shock from the dyes, except to say patients who have already experienced an adverse reaction are at greater risk.

Such people, because of the nature of their illnesses, may need to receive the dyes again, in spite of the obvious risk of a severe response. Recent studies have shown that the risk of another reaction is markedly reduced in such patients who are given antihistamines and steroids before their dye injections. The current recommendation is that people at risk of dye-induced anaphylaxis should be pretreated with a combination of both drugs.

Cold-Induced Urticaria

The development of hives in response to cold temperature has been known for years. At its most severe, cold urticaria can result in a drastic drop in blood pressure, shock, and even death.

The exact cause or causes of the disorder remain unknown. In some people, cold urticaria is an IgE-mediated reaction; in others, it may result from some other mechanism. Only recently have scientists discovered that histamine and other mediators released by mast cells play a major role in cold urticaria.

Physicians now treat cold urticaria patients vigorously with antihistamines. Certain antihistamines seem particularly adept at battling certain symptoms of the ailment. Cyproheptadine, for example, effectively prevents the welts that result from contact with ice. Unfortunately, in some patients, the amount of antihistamine needed for prevention may be greater than the person's tolerance for the drug.

Transfusion Reactions

The transfusion of blood or blood products can trigger several types of acute reactions.

An anaphylactic reaction may follow a transfusion. This response most often occurs in people who are born without IgA antibodies, as is true in roughly 1 in every 700 persons. When such an IgA-deficient patient is given blood, his body makes IgE antibodies against the IgA antibodies he receives in the transfusion. If the patient is transfused again, these IgE antibodies rapidly attack the IgA antibodies in the serum of the new blood, resulting in life-threatening anaphylaxis.

Another type of reaction—which varies from mild to severe—occurs in patients who are transfused with whole blood or red blood cells that are incompatible with their own. This is not an immediate IgE-mediated reaction, but it develops rapidly, either while receiving the blood or shortly thereafter.

Symptoms include a feeling of warmth in the arm or along the vein being transfused, rapid heart beat, facial flushing, headache, pain in the lower back, chest pains, chills followed by fever, hives, vomiting, and diarrhea. In severe cases, a drastic drop in blood pressure may occur, as well as widespread blood clots, bleeding, and kidney failure. Rarely are all these symptoms seen in the same patient. Indeed, often only a few mild symptoms appear in patients transfused with mismatched blood. This is a type II reaction, in which IgG antibodies react against the incompatible blood cells.

Aspirin Reactions

Aspirin, known scientifically as acetylsalicylic acid, may induce severe, even life-threatening reactions that closely resemble anaphylaxis.

Hives and swelling of the upper airway, which may require emergency action to restore breathing, may also follow the drug's use. Aspirin is extensively used, and it ranks with penicillin as one of the most frequent causes of adverse drug reactions.

Patients with bronchial asthma, especially those who also have nasal polyps, appear to have a relatively high reaction rate to aspirin. Estimates run as high as 7 percent, and the risk of suffering an aspirin reaction increases with age in asthma patients.

The onset of severe symptoms may come within 15 minutes after taking aspirin, or it may not occur for hours. In such cases, it is often difficult to relate the use of aspirin to the reaction. Clinically, the symptoms of aspirin sensitivity are indistinguishable from those of anaphylaxis and they call for rapid and sometimes drastic measures to save the patient's life.

The exact mechanism of the aspirin reaction remains uncertain. So far, no antibodies to aspirin have been found. This failure has led to the search for other mechanisms. Several theories exist, but strong evidence to support any of them is lacking. Unfortunately, identification of aspirin-sensitive patients is not possible with skin tests or simple laboratory tests.

Hereditary Angioedema

This is an inherited disease that produces episodic swelling. Under most circumstances, the disorder is uncomfortable, but not dangerous; swelling occurs mostly in the face and extremities. However, in some patients severe swelling may develop in the tongue, throat, or larynx. Unless this is recognized and corrected, the airway may be blocked and suffocation may result.

The disease results from a deficiency in a blood protein involved in the complement system. Frequently, a life-threatening attack follows injury to the mouth, dental surgery, or a tooth extraction. Swelling increases in the hours that follow, and the patient develops breathing difficulties.

Most non-inherited swellings respond to drug therapy: epinephrine, antihistamines, and corticosteroids. However, hereditary angioedema does not respond well to these medications. Attacks can be prevented in many patients with modified male hormones and with the drug epsilon aminocaproic acid. Physicians sometimes give these medications during an acute attack, although it is not clear how effective they are when a patient is in the midst of severe swelling. In some cases, an opening must be made in the patient's throat and a tube inserted to enable the patient to breathe.

Swelling episodes generally last only a few days. If patients are treated properly, even in the most severe cases, they usually recover unharmed. However, the danger of another attack exists. People with hereditary angioedema should take prophylactic drugs to prevent further life-threatening swelling episodes.

Chapter 14

Holiday Allergies: 'Tis the Season!

For people with asthma and allergies, the holidays present health challenges unique to the winter season. Busier-than-usual social schedules, chilly weather, and cherished family customs combine to make staying healthy a daily priority for asthma and allergy sufferers.

Surviving, and enjoying, the holidays is easier when you plan ahead and take preventive action. Here are some tips to help you combat potential holiday hazards so that you'll look back on this season with joy instead of relief.

Holiday Indulgence?

From Halloween through New Year's day, the holidays are fraught with foods to be avoided by people with food allergies. Children, especially, need to be protected from certain candies and foods that cause allergic reactions. Inform family members and friends of special diet restrictions so that there'll be plenty of "safe" food to eat at holiday get-togethers. Prepare allergy-free snacks and meals in advance; freeze or store as much as possible so that hectic work and school schedules don't erode healthy eating habits.

Eating away from home requires advance planning to prevent potential allergic reactions. Take the time to check restaurant menus before eating out; call the hostess or manager and have them help you identify menu items the allergic person can safely eat. Offer to bring allergen free dishes that compliment meals hosted by friends or relatives to ensure that everyone enjoys these special events.

If you or a family member are predisposed to food allergies, have an epinephrine injection kit with you at all times because this busy season includes events which almost always feature food too tempting to resist.

When the Weather Outside Is Frightful...

Mold can be less than delightful. From raking wet leaves to choosing logs for the fireplace, allergy sufferers need to be prepared. Remove wet dirt and leaves from around the foundation and gutters of your house to prevent outdoor mold from accumulating near windows and doors. Stack all firewood outside, bringing new logs in only for immediate use in your fireplace or wood-burning stove.

Ideally, someone without outdoor mold allergy should perform outdoor activities where mold poses a threat. If you have to perform these chores, be sure to dress appropriately (i.e., wearing protective items such as gloves, face mask etc.) and keep preventive and/or treatment medication readily available.

Mold can also flourish indoors if the humidity is too high. When the heat is on, check humidity levels in those rooms where you'll spend most of your time, including bathrooms and basement living areas. Keep indoor humidity below 50 percent, as long as you're comfortable and allergy symptoms are minimal. Consider a dehumidifier, if necessary.

The cold, too, can be less than delightful for people with asthma. Block brisk winter winds from your face with a scarf or muffler. If these don't protect against asthma episodes, consider buying a warming mask available at most medical supply stores.

If you regularly work, play or exercise outdoors, you may need medication to prevent asthma induced by cold-weather activity. With the help of your physician, identify the best preventive medication for your condition and have an adequate supply on hand. Use this preventive medication at least 15 to 30 minutes before heading outdoors.

Chestnuts Roasting on an Open Fire...

And unseen particles nipping at your nose, eyes, and throat...clean your chimney before that first holiday fire and be sure the fireplace flue works properly. Check fireplace vents and keep the fireplace doors closed to eliminate as much smoke as possible. Replace fireplace screen with a door.

If you use a wood-burning stove, talk with your allergist or family physician about ways to reduce irritants caused by smoldering embers and other combustible materials.

Dusty Decor

Decorations and ornaments stored in the attic, basement, or garage can become coated with dust. Proper storage is the key to making future festivities fun instead of frustrating. Thoroughly clean and dry all decorations, seal them in plastic bags and store the bagged items in airtight containers or clean boxes.

If you are extremely sensitive to dust, consider buying a dust mask to wear over your nose and mouth. For about $15-20, a very good mask can be purchased from most medical supply stores (make sure it fits firmly around your face).

Heating vents can blow accumulated dust and debris throughout your home. Clean or replace filters in your furnace before turning your home heating system on. Pay special attention to any attached humidifiers. Placing a nonflammable filtering material (such as cheesecloth) over heating vents can help catch dust particles. Check and replace such homemade filters frequently.

Inspect the filters in any portable air cleaners you plan to use and clean or replace them as necessary. Running air cleaners at the highest setting during winter months can help reduce allergic reactions to indoor dust and mold.

'O, Christmas Tree!

If a live evergreen tree is a tradition you cannot live without, the following tips should help make this year's tree a treasure rather than trouble. Wipe the trunk thoroughly with a solution of lukewarm water and diluted bleach (1 part bleach to 20 parts water) to eliminate any mold. Some evergreens, particularly junipers and cedar, may be pollinating even in winter—look for a yellowish tinge on the trunk and needles. Before bringing the tree inside, use a leaf blower (in a well-ventilated area away from the house or garage) to remove visible pollen grains.

Artificial Christmas trees are suitable substitutes for live trees as long as they're not coated with sprayed-on "snow." Such additions (including pine-scented sprays or oils) can aggravate asthmatic or allergic symptoms in some people.

Over the River and Through the Woods

When visiting family or friends, be prepared for possible reactions to everything, from pets to food to perfume. Never leave home without the appropriate medication(s), equipment, and a written action plan so that the proper steps can be taken in case of an emergency.

Common "Sense" of the Season

Limit (or eliminate) scented candles, potpourri, air fresheners, plant arrangements, and frequent pungent holiday baking that can cause discomfort for asthmatics or those sensitive to strong odors.

Stay Healthy, Stay Happy

If you or another family member has moderate or severe asthma, ask your physician about the need for a flu shot. Your physician may recommend that everyone in the family be immunized to protect the more vulnerable family member (particularly if that member is a child with asthma or allergy).

Respiratory infections such as chicken pox, colds and the flu abound this time of year, and children are particularly susceptible. Children with asthma receiving regular steroid therapy should be carefully monitored, because chicken pox can be a serious illness for a child on steroids. If asthma symptoms persist throughout the season, consider purchasing a peak flow meter to help monitor changes in the airways. You and your doctor can develop a written action plan for medication based on the meter's readings. Keep it with you at all times. Highlight your physician's name and phone number for quick reference in case of an emergency.

At any time of the year, it's a good idea to develop a written asthma or allergy action plan, prepared with the help of your physician. This plan can be used to monitor symptoms and prevent attacks at home, work, school or on vacation.

Happy Holidays

AAFA extends seasonably warm appreciation to Ann Munoz-Furlong, Founder of the Food Allergy Network for her contributions to this article.

This information should not substitute for seeking responsible professional care.

And Don't Forget Those Other Holidays

Doris J. Rapp, in *Allergies and Your Family* outlines some sensible precautions particularly for the allergic child for several common holiday occasions.

Easter

Be careful of eggs, nuts in chocolate, or sensitivity to specific brands or types of chocolate.

Eggs: Some children can still enjoy hard-boiled eggs even though they cannot eat less thoroughly cooked eggs.

Chocolate: Some chocolates contain almond flavoring which can trigger an allergic reaction. Colored chocolate will cause the same reactions as ordinary chocolate. Some chocolate brands cause reactions, while others do not, according to parents.

Candies: Some candies like jelly beans or other coated confections may use dyes or spices that can cause an allergic response.
Licorice, since it is a legume, can cause problems for children allergic to peanuts.

Halloween

Candies: The same difficulties with candies haunt the Halloween festival as well but parents should also watch for candied apples that may not have been thoroughly cleansed of pesticides and preservatives or may have cinnamon in the glaze.

Masks: Plastic masks can irritate a chemical or latex sensitivity.

177

Rosh Hashanah, Yom Kippur, Chanukah, Purim, and Passover

Traditional foods often contain eggs, spices, nuts, poppy seeds, chicken, wheat, and fish. The nuts and fruits of the ritual passover dish should be carefully washed to remove insecticides. Any of these can trigger food allergies. Also consider *lox* (smoked salmon) a prime cause of fish allergies, and wine often causes problems. In addition, candle smoke can bring on an asthmatic episode and the holiday decorations themselves, usually stored for the occasion, may have dust and mold.

Thanksgiving

The main culprits are the obvious chestnuts, spices, and wine but for some children, cranberries and squash are also intolerable.

Mother's Day

An allergic child might have difficulty with some flowers and some chocolates.

Fourth of July

Firecracker fumes can irritate sensitive respiratory systems triggering asthma, hay fever, or milder allergic reactions.

Birthday Parties

For an asthmatic child, a birthday can be too much. Give asthma medication the day before and on the day as well if wheezing seems common.

The usual allergic problems here: egg-whites, nuts or nut flavoring, ice cream, chocolate, cinnamon or glazed apples, and candle smoke.

—by Allan R. Cook

Chapter 15

Allergic and Immunologic Aspects of Other Diseases

The Problem

Our knowledge of the immune system, and its relation to allergic diseases, has exploded within the past two decades. With these new insights, our understanding of the mechanisms underlying many other diseases has expanded as well. Many disorders that long mystified physicians are now known to relate to responses of the immune system. Immune deficiency diseases and the rejection of transplanted organs are almost exclusively problems of immunology, for example. Many other ailments including some skin, joint, kidney, lung, intestinal, parasitic, glandular, blood, infectious, and malignant disorders have important allergic and immunologic components. As science continues to explore the intricate workings of the immune system, other diseases undoubtedly will be discovered to have an immunologic or allergic origin.

The physical, psychological, economic, and social costs of these immune- and allergy-related diseases are immense. **Rheumatoid arthritis,** for example, afflicts more than five million Americans. **Crohn's disease** and **ulcerative colitis,** two gastrointestinal disorders, have a prevalence of 9.3 per 100,000 persons. **Multiple sclerosis** afflicts 250,000 Americans, mostly young adults, at an annual estimated cost of $1.25 billion. **Systemic lupus erythematosus,** a sometimes fatal disease of the connective tissue, strikes 50,000 new

Extracted from NIH Publication No. 80-388.

victims each year. And **parasitic diseases,** a worldwide health problem, affect millions of Americans.

This chapter is devoted to a brief discussion of some of these diseases. Each poses an important health hazard, with important social and economic ramifications. Each disease also serves as a model, which could lead to understanding and perhaps control of similar diseases through immunologic manipulation. For a more detailed discussion of immunological implications, see Omnigraphics' *Immune System Disorders Sourcebook*.

Rheumatoid Arthritis

Although rheumatoid arthritis is predominantly a chronic inflammation of the joints, it may affect the entire body, particularly the connective tissue. It is painful, often debilitating, and sometimes crippling. It may appear suddenly, with acute fever, pain, swelling, and disability in many joints; or it may develop gradually, often starting with slight pain and weakness in the joints of the hand. The disease tends to grow progressively worse, although it sometimes disappears spontaneously. Women are about three times as likely as men to develop rheumatoid arthritis. There is no cure; but a number of treatments, including drugs and physical therapy, can greatly ease the problems of patients.

The cause of rheumatoid arthritis remains unknown, but strong evidence indicates some immunological phenomena contribute to its origin and development. The most striking finding is that most rheumatoid arthritis patients have a substance in their blood called **rheumatoid factor**. This is an autoantibody, an antibody that attacks a person's own tissue. Most rheumatoid factor is IgM, but it may also occur as IgA and IgG.

Despite its presence in most rheumatoid arthritis sufferers, however, evidence suggests that rheumatoid factor alone does not cause the disease. For one thing, many people, especially older ones, have rheumatoid factor and yet do not have symptoms of rheumatoid arthritis. Moreover, blood transfusions containing the autoantibody have been given to people without their developing rheumatoid arthritis. Further studies are needed to determine what stimulates the production of rheumatoid factor and its role in rheumatoid arthritis.

Some authorities believe rheumatoid factor may be stimulated by some infectious agent, since the factor may be found in association with a variety of infectious diseases. In rheumatoid arthritis, environmental factors or differences in body chemistry may determine who develops the disease and its severity. Studies to date have failed to identify any specific environmental factors. The evidence for or against any genetic predisposition to the disease is conflicting. Given the frequency, severity, and socioeconomic impact of rheumatoid arthritis, NIAID's task force considers further research vital to understanding its cause and development, and to finding more effective ways to treat or prevent it.

Liver Diseases

Immunologic research has provided critical new insights into the cause and development of viral hepatitis. This liver inflammation afflicts more than 60,000 Americans each year. Traditionally, physicians have spoken of infectious hepatitis (caused generally by contaminated foods or water) and serum hepatitis (caused generally by contaminated blood transfusions).

It is now known that either type of the disease can be passed by either route of exposure. In the 1960s, immunologists identified two separate hepatitis viruses: Type A which causes infectious hepatitis and type B which causes serum hepatitis. However, scientists now know that one or more additional hepatitis-causing viruses, designated non-A/non-B, exist and can be transmitted through blood transfusions. A vaccine against type B hepatitis is being developed, but vaccines against the type A and non-A/non-B viruses will require further research.

Most cases of hepatitis are relatively mild; indeed some people never realize they have the disease. Patients generally recover with no ill effects. However, in some patients, hepatitis becomes a chronic active disease. At least two immunologic mechanisms appear to play a role in chronic active hepatitis. In the first, the type B virus alters the surface of liver cells in such a way that the immune system no longer recognizes these cells as "self;" therefore, the body mounts an immune attack against its own liver cells. The second mechanism involves an autoantibody response. The body produces IgG autoantibodies against a specific molecule found normally on the surface of liver cells.

A small percentage of both men and women who develop serum hepatitis become carriers. Although they show no symptoms of the disease, the type B virus remains active in their bodies, and they can pass it on to others, if their blood is used for transfusions. Hepatitis

B virus can also be transmitted from a mother to an infant at delivery or during early infancy. A study of 8,000 pregnant women seen in Denver over a 2-year period showed 0.3 percent had hepatitis B infections, and, of these, all were asymptomatic carriers. Studies in Asia, where the carrier rate is much higher, indicate that about half the babies of carrier mothers are born infected. The long-term consequences of being a carrier remain uncertain. But Asian studies suggest that this state leads to an increased risk of liver failure in later life, and a greater risk of developing a rare form of liver cancer.

Gastrointestinal Diseases

Several gastrointestinal (GI) ailments involve the immune system, including inflammatory-bowel diseases and some malabsorption syndromes.

The term, malabsorption describes an inability of the gastrointestinal tract to absorb certain nutrients from food. Malabsorption is a frequently overlooked complication in patients suffering from antibody deficiencies. Because such people have deficient immune systems they are unable to produce certain protective antibodies and they may be predisposed to infections. The most common antibody-deficiency syndrome is isolated IgA deficiency, which occurs in about 1 out of 700 persons. In some of these people, the lack of IgA results in increased numbers of gastrointestinal and respiratory infections.

Recent research indicates that antibodies present in the GI tract serve several important functions:

1. they defend against infectious germs and microbial toxins;
2. IgE-mediated reactions may be important in ridding the body of parasitic worms; and
3. immunoglobulins may help control the absorption of certain antigens across the intestinal wall and into the body.

Evidence strongly suggests that immune mechanisms play a role in ulcerative colitis and Crohn's disease. Ulcerative colitis is a chronic, recurrent ulceration of the colon; Crohn's disease, or regional ileitis, is a chronic inflammation of the ileum, a section of the small intestine. Patients with these two disorders frequently have antibodies and white cells that will react against the cells that line their GI tracts. Whether these immune reactions are the cause of the diseases, or the result of the bowel inflammation is unclear. Recent work suggests, however, that ulcerative colitis and Crohn's disease may result from the interaction of some infectious agent or agents and an altered immune response that develops in certain people. NIAID's task force recommends that this lead be vigorously pursued, as should further studies of antibody- and cell-mediated immunity in the gastrointestinal tract.

Neurological Diseases

Advances in immunology have proved extraordinarily valuable in helping to understand the causes of certain diseases of the nervous system and in providing some effective new treatments. Immune mechanisms apparently play major roles in **myasthenia gravis, multiple sclerosis, Guillain-Barré syndrome, chronic inflammatory neuropathy,** and **polymyositis,** and lesser roles in a number of other neurological diseases.

Myasthenia gravis. Myasthenia gravis causes fatigue and muscular weakness that may produce a life-threatening interference with breathing and swallowing. About 1 American in 10,000 develops the disorder. The ailment results from a reduction of acetylcholine activity in the body. Acetylcholine is one of the chemicals that carries messages, in the form of electrical signals, from one nerve cell to another. Evidence strongly suggests that myasthenia gravis is an autoimmune disease. Recent work shows that most myasthenia gravis patients have antibodies that attack acetylcholine receptors—places on a cell where the acetylcholine attaches to transmit its messages. As a result, there is interference with muscle activity.

What triggers this autoimmune response in myasthenia gravis remains unknown, but using the knowledge that the disease involves the immune system, researchers have devised more effective treatments. The most successful involves the use of immunosuppressive drugs and the removal of the antibodies by plasma exchange, a technique that may be lifesaving.

Guillain-Barré syndrome. Guillain-Barré syndrome, a paralysis of the nervous system, and chronic inflammatory neuropathy, a closely related disorder, both appear to be autoimmune diseases. More work is needed to determine the antibody or cellular-immune mechanisms involved.

Polymyositis. Polymyositis, a painful muscle inflammation that is accompanied by swelling; and dermatomyositis, a form of polymyositis in which the skin is also involved are both thought to be autoimmune diseases. They usually occur in people with other autoimmune diseases and in certain cancer patients. The use of immunosuppressive drugs often produces dramatic improvements in patients suffering from these disorders.

Multiple sclerosis. Multiple sclerosis, a relatively common disorder of the central nervous system, results in the degeneration of the protective myelin sheath that coats nerve fibers. This causes a decline in muscle coordination. The disease usually occurs in young adults. Its cause continues to elude researchers, but a number of clues suggest that an immune mechanism may be responsible, possibly acting together with a viral infection.

Scientists also suspect that the immune system may contribute to such neurological ills as **Parkinson's disease** and **amyotrophic lateral sclerosis (Lou Gehrig's disease).** Finally, immunodeficiencies appear likely causes or contributors to other neurological disorders.

Blood Disorders

The techniques and concepts of immunology contribute greatly to modern hematology. With immunologic techniques, researchers have studied the causes of many blood disorders, and developed valuable diagnostic and treatment methods.

For example, immunologic techniques demonstrate the antigenic differences in blood of different people. This was initially important in the discovery of the various blood groups, allowing physicians to determine which people are compatible so that blood transfusions can be carried out safely. Transfusion therapy is vital in the treatment of some diseases, in replacing blood lost through injury, and in certain surgical procedures. One of the major triumphs of recent medical history is a way to prevent *erythroblastosis fetalis,* or Rh factor disease in newborns. This has saved the lives of many babies.

Rh factor, so named because it was first discovered in the red blood cells of rhesus monkeys, exists in the blood of about 85 percent of all humans. These people are Rh positive; those without the factor are Rh negative. An Rh negative person transfused with Rh positive blood can develop serious, possibly fatal reactions. These result from antibodies produced against red cells with the Rh factor, and a cytotoxic (type II) allergic reaction results. The transfused Rh positive blood cells clump, and are destroyed.

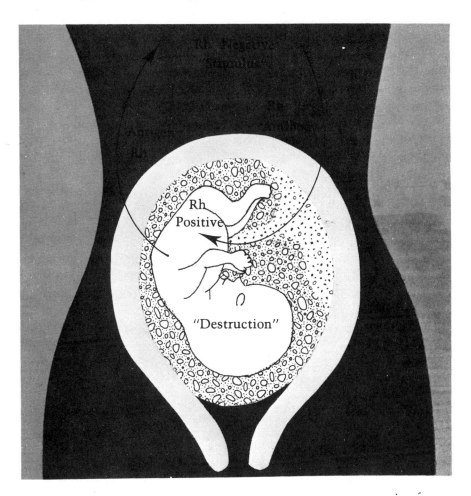

Figure 15.1. _Erythroblastosis fetalis can affect children born to an Rh positive father and an Rh negative mother. If their baby is Rh positive, as a result of inheriting the Rh factor from the father, the mother may develop antibodies against the baby's blood. There is no danger to the first such baby of these parents, but each subsequent pregnancy increases the risk that the mother's antibodies will destroy the baby's blood. Now, however, mothers with this incompatibility can, after the birth of their first and each subsequent Rh positive child, receive injections that prevent the production of the harmful antibodies. To be effective, this injection must also be administered to the mother after any spontaneous or elective abortions._

A similar situation may occur during pregnancy. If the mother is Rh negative and the baby is Rh positive, as a result of inheriting the Rh factor from the father, the mother may develop antibodies against the baby's blood. No harm comes to the mother, but the antibodies may cross the placenta and destroy the blood of a fetus (developing infant) in a later pregnancy. No damage befalls the first infant, because a previous exposure is required to develop anti-Rh antibodies. Second and third pregnancies may also be unaffected; but the more children an Rh negative mother has by an Rh positive father, the greater the risk to the next child.

Until 1968, thousands of infants died each year as the result of erythroblastosis fetalis. Then, immunology provided the key to preventing such deaths. The treatment stems from the finding that antibodies suppress themselves; they are self-regulating to some extent. Therapy consists of giving an Rh negative mother a substance called Rh-immune globulin within 72 hours after the birth of her first Rh positive child or after the loss of an unborn child, and after the birth of each subsequent Rh positive infant. An antibody in this injection prevents the production of harmful antibodies, and in virtually all cases ensures her next child won't develop erythroblastosis fetalis.

Systemic Lupus Erythematosus

This is usually a disease of young women. SLE is a debilitating and potentially fatal disease of the connective tissue that may involve many different parts of the body, with the most serious damage done in the kidneys and brain. Kidney failure, seizures, personality disorders, arthritis, joint pain, skin rashes, pleurisy, and an increase in infections may accompany the disease.

Genetic, immunologic, and viral factors may all play roles in the origin and development of SLE. It appears that a genetic susceptibility, possibly coupled with a virus, creates disorder in the immune system. The system's regulatory mechanisms appear uncontrolled, and white cells capable of mounting an autoimmune attack are activated.

Immunologists are currently focusing their research on two factors that may be involved in this disease. The first suggests that an abnormality in the differentiation and function of certain T cells is an underlying cause of SLE. The second suggests that certain viruses, called C-type viruses, may trigger the autoimmune response in susceptible individuals.

Recent research attributes the predominance of SLE in females to the effects of sex hormones. Animal studies show that male sex hormones suppress the disease in mice and female sex hormones accelerate it. The sex hormones may exert their modulating effects in SLE through action on certain T cells. The possible use of male sex hormones to treat SLE is currently being investigated.

Kidney Disease

Kidney failure is a major cause of death, and evidence indicates that immune reactions are involved in several types of kidney disease, notably **glomerulonephritis.** This disorder is an inflammation of the capillaries that form loops in a section of the kidney called the glomeruli. It accounts for over half of the 42,000 annual kidney-failure deaths in the United States.

Two separate immune responses may cause glomerulonephritis. The more common from appears to involve immune complexes and is, thus, called **immune complex glomerulonephritis (ICGN);** the rarer, called **antiglomerular basement membrane antibody disease,** or **anti-GBM disease,** apparently results from autoantibodies.

Although increasing evidence implicates immune complexes in ICGN, conclusive proof continues to elude scientists, except in a small percentage of cases. Nor have efforts to identify antigens involved in ICGN made much progress. Recently, however, a series of findings suggested that the hepatitis B virus is involved in the origin and development of a number of immune-complex mediated diseases, including glomerulonephritis.

Anti-GBM disease is responsible for only a small percentage of glomerulonephritis cases. In this form, autoantibodies attack a delicate layer of connective tissue in the kidney called the basement membrane. The disease progresses rapidly, and frequently it is accompanied by lung involvement. In most patients, there are no clues to what caused the formation of the autoantibodies. A few cases, however, have developed shortly after the inhalation of a hydrocarbon solvent. Recently, physicians have successfully treated some anti-GBM patients with immunosuppressive drugs and plasmapheresis, a technique that can remove some of the autoantibodies from the blood.

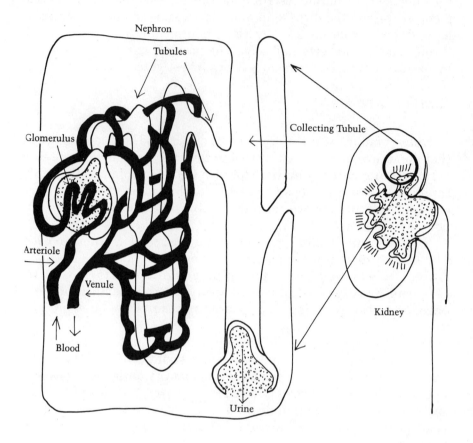

Figure 15.2. *The basic unit of the kidney, the nephron, removes unwanted substances from the blood. After entering the glomerulus (a network of many parallel blood vessels) by way of a small artery known as an arteriole, the blood is cleansed through a filtration process. The tubules complete the process by excreting the unwanted materials as urine and returning the remaining substances to the blood.*

Organ Transplants

The immune system reacts to a lifesaving organ transplant the way it responds to an infection: it tries to destroy the foreign cells. Successful organ transplants, notably kidneys, have resulted from the increasing ability of physicians to match organ donors and recipients, and to suppress what is a natural immune response to rid the body of a foreign object.

The body can mount at least three distinct rejection responses:

- hyperacute,
- acute, and
- chronic.

Hyperacute. Hyperacute rejection occurs within hours of a transplant because antibodies that attack the donated organ already exist in the patient.

Acute. Acute rejection occurs days or weeks after surgery and is a cell-mediated reaction that takes place primarily because the grafted organ activates T cells.

Chronic. Chronic rejection, a slow progressive process, may take months or years. Its mechanisms are poorly understood, but it appears due to T-cell activity. In both acute and chronic cases, death of the transplanted organ occurs because the immune response destroys blood vessels that feed the transplanted organ.

Although graft rejection results primarily from T cell attacks, the process involves a complex interaction of both cell-mediated and antibody-mediated activity.

One way of avoiding rejection is by histocompatibility matching. The cells of each human contain histocompatibility (HLA) antigens inherited from the mother and father. These chemical complexes are what the immune system "reads" to determine if a cell is "self" or "nonself." If the histocompatibility antigens spell "nonself," the immune system attacks.

There are two ways to test for these antigens. By means of a blood test using the patient's serum, physicians can now classify people according to some of their histocompatibility antigens, much as they group people by blood types. The other, more definitive test, takes longer because culture of living blood cells is required. The closer two people match according to this test, the greater the chances of success in transplanting an organ from one to the other. Anticipated advances in these tissue-typing techniques will improve current transplant successes.

Currently, an equally important factor in the success of transplants is the increasingly sophisticated use of immunosuppressive drugs to control rejection. It is not merely the drugs themselves, but the careful control of their amount and the timing of their administration that has reduced the risk of rejection.

Parasitic Diseases

Parasitic diseases are a worldwide problem; they afflict millions, particularly in the developing nations. Yet while science has intensely pursued the role of immunology in viral and bacterial infections, investigations of its defensive activity in parasitic diseases has lagged. Now, both for humanitarian and scientific reasons, there is a burgeoning interest. This has been stimulated by the realization that immunology offers an unusual opportunity to make rapid progress against many parasitic disorders.

There is some evidence that **schistosomiasis,** a serious health problem that infects some 200 million people, mostly in Asian and tropical countries, is essentially an immunologic disease. Much of the disease's damage apparently results from an immune response to the worms' eggs.

Pinworm afflicts 45 million Americans; it appears that the anal itching that accompanies this parasitic infection results from an immune reaction to pinworm secretions.

Some scientists now suggest that IgE antibodies may play a role in protecting against hookworm, a parasite that penetrates the skin of the feet and eventually reaches the lining of the intestine. This statement is based on the observation that people with high IgE levels have a low incidence of hookworm compared to people with normal amounts of the antibody.

Work with Chagas' disease, a parasitic infection found mostly in South America, suggests that heart damage accompanying the ailment results from T-cell attacks, and perhaps an autoantibody response as well.

Contrary to general belief, most parasitic infections are not controlled. Therefore, an understanding of their origin and development is vital to finding immunologic means of preventing or curing these devastating and debilitating diseases.

Cancer

Immunologic research has found that malfunctions in the regulation and expression of genes are common in malignant cells. The result is that cancer cells may have different chemicals (antigens) on their surfaces than normal cells. Some of these antigens are unique to individual patients, but many patients apparently share others. Efforts are under way to find antigens that are specific to certain cancers and found universally in patients suffering those cancers. Such antigens could serve as a means of early cancer diagnosis.

Normally, the immune system recognizes and attacks cancer cells before they do damage. When this immuno-surveillance fails, cancers can grow and spread. Patients with immune-deficiency diseases are highly susceptible to malignancies. The question that puzzles researchers is why people with apparently normal immune systems develop cancer. What weakness or defect lets cancer flourish?

Human studies do reveal that most cancers profoundly depress the body's cell-mediated immunity. Moreover, the inflammatory process, which helps amplify our immunologic protection, is also depressed. This suggests that one way to treat cancer is to stimulate or restore the immune responses. Some experimental successes have been achieved using this approach. But far more research is needed to devise effective immunologic therapies and diagnostic techniques and to understand the interaction of malignancies and the immune system.

Part Three

Food Allergens

Chapter 16

Food Allergies and Intolerances

Allergies versus Intolerances

Food allergies or food intolerances affect the lives of virtually everyone at some point. People often may have an unpleasant reaction to something they ate and wonder if they have a food allergy. Almost one out of three people either say that they themselves have a food allergy or that they modify the family diet because a family member is suspected of having a food allergy. But only about 3 percent of children have clinically proven allergic reactions to foods. In adults, the prevalence of food allergy drops to about 1 percent of the total population.

This difference between the clinically proven prevalence of food allergy and the public perception is, in part, due to reactions that are termed "food intolerances" and not food allergies. A food allergy, or hypersensitivity, is an abnormal response to a food that is triggered by the immune system. The immune system is not responsible for the symptoms of a food intolerance, even though these symptoms can resemble those of a food allergy.

It is extremely important for people who have true food allergies to identify them and prevent allergic reactions to food because these reactions can cause devastating illness and, in some cases, be fatal.

NIH Publication No. 93-3469.

Allergy Symptoms

There is a wide range of food allergy symptoms. This variability of symptoms stems from the large number of tissues in the body which can be affected by an immune reaction to food.

Frequently the first part of the body to react to food is the gastrointestinal tract. The allergic reaction in this portion of the body can cause vomiting, abdominal pain, and diarrhea. As the immune response to food affects other areas of the body, a person may develop hives (urticaria), swelling, sneezing and a runny nose, asthma or difficulty breathing. The most severe food allergy reaction is anaphylaxis—a systemic, life-threatening shock that can occur minutes after a person eats a food to which they are allergic. Anaphylactic reactions to food probably result in as many as 50 deaths a year in the United States. One of the characteristic features of this kind of reaction is trouble breathing caused by edema (swelling) of the throat or bronchi; it can also cause severe asthma, hives, a drop in blood pressure and loss of consciousness, and death, if not treated immediately.

Eczema due to food allergy is a different kind of reaction in which the target organ is the skin, which becomes crusty, red, scaly, and itchy. In children, eczema is frequently due to foods, but it can also be a preexisting condition made worse by certain foods. Probably fewer than one in twenty adults with eczema has an associated food allergy.

How Allergic Reactions Work

The mechanism behind an allergic reaction involves two features of the human immune response. One is the production of immunoglobulin E (IgE), a type of protein called an antibody that circulates through the blood. The other feature of the immune response is the mast cell, a specific cell that occurs in all body tissues but is especially common in areas of the body that are typical sites of allergic reactions, including the nose and throat, lungs, skin, and gastrointestinal tract.

The ability of a given individual to form IgE against something as benign as food is an inherited predisposition. Generally, such people come from families in which allergies are common, not necessarily food allergies but perhaps hay fever, asthma, or hives. Someone with two allergic parents is more likely to develop food allergies than someone with one allergic parent.

Before an allergic reaction can occur, a person who is predisposed to form IgE to foods first has to be exposed to the food. As this food is digested, it triggers certain cells to produce specific IgE in large amounts. The IgE is then released and attaches to the surface of mast cells. The next time the person eats that food, it interacts with specific IgE on the surface of the mast cells and triggers the cells to release chemicals such as histamine. Depending upon the tissue in which they are released, these chemicals will cause a person to have various symptoms of food allergy.

If the mast cells release chemicals in the ears, nose, and throat, a person may feel an itching in the mouth, and may have trouble breathing or swallowing. If the affected mast cells are in the gastrointestinal tract, the person may have abdominal pain or diarrhea. The chemicals released by skin mast cells, in contrast, can prompt hives.

Food allergens (the food fragments responsible for an allergic reaction) are proteins within the food that usually are not broken down by the heat of cooking or by stomach acids or enzymes that digest food. As a result, they survive to cross the gastrointestinal lining, enter the bloodstream, and go to target organs, causing allergic reactions throughout the body.

The complex process of digestion affects the timing and the location of a reaction. If people are allergic to a particular food, for example, they may first experience itching in the mouth as they start to eat the food. After the food is digested in the stomach, abdominal symptoms such as vomiting, diarrhea or pain may start.

When the food allergens enter and travel through the bloodstream, they can cause a drop in blood pressure. As the allergens reach the skin, finally, they can induce hives or eczema. All of this takes place within a few minutes to an hour.

Common Food Allergies

In adults, the most common foods to cause allergic reactions include: shellfish, such as shrimp, crayfish, lobster, and crab; peanuts, which is one of the chief foods to cause severe anaphylactic reactions; tree nuts, such as walnuts; fish; and egg.

In children, the pattern is somewhat different. The most common food allergens that cause problems in children are egg, milk, and peanuts.

The foods that adults or children react to are those foods they eat often. In Japan, for example, rice allergy is more frequent. In Scandinavia, codfish allergy is common.

Cross Reactivity

If someone has a life-threatening reaction to a certain food, the doctor will counsel the patient to avoid similar foods that might trigger this reaction. For example, if someone has a history of allergy to shrimp, testing will usually show that the person is not only allergic to shrimp, but also to crab, lobster, and crayfish, as well. This is called cross reactivity.

Another interesting example of cross reactivity occurs in people who are highly sensitive to ragweed. During ragweed pollination season, these people sometimes find that when they try to eat melons, in particular cantaloupe, they have itching in their mouths and they simply cannot eat the melon. Similarly, people who have severe birch pollen allergy also may react to the peel of apples.

Adults usually do not lose their allergies, but children can sometimes outgrow them. Children are more likely to outgrow allergies to milk or soy than allergies to peanuts, fish or shrimp.

Differential Diagnoses

A differential diagnosis means distinguishing food allergy from food intolerance or other illnesses. If a patient goes to the doctor's office and says, "I think I have a food allergy," the doctor has to consider the list of other possibilities that may lead to symptoms that could be confused with food allergy.

One possibility is the contamination of foods with microorganisms, such as bacteria, and their products, such as toxins. Contaminated meat sometimes mimics a food reaction when it is really a type of food poisoning. There are also natural substances, such as histamine, that can occur in foods and stimulate a reaction similar to an allergic reaction. For example, histamine can reach high levels in cheese, some wines, and in certain kinds of fish, particularly tuna and mackerel. In fish, histamine is believed to stem from bacterial contamination, particularly in fish that hasn't been refrigerated properly. If someone eats one of these foods with a high level of histamine, that person may have a reaction that strongly resembles an allergic reaction to food. This reaction is called histamine toxicity.

Another cause of food intolerance that is often confused with a food allergy is lactase deficiency. This most common food intolerance affects at least one out of ten people. Lactase is an enzyme that is in the lining of the gut. This enzyme degrades lactose, which is in milk.

If a person does not have enough lactase, the body cannot digest the lactose in most milk products. Instead, the lactose is used by bacteria, gas is formed, and the person experiences bloating, abdominal pain, and sometimes diarrhea.

Another type of food intolerance is an adverse reaction to certain products that are added to food to enhance taste, provide color, or protect against growth of microorganisms. Compounds that are most frequently tied to adverse reactions that can be confused with food allergy are yellow dye number 5, monosodium glutamate, and sulfites. Yellow dye number 5 can cause hives, although rarely. Monosodium glutamate (MSG) is a flavor enhancer, and, when consumed in large amounts, can cause flushing, sensations of warmth, headache, facial pressure, chest pain or feelings of detachment in some people. These transient reactions occur rapidly after eating large amounts of food to which MSG has been added. Sulfites can occur naturally in foods or are added to enhance crispness or prevent mold growth. Sulfites in high concentrations sometimes pose problems for people with severe asthma. Sulfites can give off a gas called sulfur dioxide, which the asthmatic inhales while eating the sulfited food. This irritates the lungs and can send an asthmatic into severe bronchospasm, a constriction of the lungs. Such reactions led the U.S. Food and Drug Administration (FDA) to ban sulfites as spray-on preservatives in fresh fruits and vegetables. But they are still used in some foods and are made naturally, during the fermentation of wine for example.

There are a number of other diseases that share symptoms with food allergies including ulcers and cancers of the gastrointestinal tract. These disorders can be associated with vomiting, diarrhea or cramping abdominal pain exacerbated by eating.

Some people may have a food intolerance that has a psychological trigger. In selected cases, a careful psychiatric evaluation may identify an unpleasant event in that person's life, often during childhood, tied to eating a particular food. The eating of that food years later, even as an adult, is associated with a rush of unpleasant sensations that can resemble an allergic reaction to food.

Diagnosis

To diagnose food allergy a doctor must first determine if the patient is having an adverse reaction to specific foods. This assessment is made with the help of a detailed patient history, the patient's diet diary, or an elimination diet.

The first of these techniques is the most valuable. The physician sits down with the person suspected of having a food allergy and takes a history to determine if the facts are consistent with a food allergy. The doctor asks such questions as:

- What was the timing of the reaction? Did the reaction come on quickly, usually within an hour after eating the food?

- Was allergy treatment successful? (Antihistamines should relieve hives, for example, if they stem from a food allergy.)

- Is the reaction always associated with a certain food?

- Did anyone else get sick? For example, if the person has eaten fish contaminated with histamine, everybody who ate the fish should be sick. However, in an allergic reaction, only the person allergic to the fish becomes ill.

- How much did the patient eat before experiencing a reaction? The doctor will want to know how much you ate each time and try to relate it to the severity of the reaction.

- How was the food prepared? Some people will have a violent allergic reaction only to raw or undercooked fish. Complete cooking of the fish destroys those allergens in the fish to which they react. If the fish is cooked thoroughly, they can eat it with no allergic reaction.

- Were other foods ingested at the same time of the allergic reaction? Some foods may delay digestion and thus delay the onset of the allergic reaction.

Sometimes a diagnosis cannot be made solely on the basis of history. The doctor may also ask the patient to go back and keep a record of the contents of each meal and whether he or she had a reaction. This gives more detail from which the doctor and the patient can determine if there is consistency in the reactions.

The next step some doctors use is an elimination diet. Under the doctor's direction, the patient does not eat a food suspected of causing the allergy, like eggs, and substitutes another food, in this case another source of protein. If the patient removes the food and the symptoms go away, a diagnosis can almost be made. If the patient then eats the food (under the doctor's direction) and the symptoms come back, then the diagnosis is confirmed. This technique cannot be used, however, if the reactions are severe (in which case the patient should not resume eating the food) or infrequent.

If the patient's history, diet diary or elimination diet suggest a specific food allergy is likely, the doctor will then use tests that can more objectively measure an allergic response to food. One of these is a scratch skin test, during which a dilute extract of the food is placed on the skin of the forearm or back. This portion of the skin is then scratched with a needle and observed for swelling or redness that would indicate a local allergic reaction. If the scratch test is positive, the patient has IgE on the skin's mast cells that is specific to the food being tested.

Skin tests are rapid, simple and relatively safe. But a patient can have a positive skin test to a food allergen without experiencing allergic reactions to that food. A diagnosis of food allergy is made only when a patient has a positive skin test to a specific allergen and the history of their reactions also suggests an allergy to the same food.

In some extremely allergic patients who have severe anaphylactic reactions, skin testing can't be used because it could evoke a dangerous reaction. Skin testing also cannot be done on patients with extensive eczema. For these patients a doctor may use one of two blood tests called RAST and ELISA. These tests measure the presence of food-specific IgE in the blood of patients. These tests may cost more than skin tests and results are not immediately available. As with skin testing, positive tests do not necessarily make the diagnosis.

The final method used to objectively diagnose food allergy is double blind food challenge. This testing has come into vogue over the last few years as the "gold standard" of allergy testing. For this food challenge, various foods, some of which are suspected of inducing an allergic reaction, are each placed in individual opaque capsules. The patient is asked to swallow a capsule and is then watched to see if a reaction occurs. This process is repeated until all the capsules have been swallowed. In a true double-blind test, the doctor is also "blinded," the capsules having been made up by some other medical person, so that neither the patient nor the doctor knows which capsule contains the allergen.

The one strong advantage of such a challenge is that, if the patient has a reaction only to suspected foods and not to other foods tested, it confirms the diagnosis. However, someone with a history of severe reactions cannot be tested this way. In addition, this testing is expensive because it takes a lot of time to perform. Multiple food allergies are also difficult to evaluate with this procedure. Consequently, double-blind food challenges are not done often. This type of testing is most commonly used when the doctor believes that the reaction a person is describing is not due to a specific food and wishes to obtain evidence to support this judgment so that additional efforts may be directed at finding the real cause of the reaction.

Exercise Induced Food Allergy

There is at least one situation where more than the simple ingestion of a food to which a person is sensitive is required to provoke a reaction, and that is in exercise-induced food allergy. People who experience this reaction eat a specific food before exercising. As they exercise and their body temperature goes up, they begin to itch, get light-headed, and soon have a full-blown allergic reaction such as hives. The cure for exercise-induced food allergy is simple: not eating for a couple of hours before exercising.

Treatment

Food allergy is treated by dietary avoidance. Once a patient and the patient's doctor have identified the food to which the patient is sensitive, the food must be removed from the patient's diet. To do this, patients must read lengthy, detailed ingredient lists on each food they are considering eating. Many allergy-producing foods such as peanuts, eggs, and milk, appear in foods one normally wouldn't associate them with. Peanuts, for example, are often used as a protein source and eggs are used in some salad dressings. The FDA requires ingredients in a food to appear on its label. People can avoid most of the things to which they are sensitive, if they read food labels carefully and avoid restaurant-prepared foods that might have ingredients to which they are allergic.

In highly allergic people even minuscule amounts of a food allergen (1/44,000 of a peanut kernel for example) can prompt an allergic reaction. Other less sensitive people may be able to tolerate small amounts of a food to which they're allergic.

Patients with severe food allergies must be prepared to treat an inadvertent exposure. Even people who are very knowledgeable about what they are sensitive to occasionally make a mistake. In order to protect themselves, people who have had anaphylactic reactions to a food should wear medical alert bracelets or necklaces, available at most pharmacies, stating that they have a food allergy and that they are subject to severe reactions. Such people also should always carry a syringe of adrenaline (epinephrine), obtained by prescription from their doctors, and be prepared to self-administer it if they think they are getting a food allergic reaction. They should then immediately seek medical help by either calling the rescue squad or by having themselves transported to an emergency room. Anaphylactic allergic reactions can be fatal even when they start off with mild symptoms such as a tingling in the mouth and throat or gastrointestinal discomfort.

There are several medications that can be taken to relieve food allergy symptoms that aren't part of an anaphylactic reaction. These include antihistamines to relieve gastrointestinal symptoms, hives, or sneezing and a runny nose. Bronchodilators can relieve asthma symptoms. These medications are taken after people have inadvertently ingested a food to which they are allergic but are not effective in preventing an allergic reaction when taken prior to eating the food. No medication in any form can be taken before eating a certain food that will reliably prevent an allergic reaction to that food.

There are a few unproven treatments for food allergies. One involves injections containing small quantities of the food extracts, to which the patient is allergic. These shots are given on a regular basis for a long period of time with the aim of "desensitizing" the patient to the food allergen. Allergy shots have not yet been proven to relieve food allergies.

Infants and Children

Milk and soy allergies are particularly common in infants and children. These allergies sometimes do not involve hives and asthma, but rather lead to colic, and perhaps blood in the stool or poor growth. Infants and children are thought to be particularly susceptible to this allergic syndrome because of the immaturity of their immune and digestive systems.

Milk or soy allergies in infants can develop within days to months of birth. Sometimes there is a family history of allergies or feeding problems. The clinical picture is one of a very unhappy colicky child who may not sleep well at night. The diagnosis is based in part on changing the child's diet. Rarely, food challenge is used.

If the baby is on cow's milk, the doctor may suggest a change to soy formula or exclusive breast milk, if possible. If soy formula causes an allergic reaction, parents should try feeding the baby with elemental formulas, which are processed proteins (basically sugars and amino acids). There are few if any allergens within these materials. Corticosteroids are also sometimes used to treat infants with severe food allergies. Fortunately, time usually heals this particular gastrointestinal disease. It tends to resolve within the first few years of life.

Exclusive breast feeding (excluding all other foods) of infants for the first 6 to 12 months of life is often suggested to avoid milk or soy allergies from developing within that time frame. Such breast feeding often allows parents to avoid infant-feeding problems, especially if the parents are allergic (and the infant therefore is likely to be allergic).

There are some children who are so sensitive to a certain food, however, that if the food is eaten by the mother, sufficient quantities enter the breast milk to cause a food reaction in the child. Mothers sometimes must themselves avoid eating those foods to which the baby is allergic.

There is no conclusive evidence that breast feeding prevents the development of allergies later in life. It does, however, delay the onset of food allergies by delaying the infant's exposure to those foods that can prompt allergies and may avoid altogether those feeding problems seen in infants. By delaying the introduction of solid foods until the infant is 6 months old or older, parents can also prolong the child's allergy-free period.

Controversial Issues

There are several disorders thought by some to be caused by food allergies, but the evidence is currently insufficient or contrary to such claims. It is controversial, for example, whether migraine headaches can be caused by food allergies. There are studies showing that people who are prone to migraines can have their headaches brought on by histamines and other substances in foods. The more difficult issue is whether food allergies actually cause migraines in such people.

There is virtually no evidence that rheumatoid arthritis or osteoarthritis can be made worse by foods, despite claims to the contrary.

There is also no evidence that food allergies can cause a disorder called the allergic tension fatigue syndrome, in which people are tired, nervous, and may have problems concentrating, or have headaches. Cerebral allergy is a term that has been applied to people who have trouble concentrating and have headaches, as well as other complaints. This is sometimes attributed to mast cells degranulating in the brain, but no other place in the body. There is no evidence that such a scenario can happen, and cerebral allergy is not currently recognized by allergists.

Another controversial topic is environmental illness. In a seemingly pristine environment, some people have many non-specific complaints such as problems concentrating or depression. Sometimes this is attributed to small amounts of allergens or toxins in the environment. There is no evidence that such problems are due to food allergies.

Some people believe hyperactivity in children is caused by food allergies. But this behavioral disorder has only been suggested to be associated with food additives occasionally in children, and then only when such additives are consumed in large amounts. There is no evidence that a true food allergy can affect a child's activity except for the proviso that if a child itches and sneezes and wheezes a lot, the child may be miserable and therefore more difficult to control. Also, children who are on anti-allergy medicines that can cause drowsiness may get sleepy in school or at home.

Controversial Diagnostic Techniques

Just as there are controversial food allergy syndromes and treatments there are also controversial ways of diagnosing food allergies. One of these is cytotoxicity testing, in which a food allergen is added to a patient's blood sample. A technician then examines the sample under the microscope to see if white cells in the blood "die." This technique has been evaluated in a number of studies and has not been found to effectively diagnose food allergy.

Another controversial approach is called sublingual or, if it is injected under the skin, subcutaneous provocative challenge. In this procedure, dilute food allergen is administered under the tongue of the person who may feel that his or her arthritis, for instance, is due to foods. The technician then asks the patient if the food allergen has aggravated the arthritis symptoms. In clinical studies, this procedure has not been shown to effectively diagnose food allergies.

An immune complex assay is sometimes done on patients suspected of having food allergies to see if there are complexes of certain antibodies bound to the food allergen in the bloodstream. It is said that these immune complexes correlate with food allergies. But the formation of such immune complexes is a normal offshoot of food digestion and everyone, if tested with a sensitive enough measurement, has them. To date, no one has conclusively shown that this test correlates with allergies to foods.

Another test is the IgG subclass assay, which looks specifically for certain kinds of IgG antibody. Again, there is no evidence that this diagnoses food allergy.

Controversial Treatments

Controversial treatments include putting a dilute solution of a particular food under the tongue about a half hour before the patient eats that food. This is an attempt to "neutralize" the subsequent exposure to the food that the patient believes is harmful. As the results of a well-conducted clinical study show, this procedure is not effective in preventing an allergic reaction.

Summary

Food allergies are caused by immunologic reactions to foods. There actually are several discrete diseases under this category and a number of foods that can cause these problems.

A medical evaluation after one suspects a food allergy is the key to proper management. Treatment is basically avoidance of the food(s) after they are identified. People with food allergies should become knowledgeable about allergies and how they are treated and should work with their physicians.

The National Institutes of Health supports research on food allergies through grants that it provides to research institutions throughout the world. Understanding the cause of an immune system dysfunction in allergy will ultimately lead to better methods of diagnosing, treating and preventing allergic diseases.

Questions and Answers

Would you discuss what common substances are in both peanuts and other kinds of nuts? The response I often get when I tell people that I am severely allergic to both peanuts and nuts is that I cannot be because peanuts are a legume, unlike nuts.

First of all, it is possible to be allergic to two distinct foods. It is interesting that both peanuts and nuts are concentrated sources of protein, which is probably one reason why reactions to both these foods are so frequent. But you can have cross reactions between tree nuts and peanuts, or you could develop allergies to both.

I would like to ask about diet during pregnancy. I have heard some talk about avoiding certain foods during your last trimester.

There is no evidence that avoidance of foods in the last trimester can prevent food allergies. In fact, some experimental evidence suggests this is harmful.

Would gross swelling of the lips be indicative of a food allergy?

Well, it can be, but you can also have something called idiopathic angioedema, which can cause swelling of the lips. This disorder is not caused by food allergies. If you have such a problem, talk it over with your doctor. If there is any chance that it might be a food allergy, the doctor can place you on an elemental diet for ten days. If the problem does not go away, you have ruled out food allergy.

Is intolerance a disease entity?

Food intolerance is not a distinct entity. It is a term used to cover any adverse reaction to a food that doesn't have an immunologic basis.

I have a 14-year-old daughter who has developed chronic hives in the past nine months. She has swelling and hives on the bottom of her feet to the point where she cannot walk; her fingers swell and she cannot write. She has been skin tested for food allergies, and it was negative. We are going through the elimination diet process now and seeing some improvement, but not a whole lot. The only thing that controls it is prednisone. What would you suggest as the next step?

Sometimes there is a non-specific improvement as you manipulate the diet. But chronic hives and angioedema, especially of that duration are almost never due to food allergies. Unfortunately, no cause is usually found. There is hope that they will resolve with time. I'd advise you to limit the use of steroids because steroids can do more damage than if you just use antihistamines.

Is there any hope of better management of lactose intolerance than chewing tablets that help dissolve lactose during the meal?

Probably not, other than avoidance of foods that have lactose.

What is the best way to diagnose lactose deficiency?

There are a couple of tests that involve ingesting a specific amount of lactose and then measuring the body's response. Such blood tests are done by physicians.

Can you tell us anything about gluten intolerance?

Gluten intolerance is associated with the disease called gluten-sensitive enteropathy or celiac disease. It is due to an abnormal immune response to gluten, which is a component of wheat and some other grains.

Is it possible that many people who were given the diagnosis of irritable bowel syndrome in the past are turning out to actually have allergies?

There is no good evidence that irritable bowel syndrome is due to food allergies in most instances.

This summer I had lunch at a fast food restaurant for the first time and I broke out in hives. The doctor seemed to think maybe it was the sulfites in the food. Now you said there had been regulations for salad bars and sulfites, but in the whole food industry are there regulations for the use of sulfites?

Yes, there are industry-wide regulations covering the use of sulfites. Now I do not know anything about the restaurant you ate at, but it is more likely that you ate something else you are allergic to because sulfites rarely cause hives.

Chapter 17

A Fresh Look at Food Preservatives

Unless you grow all your food in your own garden and prepare all your meals from scratch, it's almost impossible to eat food without preservatives added by manufacturers during processing. Without such preservatives, food safety problems would get out of hand, to say nothing of the grocery bills. Bread would get moldy, and salad oil would go rancid before it's used up.

Food law says preservatives must be listed by their common or usual names on ingredient labels of all foods that contain them—which is most processed food. You'll see calcium propionate on most bread labels, disodium EDTA on canned kidney beans, and BHA on shortening, just to name a few. Even snack foods—dried fruit, potato chips, and trail mix—contain sulfur-based preservatives.

Manufacturers add preservatives mostly to prevent spoilage during the time it takes to transport foods over long distances to stores and then our kitchens.

It's not unusual for sourdough bread manufactured in California to be eaten in Maine, or for olive oil manufactured in Spain to be used on a California salad. Rapid transport systems and ideal storage conditions help keep foods fresh and nutritionally stable. But breads, cooking oils, and other foods, including the complex, high-quality convenience products consumers and food services have come to expect, usually need more help.

Preservatives serve as either antimicrobials or antioxidants—or both. As antimicrobials, they prevent the growth of molds, yeasts and

FDA Consumer, October 1993.

bacteria. As antioxidants, they keep foods from becoming rancid, browning, or developing black spots. Rancid foods may not make you sick, but they smell and taste bad. Antioxidants suppress the reaction that occurs when foods combine with oxygen in the presence of light, heat, and some metals. Antioxidants also minimize the damage to some essential amino acids— the building blocks of proteins— and the loss of some vitamins.

Safety Questions

Consumers often ask the Food and Drug Administration about the safety of preservatives, and if there's a system in place to make sure preservatives are safe.

Many preservatives are regulated under the food additives amendment, added to the Federal Food, Drug, and Cosmetic Act in 1958. The amendment strengthened the law to ensure the safety of all new ingredients that manufacturers add to foods. Under these rules, a food manufacturer must get FDA approval before using a new preservative, or before using a previously approved preservative in a new way or in a different amount. In its petition for approval, the manufacturer must demonstrate to FDA that the preservative is safe for consumers, considering:

- the probable amount of the preservative that will be consumed with the food product, or the amount of any substance formed in or on the food resulting from use of the preservative;

- the cumulative effect of the preservative in the diet; and

- the potential toxicity (including cancer-causing) of the preservative when ingested by humans or animals.

Also, a preservative may not be used to deceive a consumer by changing the food to make it appear other than it is. For example, preservatives that contain sulfites are prohibited on meats because they restore the red color, giving meat a false appearance of freshness. (The U.S. Department of Agriculture regulates meats, but depends on the FDA regulation to prohibit sulfites in meats.)

The food additive regulations require the preservative to be of food grade and be prepared and handled as a food ingredient. Also, the quantity added to food must not exceed the amount needed to achieve the manufacturer's intended effect.

Regulations about the use of nitrites demonstrate the scrutiny given to the use of additives. Nitrites, used in combination with salt, serve as antimicrobials in meat to inhibit the growth of bacterial spores that cause botulism, a deadly food-borne illness. Nitrites are also used as preservatives and for flavoring and fixing color in a number of red meat, poultry, and fish products.

Since the original approvals were granted for specific uses of sodium nitrite, safety concerns have arisen. Nitrite salts can react with certain amines (derivatives of ammonia) in food to produce nitrosamines, many of which are known to cause cancer. A food manufacturer wanting to use sodium nitrites must show that nitrosamines will not form in hazardous amounts in the product under the additive's intended conditions of use. For example, regulations specify that sodium nitrite, used as an antimicrobial against the formation of botulinum toxin in smoked fish, must be present in 100 to 200 parts per million. In addition, other antioxidants, such as sodium ascorbate or sodium erythorbate, may be added to inhibit the formation of nitrosamines.

As scientists learn more about the action of certain chemicals in our bodies, FDA uses the new data to reevaluate the permitted uses of preservatives. Two examples are the commonly used preservatives butylated hydroxyanisole (BHA) and sulfites.

BHA

BHA and the related compound butylated hydroxytoluene (BHT) have been used for years, mostly in foods that are high in fats and oils. They slow the development of off-flavors, odors, and color changes caused by oxidation. When the food additives amendment was enacted, BHA and BHT were listed as common preservatives considered *generally recognized as safe* (GRAS). GRAS regulations limit BHA and BHT to 0.02 percent or 200 parts per million (ppm) of the fat or oil content of the food product.

Lawrence Lin, Ph.D., of FDA's Center for Food Safety and Applied Nutrition, explains, "The 0.02 percent allowed relates only to the product's fat content. For example, if a product weighs 100 grams and one of those grams is fat, the quantity of BHA in the product cannot exceed 0.02 percent of that one gram of fat."

BHA is also used as a preservative for dry foods, such as cereals. But because such foods contain so little fat, the amount of BHA allowed cannot be measured against the percentage of fat, explains Lin. Therefore, as manufacturers petitioned FDA for approvals for this use, the agency set limits for each type of food. On cereals, for example, FDA limited BHA to 50 ppm of the total product.

In 1978, under contract with FDA, the Life Sciences Research Office of the Federation of American Societies for Experimental Biology (FASEB) examined the health aspects of BHA as part of FDA's comprehensive review of GRAS safety assessments. FASEB concluded that although BHA was safe at permitted levels, additional studies were needed.

Since that evaluation, other studies suggested that at very high levels in the diets of laboratory animals, BHA could cause tumors in the forestomach of rats, mice and hamsters, and liver tumors in fish. Many experts examined the data and concluded the tests did not establish that such problems could exist in humans, mostly because humans do not have forestomachs. Other studies showed that BHA was protective, inhibiting the effect of some chemical carcinogens, depending on the conditions of the tests.

Studies on BHA were reviewed by scientists from the United Kingdom, Canada, Japan, and the United States. Their findings were published in 1983 in the *Report of the Working Group on the Toxicology and Metabolism of Antioxidants* and reviewed in the *1990 Annual Review of Pharmacology and Toxicology*. The 1983 report stated that data from a Japanese study showed a high incidence of cancerous tumors and papillomas (benign tumors of the skin or mucous membranes) of the forestomach of treated rats and that the effect was dose-related. The report also mentioned the possible existence of a no-effect level, based on dose response, and noted that the level which produced cancer in this study was many thousands of times higher than the level to which humans are exposed.

In November 1990, Glenn Scott, M.D., a physician then living in New York who has since moved to Cincinnati, filed a petition with FDA, asking the agency to prohibit the use of BHA in food. Scott cited animal studies to support his request. Before acting on Scott's petition, however, FDA asked FASEB to re-examine the scientific data on BHA. By March 1994, FASEB is scheduled to provide FDA with a report on the most current scientific information bearing on the relationship of BHA ingestion to cancer in animals.

Sulfites

Sulfites are used primarily as antioxidants to prevent or reduce discoloration of light-colored fruits and vegetables, such as dried apples and dehydrated potatoes. They are also used in wine-making because they inhibit bacterial growth but do not interfere with the desired development of yeast.

Sulfites are also used in other ways, such as for bleaching food starches and as preventives against rust and scale in boiler water used in making steam that will come in contact with food. Some sulfites are used in the production of cellophane for food packaging.

FDA prohibits the use of sulfites in foods that are important sources of thiamin (vitamin B_1), such as enriched flour, because sulfites destroy the nutrient.

Though most people don't have a problem with sulfites, some do.

FDA's sulfite specialist, consumer safety officer Joann Ziyad, Ph.D., points to a bookcase full of binders and says, "Those are the case histories of adverse reactions to sulfites that have been reported to FDA. Since 1985, when the agency started reporting on sulfites through the Adverse Reaction Monitoring System, over 1,000 adverse reactions have been recorded."

As reports of adverse reactions mounted, FDA asked FASEB to re-examine the use of sulfites. FASEB's report, released in 1985, concluded that sulfites posed no hazard to most Americans, but that they were a hazard of unpredictable severity to people who were sensitive to the substance. Based on the FASEB study, FDA estimated that more than 1 million asthmatics are sensitive or allergic to the substance.

In 1986, FDA ruled that sulfites used specifically as preservatives must be listed on the label, regardless of the amount in the finished product. Sulfites used in food processing but not serving as preservatives in the final food must be listed on the label if present at levels of 10 parts per million or higher. Regulations issued in 1990 extended these required listings to standardized foods.

Also in 1986, FDA banned the use of sulfites on fruits and vegetables intended to be eaten raw, such as in salad bars and grocery store produce sections. Grocers and restaurateurs were using them to maintain the color and crispness of fresh produce. (Even before the FDA ban, industry trade groups had persuaded many of their members to stop using sulfites on fresh produce.)

FDA plans to re-propose a ban for sulfites on fresh, peeled potatoes served or sold unpackaged and unlabeled, such as for french fries in restaurants. An earlier FDA rule dealing with sulfites on potatoes was invalidated by the court in 1990 on procedural grounds.

In addition, sulfite-sensitive consumers are learning how to avoid sulfites. Consumer awareness combined with FDA actions have slowed the number of adverse reaction reports. Ziyad says that from 1990 to 1992, fewer than 40 were reported, and at press time, there had been only three reports in 1993.

Ziyad says the only way FDA can know about sulfite-sensitivity problems is through consumer and physician reports. Adverse reaction reporting is totally voluntary, and FDA encourages physicians to report patients' reactions to sulfites. But there are times when such reactions are not medically treated because the individual doesn't go to the doctor with the condition or the symptoms are not recognized. Such information would help FDA evaluate the current status of problems with foods among sulfite-sensitive individuals.

The agency's Adverse Reaction Monitoring System collects and acts on complaints concerning all food ingredients, including preservatives. If you have an adverse reaction from eating a food that contains sulfites, describe the circumstances and your reaction to the FDA district office in your area (see local phone directory) and send a report in writing to:

Adverse Reaction Monitoring System (HFS-636)
200 C St., S.W.
Washington, DC 20204

Puzzling It Out

Preservatives are a puzzle for many consumers that can sometimes raise safety concerns. Even though these concerns are usually unfounded, some industry publications are reporting attempts to find naturally occurring substitutes for synthetic antioxidants.

In a 1990 article, one such publication, *Inform*, says alternatives to synthetics are commercially available in the United States, although most are generally more costly or have other drawbacks. For example, tocopherol (vitamin E), generally is not as effective in vegetable fats and oils as it is in animal fats. Also, some herbs and herb extracts, such as rosemary and sage, can do the work of antioxidants, but they impart strong color or flavors. And just because these are plant-derived doesn't necessarily mean they are always safe. *Inform* points to the FDA rule that newly identified natural antioxidants, like other new food additives, must undergo rigorous toxicological tests before they can be approved.

As an additional alternative to synthetic antioxidants, the edible oil industry is increasingly using ultraviolet-barrier packaging and filling under nitrogen to protect the product's stability.

FDA scientists will continue to carefully evaluate all research presented to the agency on new preservatives to ensure that substances added to food to preserve quality and safety are themselves safe.

A Sulfite by Any Other Name

People who are sulfite-sensitive should know which foods may possibly contain sulfites. But it's not always obvious by the chemical names on the label which ingredients are sulfites. Currently, there are six sulfiting agents allowed in packaged foods. The names by which they are listed on food labels are:

- sulfur dioxide
- sodium sulfite
- sodium and potassium bisulfite
- sodium and potassium metabisulfite

They are used in the following food categories at these typical maximum residual sulfur dioxide equivalent levels:

baked goods, 30 ppm
beer, 25 ppm
wine, 275 ppm
tea, 90 ppm
condiments and relishes, 30 ppm
vinegar, 75 ppm
dairy products, 200 ppm
processed seafood products, other than dried or frozen, 25 ppm
shrimp, fresh and frozen, 100 ppm
lobster, frozen, 100 ppm
gelatin, 40 ppm
grain products, 200 ppm
gravies and sauces, 75 ppm
jams and jellies, 30 ppm

nut products, 25 ppm
plant protein isolates, 110 ppm
dried fruit, 2,000 ppm
fruit juices: concentrates, 1,000 ppm; regular-strength, 300 ppm
glacé fruit, 150 ppm
maraschino cherries, 150 ppm
dehydrated vegetables, 200 ppm
dehydrated potatoes, 500 ppm
canned vegetables, 30 ppm
frozen potatoes, 50 ppm
vegetable juice, 100 ppm
filled crackers, 75 ppm
dry mix soup mixes, 20 ppm
sugar, 20 ppm
sweet sauces and syrups, 60 ppm
molasses, 300 ppm

The symptom most reported by sulfite-sensitive people is difficulty breathing. Other problems range from stomach-ache and hives to anaphylactic shock. In addition to knowing which food preservatives are sulfites and which foods are likely to contain them, sulfite-sensitive consumers can help themselves avoid health problems by following these suggestions:

• Read food labels and choose foods that don't contain sulfites.

• Be aware that foods served in restaurants, especially potato products and some canned foods, could contain sulfites. Ask the waiter if sulfites are used in what you plan to order.

For example, lemon juice in your tea or splashed on your salad could be a source of sulfites. Fresh-squeezed lemon is OK, but bottled lemon juice often contains sodium bisulfite.

—by Judith E. Foulke

Judith E. Foulke is a staff writer for FDA Consumer.

Chapter 18

From Shampoo to Cereal: Seeing to the Safety of Color Additives

It starts when you get up in the morning.

You snatch a bar of soap and scrub your face. That's likely your first dab into the palette of added tints and hues that will color much of your day. Most of us hardly notice them, but color additives surround us. They're in shampoos, in shaving cream, toothpaste, deodorant, contact lenses, lipstick, eyeliner, and mascara. At breakfast, the colors keep coming. Juice, cereal, pastry, coffee creamer, vitamins all are likely to have added colors.

Color additives make things attractive, appealing, appetizing. They also serve as a code of sorts, allowing us to identify products on sight, like medicine dosages and candy flavors. We might reason, for example, that a pale green candy is mint flavored, while a darker green one is lime. Based on our color analysis alone, there will probably be no surprises when we pop the candy into our mouths.

With this rainbow hodgepodge bombarding us daily, it's only natural that consumers might wonder: Just how safe are all these colors? "Very," says John E. Bailey, Ph.D., acting director of FDA's Office of Cosmetics and Colors.

He explains that FDA has, over nearly a century, refined its process of monitoring and controlling color additive use. By law, industry must prove the safety of colors it sells. FDA ensures that colors on the market are safe for their intended purposes and do not cover up product inferiority or otherwise deceive consumers. FDA watches domestic color use closely, seizing products found unsafe.

FDA Consumer, December 1993.

Still, Bailey says, some consumers believe color additives can cause health problems or even be hazardous. This notion stems, he says, from persistent public attitudes about colors banned in the past. He says consumer confidence in the safety of all colors can be shaken when FDA removes a color from the market. But he emphasizes: "I think we can say with assurance that today's colors are safe if used properly and that consumers need not be worried."

Yellow Means Caution

Two categories make up FDA's list of permitted colors: those the agency certifies by batch (derived primarily from petroleum and coal sources) and ones exempt from batch certification (obtained largely from plant, animal, or other mineral sources: fruit juice, carmine, and titanium dioxide, for example). Colors found to be potentially hazardous have been purged from the list of permissible additives. What remains is a wide color spectrum approved for use in foods, over-the-counter and prescription drugs, cosmetics, or in medical devices such as surgical sutures and contact lenses.

Though these colors have a good safety record, one commonly used additive reportedly has prompted minor adverse reactions in some people. It is FD&C Yellow No. 5, listed as tartrazine on medicine labels, a color found widely in beverages, desserts, processed vegetables, drugs, makeup, and many other products. FDA certifies more than 2 million pounds of it yearly.

In 1986, an FDA advisory committee concluded that Yellow No. 5 may cause itching or hives in a small population subgroup. This kind of skin reaction usually is not a serious one, says Linda Tollefson, D.V.M., an FDA epidemiologist. "Reactions are classified as hypersensitive and are not true allergic reactions, which would be more severe."

Nonetheless, since 1980 (for drugs) and 1981 (for foods), FDA has required all products containing Yellow No. 5 to list the color on their labels so consumers sensitive to the dye can avoid it. (As of May 8, 1993, labels must list all certified colors as part of the requirements of the Nutrition Labeling and Education Act of 1990.)

A Certified Success

FDA requires domestic and foreign certifiable color manufacturers to submit samples taken from every batch of color produced. The agency has listed each certifiable color based on a specific chemical formula shown to produce no harmful effects in laboratory animals.

Each color has chemical "specifications" that place restrictions on the levels of impurities allowed in the additive. In some cases, these limitations are designed to ensure that the color contains no cancer-causing substances. Using chromatography and other sophisticated analytical techniques, FDA scientists probe sample compositions to confirm that each batch is within these limitations.

"We analyze every batch because every batch is a little different from the one before it," says Bailey. He explains that complex organic chemical reactions occurring during manufacturing can throw off a sample's composition. It's like baking a cake: Even though you follow a recipe closely, the cake turns out just a little different each time.

With certifiable colors, a shift in composition can mean rejection of an entire batch. In fiscal year 1992, of 3,943 batches tested, the agency rejected 40. FDA also regularly inspects color manufacturers and end-users such as candy makers.

FDA is especially vigilant in monitoring products from foreign countries, which may contain color additives that are illegal domestically. The agency regularly seizes entire product shipments that contain prohibited colors. Often, this detective work comes easily. FDA, through its "import alerts," flags certain products. "You look for a pattern," says Bailey.

The batch certification program supports itself because the law requires manufacturers to pay FDA a user fee for every pound of color the agency certifies. "We like to think of [batch certification] as a government success story," Bailey says.

The Red Scare

In 1960, amendments to the Food, Drug, and Cosmetic Act of 1938 added the so-called Delaney anti-cancer clause to FDA's legal mandate. Among other things, the clause prohibits marketing any color additive the agency has found to cause cancer in animals or humans, regardless of amount.

In recent years, regulators have faced a dilemma in light of technological advances that enable scientists to identify smaller and smaller concentrations of a substance and conduct more sensitive toxicological tests. Are such tiny amounts a health threat? Scientists have yet to answer this question. Congress has held hearings to examine the pros and cons of liberalizing the Delaney clause. At press time, debates on the issue were in progress.

FDA applied the Delaney clause in 1990 when it outlawed several uses of the strawberry-toned FD&C Red No. 3. The banned uses include cosmetics and externally applied drugs, as well as all uses of the color's non-water-soluble "lakes." FDA previously had allowed these "provisional" uses while studies were in progress to evaluate the color's safety. Research later showed large amounts of the color causes thyroid tumors in male rats.

Though FDA viewed Red No. 3 cancer risks as small about 1 in 100,000 over a 70-year lifetime the agency banned provisional listings because of Delaney directives. At the same time, Red No. 3 has "permanent" listings for food and drug uses that are still allowed, although the agency has announced plans to propose revoking these uses as well. For now, Red No. 3 can be used in foods and oral medications. Products such as maraschino cherries, bubble gum, baked goods, and all sorts of snack foods and candy may contain Red No. 3.

According to the International Association of Color Manufacturers, Red No. 3 is widely used in industry and hard to replace. It makes a very close match for primary red, which is important in creating color blends. It doesn't bleed, so drug companies use it to color pills with discernible shades for identification.

If Red No. 3 joins the ranks of colors forbidden for all uses, it won't be the first FD&C red in recent years to be pulled from the market. FDA banned FD&C Red No. 2, a tint that continues to be an enigma, in 1976.

In the early 1970s, data from Russian studies raised questions about Red No. 2's safety. Several subsequent studies showed no hazards. FDA conducted its own tests, which were inclusive. The consumer-oriented Health Research Group petitioned FDA to ban the color, while congressional and public interest mounted.

FDA turned the matter over to its Toxicology Advisory Committee, which evaluated numerous reports and decided there was no evidence of a hazard. The committee then asked FDA to conduct follow-up analyses. Agency scientists evaluated biological data and concluded that "it appears that feeding FD&C Red No. 2 at a high dosage results in a statistically significant increase" in malignant tumors in female rats.

There still was no positive proof of either potential danger or safety. FDA ultimately decided to ban the color because it had not been shown to be safe. The agency based its decision in part on the presumption that the color might cause cancer.

The judgment had a profound effect on consumer attitudes toward certifiable colors, says FDA's John E. Bailey. "The Red No. 2 decision will always be with us," he says. For example, some candy manufacturers reacted by removing red-colored pieces from their products, even if there was no Red No. 2 present. They were afraid sales would plummet because of public perception that red candies were dangerous.

Though long gone from U.S. shelves, products tinted with Red No. 2 still can be found in Canada and Europe. Whether the color is gone forever in the United States remains to be seen. FDA and industry officials say it could stage a comeback. Industry could petition FDA to list Red No. 2 as a certifiable color if animal study data adequately show safety. If FDA then agrees, consumers could once again be munching on candies and using other products tinted with the deep-red dye.

Animal-less Studies?

Because of the cost, it is unlikely that industry will commission new animal studies to measure Red No. 2's safety. But advances in toxicological trial methods could enable scientists to assess potential hazards without using animals. Technology is moving toward a time when chemical substances could be evaluated accurately with a battery of short-term tests conducted in the test tube. Such analyses would greatly shorten the time and expense of evaluating not only colors but other food additives and environmental chemicals.

These test tube trials are not here yet. But if and when they arrive, they may have government and industry taking another look at certain color additives, including Red No. 2.

As for the colors that remain in use, consumers can rest assured that color additives are among the most scrutinized of all food ingredients. Next time you quaff a glass of red fruit punch or pop a blue pill, consider that those colors have been studied, studied, and restudied, sometimes dozens of times. And remember that FDA inspects every batch of certifiable colors used in consumer products.

You may, however, want to avoid consuming huge quantities of any one color additive. As Bailey says: "Good sense is the best policy. As with many other food ingredients, don't overuse any one product. Practice everything in moderation."

A Colorful History

Color additives have long been a part of human culture. Archaeologists date cosmetic colors as far back as 5000 B.C. Ancient Egyptian writings tell of drug colorants, and historians say food colors likely emerged around 1500 B.C.

Through the years, color additives typically came from substances found in nature, such as turmeric, paprika and saffron. But as the 20th century approached, new kinds of colors appeared that offered marketers wider coloring possibilities. These colors, many whipped up in the chemist's lab, also created a range of safety problems.

In the late 1800s, some manufacturers colored products with potentially poisonous mineral- and metal-based compounds. Toxic chemicals tinted certain candies and pickles, while other color additives contained arsenic or similar poisons. Historical records show that injuries, even deaths, resulted from tainted colorants. Food producers also deceived customers by employing color additives to mask poor product quality or spoiled stock.

By the turn of the century, unmonitored color additives had spread through the marketplace in all sorts of popular foods, including ketchup, mustard, jellies, and wine. Sellers at the time offered more than 80 artificial coloring agents, some intended for dyeing textiles, not foods. Many color additives had never been tested for toxicity or other adverse effects.

As the 1900s began, the bulk of chemically synthesized colors were derived from aniline, a petroleum product that in pure form is toxic. Originally, these were dubbed "coal-tar" colors because the starting materials were obtained from bituminous coal. (These formulations still are used today albeit safely for most certifiable color additives.)

Though colors from plant, animal and mineral sources (at one time the only coloring agents available) remained in use early in this century, manufacturers had strong economic incentives to phase them out. Chemically synthesized colors simply were easier to produce, less expensive, and superior in coloring properties. Only tiny amounts were needed. They blended nicely and didn't impart unwanted flavors to foods. But as their use grew, so did safety concerns.

In 1906, Congress passed the Pure Food and Drugs Act. This marked the first of several laws allowing the federal government to scrutinize and control color additive use. The act covered only food coloring. It was not until passage of the Federal Food, Drug, and Cosmetic Act of 1938 that FDA's mandate included the full range of color additives. That statute created the color designations consumers still can read on product packages: "FD&C" (permitted in food, drugs and cosmetics); "D&C" (for use only in drugs and cosmetics); and "Ext. D&C" (colors for external-use drugs and cosmetics).

Public hearings and regulations following the 1938 law gave colors the numbers that separate their hues. These letter and number combinations FD&C Blue No. 1 or D&C Red No. 17, for example make it easy to distinguish colors used in food, drugs or cosmetics from dyes made for textiles and other uses. Only FDA-certified color additives can carry these special designations.

The law also created a listing of color "lakes." These are water-insoluble forms of certain approved colors used in coated tablets, cookie fillings, candies, and other products in which color bleeding could make a mess or otherwise cause problems.

Though the 1938 law did much to bring color use under strict control, nagging questions lingered about tolerance levels for color additives. One incident in the 1950s, in which scores of children contracted diarrhea from Halloween candy and popcorn colored with large amounts of FD&C Orange No. 1, led FDA to retest food colors. As a result, in 1960, the 1938 law was amended to broaden FDA's scope and allow the agency to set limits on how much color could be safely added to products.

FDA also instituted a pre-marketing approval process, which requires color producers to ensure, before marketing, that products are safe and properly labeled. Should safety questions arise later, colors can be re-examined. The 1960 measures put color additives already on the market into a "provisional" listing. This allowed continued use of the colors pending FDA's conclusions on safety.

From the original 1960 catalog of about 200 provisionally listed colors, which included straight colors and lakes, only lakes of some colors remain on the provisional list. Industry withdrew or FDA banned many, while the rest became permanently listed and are still used. Some of these colors, derived from coal or petroleum sources, are subject to certification and carry the F, D, or C prefix. Others, exempt from certification, are pigments and colors derived from plant, animal and mineral sources. They are found in a myriad of products from the caramel that tints cola drinks to the orange annatto that gives color to cheese.

FDA certified over 11.5 million pounds of color additives last fiscal year. Of all those colors, straight dye FD&C Red No. 40 is by far the most popular. Manufacturers use this orange-red color in all sorts of gelatins, beverages, dairy products, and condiments. FDA certified more than 3 million pounds of the dye in fiscal year 1992, almost a million pounds more than the runner-up, FD&C Yellow No.5.

Color Additive Terms

Allura Red AC. The common name for uncertified FD&C Red No. 40.

Certifiable color additives. Colors manufactured from petroleum and coal sources listed in the *Code of Federal Regulations* for use in foods, drugs, cosmetics, and medical devices.

Coal-tar dyes. Coloring agents originally derived from coal sources.

D&C. A prefix designating that a certifiable color has been approved for use in drugs and cosmetics.

Erythrosine. The common name of uncertified FD&C Red No. 3.

Exempt color additives. Colors derived primarily from plant, animal and mineral (other than coal and petroleum) sources that are exempt from FDA certification

Ext. D&C. A prefix designating that a certifiable color may be used only in externally applied drugs and cosmetics.

FD&C. A prefix designating that a certified color can be used in foods, drugs or cosmetics.

Indigotine. The common name for uncertified FD&C Blue No. 2.

Lakes. Water-insoluble forms of certifiable colors that are more stable than straight dyes and ideal for products in which leaching of the color is undesirable (coated tablets and hard candies, for example)

Permanent listing. A list of allowable colors determined by tests to be safe for human consumption under regulatory provisions.

Provisional listing. A list of colors, originally numbering about 200, that FDA allows to continue to be used pending acceptable safety data.

Straight dye. Certifiable colors that dissolve in water and are manufactured as powders, granules, liquids, or other special forms (used in beverages, baked goods, and confections, for example).

Tartrazine. A common name for uncertified FD&C Yellow No.5.

For a complete list of all colors approved for use in foods, drugs, cosmetics, and medical devices, contact:

Office of Cosmetics and Colors (HFS-125)
Food and Drug Administration
200 C St.,S.W.
Washington, DC 20204
(202) 205-4143

Adverse Reactions?

Though reactions to color additives are rare, FDA wants to know about them. The agency operates the Adverse Reaction Monitoring System (ARMS) to collect and act on complaints concerning all food ingredients, including color additives. Consumers can register complaints two ways: by contacting their FDA district office (see local phone directory) or by sending written reports of adverse reactions to:

ARMS
HFS-636
Food and Drug Administration
200 C St., N.W.
Washington, DC 20204

—by John Henkel

John Henkel is a staff writer for FDA Consumer.

Chapter 19

Deadly Foods: Even a Trace Can Trigger Anaphylaxis

One spring day in 1972, Jacki Kwan was quietly working on her research calculations and munching pistachio nuts a co-worker had brought back from the Middle East. After stuffing her body full of pistachios, as she put it, she decided to take a break and go downstairs to pick up her paycheck. Kwan rode the elevator from the 4th floor to the basement and was walking down the hall when she began to feel uncomfortably warm. Then she started to itch. "At that point," she said, "I knew it was the pistachio nuts, because the reaction triggered a vague memory of a problem I had as a child once when I ate pistachio ice cream."

Kwan got her check and went back upstairs. In another 10 minutes she was back at her desk, feeling "really miserable." No wonder: "The itching had become severe and I was getting hives all over my body," Kwan said. "I was flushed and puffy, and started to vomit and have diarrhea at the same time. Everything was getting progressively worse. Finally, I could feel my throat swell up and start to close, and I was having trouble breathing."

Kwan was indeed having an allergic reaction to the pistachio nuts. But her response was not the usual runny nose, watery eyes, sneezing, or itching so many allergy sufferers endure. She was having an anaphylactic reaction: an acute, life-threatening medical emergency. Her symptoms were classic.

DHHS Publication No. (FDA)90-1161. Reprinted from *FDA Consumer*, May 1989.

227

Anaphylaxis typically comes on within minutes of exposure to the offending substance, peaks within 15 to 30 minutes, and is over within hours. The first symptom is usually a sensation of warmth followed by intense itching, especially on the soles of the feet and the palms of the hand. The skin flushes, hives may appear, and the face may swell. Breathing becomes difficult, and the patient may feel faint and anxious. It's not surprising that patients often describe, as Kwan did, a sense of impending doom. Blood pressure may drop precipitously. Convulsions, shock, unconsciousness, even death may follow. Roughly 60 percent to 80 percent of anaphylactic deaths are caused by an inability to breathe because swollen airway passages obstruct airflow to the lungs. The second most common cause of anaphylactic deaths—about 24 percent by one estimate—is shock, caused by insufficient blood circulating through the body.

In the March 1986 *Western Journal of Medicine*, Lawrence M. Lichtenstein, M.D., of Johns Hopkins University School of Medicine described anaphylaxis as "a dramatic problem which generally has a yes or no outcome: The patient either recovers completely or dies. Fortunately, death is rare."

For Kwan, it was a case of being in the right place at the right time. She was working as a medical technologist in an anesthesiology laboratory at the Washington Hospital Center in Washington, D.C. The doctors in the lab rushed her to a nearby room to lie down and gave her an injection of epinephrine (adrenalin). Kwan recovered quickly and hasn't eaten a pistachio since.

The frightening and life-threatening symptoms of anaphylaxis are caused by the release of substances known as mediators from mast cells and from basophils, a type of white blood cell. Since the skin and the respiratory and digestive tracts are rich in mast cells, the organs of these systems are the ones primarily affected in the reaction.

The cause of anaphylaxis was first explored in the 1920s when horse serum being used to make antitoxin for diphtheria, scarlet fever, tetanus, and tuberculosis was found to induce the reaction. Scientists have since discovered that the explosive reaction of anaphylaxis is the culmination of a complicated sequence of events.

Anaphylaxis, like less severe allergic reactions, is an abnormal response to an antigen (a foreign substance, usually a protein) that doesn't bother most people but elicits symptoms in those who have an inherited hypersensitivity to it. Well-known antigens that can cause anaphylaxis include penicillin, insect venom, pollen extracts, fish, shellfish and nuts.

Initial exposure to the antigen prompts the hypersensitive person to produce immunoglobulin E (IgE) antibodies. Whereas most antibodies (IgG, IgM, IgA, IgD) are primarily protective—helping to fight harmful bacteria, viruses, fungi, and other toxic substances—IgE antibodies are more likely to work against the body, "sensitizing" the affected person for a future allergic response.

IgE antibodies attach themselves to mast cells and basophils, priming the body for the allergic reaction. Subsequent exposure to the antigen completes the linkage needed to set off the sequence of events that leads to that "sense of impending doom": The antigen hooks up to the IgE antibodies bound to the mast cells, causing the cells to "degranulate"—the scientists' term for an explosive discharge of histamine and other substances from the cell granules. The released mediators cause blood vessels to dilate and leak fluid into the surrounding tissues and cause smooth muscle in the airways to contract. All this activity results in the familiar symptoms of allergy or, in extreme cases, anaphylaxis.

Since the middle of the 20th century, penicillin has been by far the most common cause of anaphylaxis. (Fortunately, most allergic responses to the drug are far less serious. Some involve only localized skin reactions: hives, rashes or inflammation caused by direct topical administration of the drug. Others are systemic reactions, with wheezing, swelling, redness, and vasculitis—inflammation of blood vessels—but not the life-threatening symptoms of anaphylaxis).

Allergic reactions to insect stings are another major cause of anaphylactic death, almost always caused by the order Hymenoptera: honeybees, bumblebees, wasps, hornets, yellow jackets, and fire ants. Nevertheless, although many millions of people in the United States are allergic to insect venom, and hundreds of thousands of them have allergic reactions to stings each year, the number of deaths reported from these reactions is estimated at only 50 to 100 per year.

Some substances can cause a reaction just like anaphylaxis, but the mast cell degranulation is triggered without IgE. (Some experts refer to these as "anaphylactoid" reactions to distinguish them from true IgE-mediated anaphylaxis. By any name, though, the outcome is the same.) Dyes used in certain diagnostic X-ray tests are the most common cause.

Anaphylactoid reactions can also be incited by physical stimuli, such as cold temperatures or exercise—good news for couch potatoes in search of an excuse to avoid jogging. The reason for mast cell degranulation in these circumstances is not thoroughly understood.

Some people with exercise-induced anaphylaxis develop symptoms only if they've eaten before exercising. This is called "food-dependent exercise-induced" anaphylaxis. Writing in the March 1986 issue of the *Western Journal of Medicine*, Gildon N. Beall, M.D., and his colleagues at Harbor UCLA Medical Center in Torrence, CA, described the case of a 25-year-old woman who had episodes of food-dependent exercise-induced anaphylaxis. The incidents "only occurred Friday evenings on the dance floor after her escort had treated her to dinner. The patient's problem resolved when she ate dinner after dancing rather than before." Some people are susceptible to this form of anaphylaxis only if they've eaten certain foods (most commonly celery or shellfish).

There are numerous other less common precipitators of anaphylactic or anaphylactoid reactions. Medical reports point to substances as varied as cancer drugs, a hair dye ingredient, topical antibiotics, cornstarch surgical glove powder, milk protein in a diaper rash ointment, cabbage, pig insulin, dextran (used in intravenous drug therapy), muscle relaxants, and wines that contain sulfites. (Because sulfites in foods, wine, beer and drugs can cause severe adverse reactions in some people, FDA has taken steps to curtail the widespread use of these preservatives and to help warn consumers about products that contain them. See "Reacting to Sulfites in the December 1985/January 1986 *FDA Consumer.*)

Despite the numerous foods, chemicals, drugs, and physical precipitators known to cause anaphylaxis, in most instances the cause of a reaction is unknown (idiopathic). Researchers at Northwestern University Medical School in Chicago recently reported on 73 patients with idiopathic anaphylaxis. "Idiopathic anaphylaxis," the researchers wrote in the February 1987 *Archives of Internal Medicine*, "can be extremely frightening to both patient and physician when no inciting source is found. Patients often attribute their symptoms to foods or food additives, and many patients become increasingly frustrated by the unpredictability of their reactions." Three patients followed by the scientists became afraid to eat because they feared it would induce anaphylaxis. Reassurance helped rid the fear in two of the three. The third patient consulted another physician who performed laboratory tests and advised her not to eat eggs, soybeans, chocolate, or fish. Despite avoiding these foods, she continued to have anaphylactic episodes and lost more than 18 pounds in two years.

In the October 1987 issue of *Obstetrics and Gynecology*, Jay E. Slater, M.D., and his colleagues at the National Institutes of Health in Bethesda, Md., reported a study of five women with recurrent idiopathic anaphylaxis whose episodes were thought to be related to secretion of the hormone progesterone. The researchers speculated that the hormone might somehow foster release of mediators from mast cells. The women were treated with a drug that lowered their progesterone levels by stopping their menstrual periods, and three of the five stopped having attacks. The researchers noted certain common characteristics among the women who responded successfully (such as a history of previous ovarian problems and diagnosis of the problem after age 36), and concluded that the drug would most likely benefit patients with similar characteristics.

When possible, the best course for preventing anaphylaxis is, obviously, to do what Jacki Kwan does: avoid the instigator—in her case, pistachios. Michael A. Kaliner, M.D., of the National Institute of Allergy and Infectious Diseases recommends, for example, that "people with known sensitivity to insect stings should avoid areas where they are likely to encounter stinging insects; always wear shoes when walking in grass; avoid smelling like a flower by using perfumes or other scented products, such as scented soaps, aftershaves, or suntan lotions; and avoid looking like a flower by wearing flowered or brightly colored clothing." (Dark colors like brown and black may provoke an attack; bees, are least attracted to white and light khaki.)

Next best is to be prepared for an attack.

Several emergency treatment kits are available by prescription and should always be carried by people who know they are prone to anaphylaxis. All the kits contain epinephrine, which stops the action of the mediators, preloaded in the injecting device. One type contains a notched syringe to ensure the correct dose is given Richard Nicklas, M.D., an allergist in FDA's Center for Drug Evaluation and Research, cautions that "The patient or another person should be fully instructed in its use by the prescribing physician." Other kits contain a spring-loaded injector that automatically injects a predetermined dose of the drug when it is pressed against the thigh.

Some kits also contain a tourniquet and an antihistamine. **But an antihistamine is not an effective emergency treatment.** It is included in the kit to reduce symptoms that may continue after treatment with epinephrine. **Anaphylaxis must be treated immediately with epinephrine.** The tourniquet is for use in the case of an insect sting on an arm or leg. First the stinger should be flicked. The tourniquet should be applied above the site of the sting and loosened every 10 minutes to allow sufficient blood circulation. If possible, a cold pack should also be applied. The cold causes the blood vessels to constrict, which slows venom getting into the bloodstream.

Emergency kits are not a substitute for professional medical help. They are intended for patients to use until they can reach a doctor or hospital. The patient should not hesitate, however, to use the medication immediately, as directed by the physician.

Finally, treatments to reduce sensitivity in a patient (allergen immunotherapy), or to completely desensitize a patient (desensitization therapy), are effective for some patients. Immunotherapy involves injecting the allergen, such as insect venom, in increasing amounts over a period of years. The injected allergen stimulates production of IgG antibodies, which confer protection from the substance.

Desensitization is done in patients who need treatment with a life-saving drug to which they are allergic, usually penicillin, and for which there is no effective substitute. Unlike allergen immunotherapy, desensitization is done in the hospital over a short period, beginning with extremely diluted solutions of the allergen. The patient is watched carefully as the dose is gradually increased and may be treated with antihistamines or other medicines if symptoms occur.

Experts disagree about whether certain individuals are predisposed to anaphylaxis. Many feel that people with a history of allergies are more likely to have an anaphylactic episode; others are unconvinced that this or other factors—such as age, sex, race or geographic location—predispose a person to it. One thing is clear, though: Previous exposure to the allergen usually precedes the anaphylactic reaction. Sometimes people will notice that an allergen makes them feel bad in some way: perhaps mild itching or upset stomach. This may indicate that future exposure will produce a more severe reaction.

Whatever the reason for anaphylaxis, as Johns Hopkins' Lichtenstein says, its outcome is generally a yes or a no. Patient awareness, preparedness, and prompt action can help raise the tally in the yes column.

—by Marian Segal

Marian Segal is a member of FDA's public affairs staff.

Chapter 20

Lactose Intolerance: Soured on Milk

What is Lactose Intolerance?

Lactose intolerance is the inability to digest significant amounts of lactose, the predominant sugar of milk. This inability results from a shortage of the enzyme lactase, which is normally produced by the cells that line the small intestine (see figure 20.1). Lactase breaks down milk sugar into simpler forms that can then be absorbed into the bloodstream. When there is not enough lactase to digest the amount of lactose consumed, the results, although not usually dangerous, may be very distressing. While not all persons deficient in lactase have symptoms, those who do are considered to be lactose intolerant.

Common symptoms include nausea, cramps, bloating, gas, and diarrhea, which begin about 30 minutes to 2 hours after eating or drinking foods containing lactose. The severity of symptoms varies depending on the amount of lactose each individual can tolerate.

Some causes of lactose intolerance are well known. For instance, certain digestive diseases and injuries to the small intestine can reduce the amount of enzymes produced. In rare cases, children are born without the ability to produce lactase. For most people, though, lactase deficiency is a condition that develops naturally over time. After about the age of two, the body begins to produce less lactase. However, many people may not experience symptoms until they are much older.

NIH Publication No. 94-2751.

233

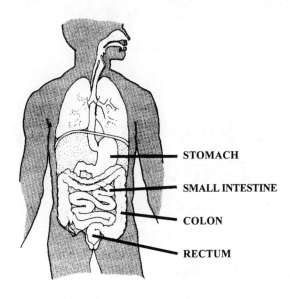

STOMACH

SMALL INTESTINE

COLON

RECTUM

Figure 20.1. The Digestive Tract

Between 30 and 50 million Americans are lactose intolerant. Certain ethnic and racial populations are more widely affected than others. As many as 75 percent of all African-Americans and Native Americans and 90 percent of Asian-Americans are lactose intolerant. The condition is least common among persons of northern European descent.

How Is Lactose Intolerance Diagnosed?

The most common tests used to measure the absorption of lactose in the digestive system are the lactose tolerance test, the hydrogen breath test, and the stool acidity test. These tests are performed on an outpatient basis at a hospital, clinic, or doctor's office.

The lactose tolerance test begins with the individual fasting (not eating) before the test and then drinking a liquid that contains lactose. Several blood samples are taken over a 2-hour period to measure the person's blood glucose (blood sugar) level, which indicates how well the body is able to digest lactose.

Normally, when lactose reaches the digestive system, the lactase enzyme breaks down lactase into glucose and galactose. The liver then changes the galactose into glucose, which enters the bloodstream and raises the person's blood glucose level. If lactose is incompletely broken down the blood glucose level does not rise, and a diagnosis of lactose intolerance is confirmed.

The hydrogen breath test measures the amount of hydrogen in the breath. Normally, very little hydrogen is detectable in the breath. However, undigested lactose in the colon is fermented by bacteria, and various gases, including hydrogen, are produced. The hydrogen is absorbed from the intestines, carried through the bloodstream to the lungs, and exhaled. In the test, the patient drinks a lactose-loaded beverage, and the breath is analyzed at regular intervals. Raised levels of hydrogen in the breath indicate improper digestion of lactose. Certain foods, medications, and cigarettes can affect the test's accuracy and should be avoided before taking the test. This test is available for children and adults.

The lactose tolerance and hydrogen breath tests are not given to infants and very young children who are suspected of having lactose intolerance. A large lactose load may be dangerous for very young individuals because they are more prone to dehydration that can result from diarrhea caused by the lactose. If a baby or young child is experiencing symptoms of lactose intolerance, many pediatricians simply recommend changing from cow's milk to soy formula and waiting for symptoms to abate.

If necessary, a stool acidity test, which measures the amount of acid in the stool, may be given to infants and young children. Undigested lactose fermented by bacteria in the colon creates lactic acid and other short-chain fatty acids that can be detected in a stool sample. In addition, glucose may be present in the sample as a result of unabsorbed lactose in the colon.

How Is Lactose Intolerance Treated?

Fortunately, lactose intolerance is relatively easy to treat. No treatment exists to improve the body's ability to produce lactase, but symptoms can be controlled through diet.

Young children with lactase deficiency should not eat any foods containing lactose. Most older children and adults need not avoid lactose completely, but individuals differ in the amounts of lactose they can handle. For example, one person may suffer symptoms after drinking a small glass of milk, while another can drink one glass but not two. Others may be able to manage ice cream and aged cheeses, such as cheddar and Swiss but not other dairy products. Dietary control of lactose intolerance depends on each person's learning through trial and error how much lactose he or she can handle.

For those who react to very small amounts of lactose or have trouble limiting their intake of foods that contain lactose, lactase enzymes are available without a prescription. One form is a liquid for use with milk. A few drops are added to a quart of milk, and after 24 hours in the refrigerator, the lactose content is reduced by 70 percent. The process works faster if the milk is heated first, and adding a double amount of lactase liquid produces milk that is 90 percent lactose free. A more recent development is a chewable lactase enzyme tablet that helps people digest solid foods that contain lactose. Three to six tablets are taken just before a meal or snack.

Lactose-reduced milk and other products are available at many supermarkets. The milk contains all of the nutrients found in regular milk and remains fresh for about the same length of time or longer if it is super-pasteurized.

How Is Nutrition Balanced?

Milk and other dairy products are a major source of nutrients in the American diet. The most important of these nutrients is calcium. Calcium is essential for the growth and repair of bones throughout life. In the middle and later years, a shortage of calcium may lead to thin, fragile bones that break easily (a condition called osteoporosis). A concern, then, for both children and adults with lactose intolerance, is getting enough calcium in a diet that includes little or no milk.

The recommended dietary allowance (RDA) for calcium, revised in 1989 by the Food and Nutrition Board of the National Academy of Sciences, varies by age group. Infants up to 5 months need 400 mg per day, and from 5 months to 1 year, 600 mg. Children 1 to 10 years need 800 mg and 11- to 24-year-olds need 1,200 mg. Pregnant and nursing women also need 1,200 mg per day, and people age 25 and older need 800 mg per day. However, the results of a 1984 conference at the National Institutes of Health (NIH) suggest that women who have not yet reached menopause and older women who are taking the hormone estrogen after menopause should consume about 1,000 mg of calcium daily (roughly the amount in a quart of milk).

In planning meals, making sure that each day's diet includes enough calcium is important, even if the diet does not contain dairy products. Many nondairy foods are high in calcium. Green vegetables, such as broccoli and kale, and fish with soft, edible bones, such as salmon and sardines, are excellent sources of calcium. To help in planning a high-calcium and low-lactose diet, Table 20.1 lists some common foods that are good sources of dietary calcium and shows about how much lactose the foods contain.

Recent research shows that yogurt with active cultures may be a good source of calcium for many people with lactose intolerance, even though it is fairly high in lactose. Evidence shows that the bacterial cultures used in making yogurt produce some of the lactase enzyme required for proper digestion.

Clearly, many foods can provide the calcium and other nutrients the body needs, even when intake of milk and dairy products is limited. However, factors other than calcium and lactose content should be kept in mind when planning a diet. Some vegetables that are high in calcium (Swiss chard, spinach, and rhubarb, for instance) are not listed in Table 20.1 because the body cannot use their calcium content. They contain substances called oxalates, which stop calcium absorption. Calcium is absorbed and used only when there is enough vitamin D in the body. A balanced diet should provide an adequate supply of vitamin D. Sources of vitamin D include eggs and liver. However, sunlight helps the body naturally absorb or synthesize vitamin D, and with enough exposure to the sun, food sources may not be necessary.

Some people with lactose intolerance may think they are not getting enough calcium and vitamin D in their diet. Consultation with a doctor or dietitian may be helpful in deciding whether any dietary supplements are needed. Taking vitamins or minerals of the wrong kind or in the wrong amounts can be harmful. A dietitian can help in planning meals that will provide the most nutrients with the least chance of causing discomfort.

What Is Hidden Lactose?

Although milk and foods made from milk are the only natural sources, lactose is often added to prepared foods. People with very low tolerance for lactose should know about the many food products that may contain lactose, even in small amounts. Food products that may contain lactose include:

237

- Bread and other baked goods.
- Processed breakfast cereals.
- Instant potatoes, soups, and breakfast drinks.
- Margarine.
- Lunch meats (other than kosher).
- Salad dressings.
- Candies and other snacks.
- Mixes for pancakes, biscuits, and cookies.

Some products labeled nondairy, such as powdered coffee creamer and whipped toppings, may also include ingredients that are derived from milk and therefore contain lactose.

Smart shoppers learn to read food labels with care, looking not only for milk and lactose among the contents but also for such words as whey, curds, milk by-products, dry milk solids, and nonfat dry milk powder. If any of these are listed on a label, the item contains lactose.

In addition, lactose is used as the base for more than 20 percent of prescription drugs and about 6 percent of over-the-counter medicines. Many types of birth control pills, for example, contain lactose, as do some tablets for stomach acid and gas. However, these products typically affect only people with severe lactose intolerance.

Summary

Even though lactose intolerance is widespread, it need not pose a serious threat to good health. People who have trouble digesting lactose can learn which dairy products and other foods they can eat without discomfort and which ones they should avoid. Many will be able to enjoy milk, ice cream, and other such products if they take them in small amounts or eat other food at the same time. Others can use lactase liquid or tablets to help digest the lactose. Even older women at risk for osteoporosis and growing children who must avoid milk and foods made with milk can meet most of their special dietary needs by eating greens, fish, and other calcium-rich foods that are free of lactose. A carefully chosen diet (with calcium supplements if the doctor or dietitian recommends them) is the key to reducing symptoms and protecting future health.

Vegetables	Calcium Content*	Lactose Content**
Broccoli (cooked), 1 cup	94 - 177 mg	0
Chinese cabbage (bok choy, cooked), 1 cup	158 mg	0
Collard greens (cooked), 1 cup	148 - 357 mg	0
Kale (cooked), 1 cup	94 - 179 mg	0
Turnip greens (cooked), 1 cup	194 - 249 mg	0
Dairy Products		
Ice cream/ice milk, 8 oz	176 mg	6 - 7 g
Milk (whole, low-fat skim, buttermilk), 8 oz	291 - 316 mg	12 - 13 g
Processed cheese, 1 oz	159 - 219 mg	2 - 3 g
Sour cream, 4 oz	134 mg	4 - 5 g
Yogurt (plain), 8 oz	274 - 415 mg	12 - 13 g
Fish/Seafood		
Oysters (raw), 1 cup	226 mg	0
Salmon with bones (canned), 3 oz	167 mg	0
Sardines, 3 oz	371 mg	0
Shrimp (canned), 3 oz	98 mg	0
Other		
Molasses, 2 tbsp	274 mg	0
Tofu (processed with calcium salts), 3 oz	225 mg	0

* Nutritive Value of Foods. Values vary with methods of processing and preparation.

** Derived from *Lactose Intolerance: A Resource Including Recipes,* Food Sensitivity Series, American Dietetic Association, 1991.

Table 20.1. *Calcium and Lactose in Common Foods*

Additional Readings

American Dietetic Association. *Lactose Intolerance: A Resource Including Recipes,* Food Sensitivity Series (1991). American Dietetic Association, 216 West Jackson Blvd. Chicago, IL 60606. (312) 899-0040. Resource book provides recipes and information about food products.

Kidder B. *The Milk-Free Kitchen: Living Well Without Dairy Products: 450 Family-Style Recipes.* New York: Henry Holt and Company, 1991. Cookbook with 450 lactose-free recipes.

Montes RG, Perman JA. Lactose intolerance: pinpointing the source of nonspecific gastrointestinal symptoms. *Postgraduate Medicine* 1991;89 (8):175-184. Article for health care professionals explains diagnosis and treatment of lactose intolerance.

Zukin J. *Dairy-Free Cookbook.* New York: St. Martin's Press, 1989. Commercial Writing Service, P.O. Box 3074, Iowa City, IA 52244. Book contains more than 150 recipes and practical information for living with lactose intolerance.

Zukin J. *The Newsletter For People With Lactose Intolerance and Milk Allergy.* Commercial Writing Service, P.O. Box 3074, Iowa City, IA 52244. Newsletter provides practical information, resources, and recipes.

Chapter 21

Allergy To Foods Containing Concealed Milk Proteins

Six children sensitive to cow's milk developed severe allergic reactions after eating foods that were labeled "nondairy" or that had no milk products listed on their labels, according to scientists at Johns Hopkins University in Baltimore, Maryland. Subsequent analysis of the foods revealed that in many instances milk proteins were used in processing the foods but were listed only as "flavoring" on the product labels.

Principal investigator Dr. Hugh A. Sampson, professor of pediatrics in the division of pediatric allergy and immunology at Johns Hopkins, applauds recent Federal regulations requiring that vegetable or animal proteins used in food processing be specifically listed on product labels. "The listing will certainly help patients with food allergies avoid foods they are sensitive to," he says.

The presumed milk-free foods included bologna, hot dogs, tuna fish, and nondairy frozen desserts. On each occasion a parent had read the product label carefully to avoid exposing the child to food containing milk or milk proteins. After eating the foods three of the children, who were 5 to 11 years old, required emergency room treatment, and one child was hospitalized. Allergic symptoms included hives; burning tongue; abdominal pain; shortness of breath; wheezing; and swelling of the lips, face, and tongue. According to Dr. Sampson, adverse reactions to cow's milk have been estimated to occur in 0.1 to 7.5 percent of children.

Research Resources Reporter, May/June 1992.

In an effort to explain the children's unexpected allergic reactions to "nondairy" foods Dr. Sampson and his colleagues analyzed the foods. They found traces of milk protein in all samples. The frozen desserts may have been contaminated when they were manufactured in dairy-processing plants, the scientists say. The processed meats contained sodium caseinate, a milk derivative that was listed as a "flavoring" on the product labels.

"There are so many products that contain milk proteins and such a huge number of prepared foods on the market that it is difficult for allergic patients or their parents to know what is in them under the old labeling guidelines," says Dr. James E. Gern, a fellow in the division of pediatric allergy and immunology at Johns Hopkins. "So much was labeled ambiguously as 'flavorings'."

To correct the confusion the two Federal agencies that oversee food labeling have taken steps to require that consumers receive more complete information on product labels. New labeling regulations from the U.S. Department of Agriculture (USDA), which regulates meat and poultry products, went into effect in September 1991. The new regulations require that meat and poultry manufacturers specifically list any vegetable or animal protein used in food processing. The U.S. Food and Drug Administration (FDA), which regulates the labeling of foods that do not contain meat or poultry, has proposed similar revisions to their labeling regulations.

"Everybody is focusing on labels that specify the cholesterol and sodium contents of foods. I am not saying that that is not important, but it is very unlikely that one serving of food with a little bit higher cholesterol content is going to kill somebody," Dr. Sampson says. "But in children with food allergy insufficient labeling could be lethal, so the new labeling requirements are very important."

Total elimination of the particular food allergen is important, according to Dr. Sampson. "When people keep getting small contaminating amounts of a food they are sensitive to, it may not be enough to give them major symptoms, but it is certainly enough to keep their immune system stimulated," he explains.

The six children were the first in a series of children with milk allergy who developed allergic symptoms after eating food presumed to contain no milk products. "We initiated this study because some of our patients were having reactions to foods that should not have caused symptoms," Dr. Sampson notes. "When any of our milk-allergic patients react to a non-suspect food we assay the food for milk protein."

Dr. Sampson and his colleagues tested the foods for contamination with cow's milk by sensitive enzyme-linked immunosorbent assays for whey, casein, and other milk proteins. Nine samples of frozen soy and rice desserts and one sample each of tuna fish and beef hot dog were analyzed.

Relatively large amounts of milk proteins were found in the two frozen nondairy desserts that had caused allergic reactions. Both had been manufactured in dairy-processing facilities, and accidental contamination was blamed for the presence of the milk proteins. The manufacturers of the hot dogs and the bologna reported that their product recipes had recently been changed to include hydrolyzed sodium caseinate (the sodium salt of casein redissolved at an alkaline pH), added to improve the texture of the processed meat. The product labels had not specifically noted the inclusion of this milk derivative in the recipe; it was considered "natural flavoring" for labeling purposes, according to the investigators. Under the USDA's new labeling regulations the presence of milk protein must be specified on the product label.

Even with improved product labels, however, tuna may continue to present risks for milk-allergic patients. Wholesalers may add casein to tuna fish before it reaches a distributor in the United States for packaging. The distributor may not even be aware of it, Dr. Sampson says.

Dr. Sampson and his colleagues are also in the middle of studies trying to define why people may react to certain foods. "Egg, peanut, and milk account for 80 to 85 percent of all reactions we can confirm in children," Dr. Sampson says. "We are breaking down these particular foods, looking at their protein fractions and antibody-binding parts to see if we can determine why people would react to eggs and not to corn, for example."

"And we are also studying why people become tolerant," he says. "We have allergic children who lose their allergy. What are the changes in their immune system that now allow them to eat foods they were previously allergic to?"

—by Maureen Curran

Additional Reading

Sampson, H. A., Bernhisel-Broadbent, J., Yang, E., and Scanlon, S. M., Safety of casein hydrolysate in children with cow's milk allergy. *Journal of Pediatrics* 118:520-525, 1991.

Gern, J. E., Yang, E., Evrard, H. M., and Sampson, H. A., Allergic reactions to milk-contaminated "nondairy" products. *New England Journal of Medicine* 324:976-979, 1991.

Pastorello, E. A., Stocchi, L., Pravettoni, V., et al., Role of the elimination diet in adults with food allergy. *Journal of Allergy and Clinical Immunology* 84:475-483, 1989.

Bock, S. A., Prospective appraisal of complaints of adverse reactions to foods in children during the first 3 years of life. *Pediatrics* 79:683-688, 1987.

Chapter 22

Childhood Atopic Dermatitis: A Result of Food Hypersensitivity

Immune Responses Linked To Food Allergy In Children With Atopic Dermatitis

In patients with food hypersensitivity the offending food causes certain types of cells to release a substance called a cytokine that induces other cells to release histamine, the chemical that causes allergic symptoms, according to investigators at the Johns Hopkins University School of Medicine in Baltimore, Maryland.

Food hypersensitivity, or allergy, often is expressed as atopic dermatitis, a skin condition that affects about one in ten children at some time during childhood. The symptoms of atopic dermatitis range from occasional mild skin irritation to an itchy, measles-like rash so unpleasant that children scratch themselves until the skin bleeds. The first signs of the disease are often reddish, bumpy patches on the face, neck, arms, and legs. In severe cases, intense scratching leads to chronic eczema as the affected skin becomes thickened, leathery, and vulnerable to infection.

Despite its prevalence atopic dermatitis is poorly understood. Many children with atopic dermatitis are hypersensitive to such foods as eggs or peanuts; they can avoid the skin reaction by following a diet that excludes the food. Although many children who are food-sensitive grow out of the problem, others carry it into adult life and must maintain a restricted diet.

Research Resources Reporter, May 1990.

245

Researchers are finding clues that help explain why eating certain foods can lead to skin reactions. The emerging picture of food-related eczema reveals a complex interplay of immune system cells and inflammatory responses within the skin. Because atopic dermatitis seems to involve so many elements of the immune system, achieving a better understanding of the disease promises to provide insights into the basic mechanisms that cause allergy, says Dr. Hugh A. Sampson, associate professor of pediatrics at the Johns Hopkins University School of Medicine in Baltimore.

One key part of an allergic reaction is the activation of mast cells in the skin. When these mast cells are exposed to a specific food allergen, they release histamine and other substances that produce inflammation. This immediate response usually subsides within about an hour and is often followed by a late-phase response as basophils, mononuclear cells, and other immune-system cells invade the inflamed area over a period of several hours.

Other researchers suspected that release of histamine by mast cells contributed to atopic dermatitis in food-sensitive children. Dr. Sampson and his coworkers confirmed this finding by measuring markedly elevated serum levels of histamine in children after allergic reactions to foods.

Although release of histamine by mast cells is clearly part of the chain of events that produces atopic dermatitis, Dr. Sampson suspected that other immunologic mechanisms were involved, mechanisms that did not depend on immediate activation of mast cells by food allergens. Certain types of white blood cells—basophils and mononuclear cells—seem to play a role in the late-phase response by gathering to the local reaction and helping maintain the inflammatory response, he explains.

In an effort to identify these immunologic factors; Dr. Sampson and his associates studied 83 atopic dermatitis patients 2 to 23 years of age. Of the 83 patients, 63 also had a food allergy; they served as the study group. Most of these food-sensitive patients had already eliminated the offending foods from their diets. The other 20 patients with atopic dermatitis but no food allergies served as control subjects, as did a group of 18 normal volunteers. The children underwent testing in the Pediatric Clinical Research Center of the Johns Hopkins University Hospital. Dr. Sampson is director of the research center, which is supported by the National Center for Research Resources.

The investigators took blood samples from the subjects and isolated their basophils in the laboratory. The spontaneous rate of histamine release by basophils *in vitro* was higher among patients with both atopic dermatitis and food allergy than it was among other subjects. The rate of histamine release was especially high in basophils from 25 food-sensitive patients who were still eating foods that caused reactions. This suggests that measurement of basophil histamine release might provide a way to monitor allergic children who are trying to eliminate troublesome foods from their diets, Dr. Sampson says.

Double-blind food challenges were used to test allergic responses in all of the study patients. Twenty-two patients showed symptoms of hypersensitivity to certain foods, but there was no immediate change in release of histamine by basophils or in the amount of histamine that basophils contained. The researchers are now investigating whether basophils become activated during the late-phase allergic response that develops several hours later.

Among patients following an elimination diet the spontaneous rate of histamine release from basophils was only slightly higher than that of control subjects. Follow-up of eight patients who stopped eating the offending foods showed a large drop in the rate of *in vitro* histamine release by basophils after four to twelve months on a restricted diet.

The tendency for elevated histamine release to persist for some time after patients had begun an elimination diet suggested that factors other than food allergens might be activating the basophils. Other investigators had earlier reported evidence of histamine-releasing factors produced by the immune system. To investigate this idea Dr. Sampson and his associates studied the patients' mononuclear cells, which belong to a class of white blood cells that includes monocytes and lymphocytes. These cells are normally found in blood and lymphatic tissue. In atopic dermatitis mononuclear cells behave abnormally: they infiltrate the inflamed skin and interact with other cells, which prolongs the inflammatory reaction. Children with atopic dermatitis generally seek medical help because of the skin problem. In addition to the dermatitis about 80 percent of affected children have other allergic symptoms that include asthma, nasal congestion, or gastrointestinal problems. In many food-sensitive children all of the allergic symptoms disappear once the offending food is removed from the diet. Thus atopic dermatitis provides a good opportunity to study allergy because it is easy to control exposure to foods that cause the skin reaction, Dr. Sampson says.

An allergic reaction to foods represents the immune system's attempt to rid the body of foreign substances, or allergens. As long as a child with food hypersensitivity keeps eating an offending food, inflammatory responses continue to occur in the skin, leading to atopic dermatitis.

The researchers cultured mononuclear cells from 13 food-hypersensitive patients, then took some of the culture solution and added it to basophils from other patients who were allergic to different foods. The result was increased histamine release by the basophils. This effect was not seen when the culture solution was taken from mononuclear cells of patients without food allergies.

It appears that mononuclear cells of food-sensitive patients produce a histamine-releasing factor (HRF) that lowers the threshold of reactivity of basophils and mast cells. Production of HRF appears to depend on activation of mononuclear cells through continued exposure to food allergens. In ten food-sensitive patients who stayed on an elimination diet for about a year, the mononuclear cells appeared to stop producing HRF. Currently, Dr. Sampson is trying to determine which kind of mononuclear cells produce HRF.

Because these studies were conducted *in vitro* the findings may not reflect what occurs in people with atopic dermatitis, Dr. Sampson notes. Yet there is strong circumstantial evidence that HRF plays a role in the skin disorder. All patients whose basophils had high rates of histamine release had mononuclear cells that produced HRF. Conversely, the factor was never produced in patients with normal rates of histamine release.

Basophils of food-sensitive patients do not seem to release histamine spontaneously in the body after exposure to an offending food. Instead, the presence of HRF seems to make basophils and mast cells prone to release histamine in response to minor, nonspecific stimuli such as heat, drying, or irritants—"like a gun with a hair trigger." This is analogous to the airway hyper-reactivity that occurs in asthma, Dr. Sampson explains. He and his associates are conducting further studies to see what role this "cutaneous hyper-reactivity" plays in atopic dermatitis.

Dr. Sampson has studied about 220 children with atopic dermatitis, most of them under age ten. The children often have severe itching and scratch themselves for an hour or two after eating a food. The scratching can lead to bleeding, oozing, and crusting of the lesions. "It's a horrible problem," Dr. Sampson says. "If you sit up all night with a crying child who scratches himself to a state of bleeding and wakes up every morning with blood on the sheets, that's incredibly disruptive to the family." Mothers whose children have both asthma and atopic dermatitis generally view the skin condition as a worse problem than the asthma.

The children are hospitalized so that diet and environmental factors can be carefully controlled. By applying skin medications and keeping the children away from certain foods, household aeroallergens, stress, and other factors that may contribute to the problem, the skin inflammation can be stopped within 3 to 4 days. This makes it possible to get clear results from food challenges.

"The children come to us with terrible skin," Dr. Sampson explains. "You can't interpret anything [from allergy testing] until you clear up the skin." Once the children stop scratching themselves, it takes several months for the hard, scaly skin to fully regain its normal consistency.

In the present study only patients with food allergies had basophils that responded to HRF. How did these basophils differ from those of patients without food hypersensitivity? Other scientists had suggested that in food-sensitive patients the cell surface of basophils contains a special kind of immunoglobulin-E, or IgE, dubbed IgE+. IgE is a type of antibody that is produced in excess in persons with allergy. IgE binds to the histamine-containing mast cells and basophils, and the bound antibody causes the cells to release histamine when the individual is exposed to the offending food allergen. Dr. Sampson and his associates hypothesized that HRF could activate basophils in food-sensitive children by binding to IgE+.

The investigators isolated basophils from six subjects without food hypersensitivity and used an acid to strip off the normal IgE from the cell surface. When serum containing IgE+ from food-sensitive children was added to the stripped basophils, the cells became responsive to HRF and released histamine. The stripped basophils did not respond to HRF after exposure to normal IgE.

These results showed that an abnormality in IgE, not in the basophils, led to release of histamine in response to HRF. Dr. Sampson and his colleagues are now trying to learn the mechanisms that lead to production of IgE+. They suspect that normal IgE undergoes different chemical changes such as glycosylation, addition of carbohydrates, in patients with atopic dermatitis.

About 60 percent of the children with atopic dermatitis who were studied by Dr. Sampson have been allergic to one or more foods. The most common food allergies—to egg, peanut, milk, fish, soy, and wheat—accounted for about 90 percent of the positive responses. Immediate allergic reactions to eating the foods include such symptoms as skin redness, itching, nausea, vomiting, diarrhea, nasal congestion, runny nose, sneezing, and wheezing.

To identify possible food allergies, small amounts of food extracts are punctured into the surface of the skin with a needle. Inflammatory responses to this skin prick test, or positive responses to other screening tests, mean that further evaluation is needed. The researchers use double-blind food challenges to confirm the presence of food allergies. The children receive capsules or juice containing a placebo or a food suspected of causing allergic symptoms.

In many of the children with food allergies the allergy had not been identified previously because standard allergy tests and trial diets are often imprecise. The only way to accurately identify the allergy is to isolate the child in the hospital and change just one dietary variable at a time, Dr. Sampson says.

In some children the atopic dermatitis appears to be food related, but the children do no show typical clinical reaction when they eat the foods in question. These children have positive skin tests to the foods, but it is not clear why they do not develop other symptoms of food allergy, according to Dr Sampson.

Some children with atopic dermatitis do not have food allergy; other allergies or immunologic abnormalities apparently cause the skin reaction. Such factors also play a role in food-sensitive children who may still have allergic symptoms even after eliminating problem foods from the diet. In these children sensitivity to food is just one of several factors that lead to atopic dermatitis, he explains.

About one in three children with atopic dermatitis loses the allergy within a year or two. Researchers do not know why this happens, especially since the change cannot be detected by standard laboratory tests. "If we understood why the allergy disappears in some children we might be able to help the others get over their allergy," Dr. Sampson says. Some children who remain allergic after two years will lose their allergy later, but there are no long-term data on how many eventually grow out of the problem.

In six breast-fed infants who Dr. Sampson evaluated, atopic dermatitis was linked to food antigens present in the mother's milk. In each case the rash disappeared when the mother stayed on an egg-free diet. As they grew older these children remained sensitive to egg but had no allergic reactions while on an egg-free diet.

The only proven treatment for food allergy is an elimination diet that strictly avoids the offending food. Such a diet is most often not hard to follow because the allergy is generally limited to just one or two foods to which the child is clearly hypersensitive. After reacting to a food challenge, the children are convinced that the food causes a problem. "This makes them try much harder to keep it out of the diet," Dr. Sampson says.

He and his associates tested the effect of an elimination diet in 22 children with food-related atopic dermatitis. During 3 to 4 years of follow-up, 17 children who maintained an elimination diet showed dramatic improvement in their symptoms. Only slight improvement was seen in the five children who did not adhere to a restricted diet.

Dr. Sampson and his colleagues are currently trying to determine the structure of HRF, which they suspect is a glycoprotein. After they obtain purified HRF the Baltimore researchers plan to make antibodies to it. Such antibodies could be used to detect HRF, to measure its concentration in tissues, and to further explore its role in atopic dermatitis. "We hope these studies will lead to a better understanding of most allergic diseases," he says.

—by Calvin Pierce

Additional Reading

Sampson, H. A., Broadbent, K. R., and Bernhisel-Broadbent, J., Spontaneous release of histamine from basophils and histamine-releasing factor in patients with atopic dermatitis and food hypersensitivity. *New England Journal of Medicine* 321:228-232, 1989.

Sampson, H. A., The role of food allergy and mediator release in atopic dermatitis. *Journal of Allergy and Clinical Immunology* 81:635-645, 1988.

Sampson, H. A., Late-phase response to food in atopic dermatitis. *Hospital Practice* Dec. 15, 1987:111-128.

Sampson, H. A., Food hypersensitivity and atopic dermatitis: Evaluation of 113 patients. *Journal of Pediatrics* 107: 669-675, 1985.

The research described in this article was supported by the National Institute of Allergy and Infectious Diseases and the General Clinical Research Centers Program of the National Center for Research Resources.

Chapter 23

Scientists Net Major Shrimp Allergen

Crab feasts, clambakes, and shrimp barbecues are among the pleasures of summer. But some individuals approach these warm-weather fetes with anxiety. These are the people who break out in hives and sneeze and wheeze when they eat seafood. And for the unlucky, hyperallergic few, shellfish are so dangerous that even minute amounts may precipitate a dangerous anaphylactic reaction.

NCRR-supported researchers in New Orleans have been fishing for clues to the causes of seafood allergies for more than a decade. These scientists and, independently, another team of investigators have now found that a protein in the muscles of shrimp is a major trigger of allergic reactions in shrimp-sensitive individuals.

Shellfish are a major cause of allergic food reactions. Dr. Samuel B. Lehrer, research professor of medicine at Tulane University in New Orleans, estimates that more than 250,000 individuals in the United States have developed or are at risk of developing an allergy to shellfish. "Some individuals have a response to shrimp as soon as it is in their mouth. They get swelling of their lips and may have swelling of the throat that makes it difficult to breathe."

To pinpoint the component of shrimp that makes hypersensitive persons ill, Dr. Lehrer, Dr. Carolyn Daul, and their colleagues made extracts of cooked shrimp meat and of water used to boil shrimp. Tiny amounts of these extracts were injected under the skin of patients who had a history of adverse reactions—including wheezing or shortness of breath, patches of itchy red skin. nausea, vomiting or diarrhea—

NCRR Reporter, September/October 1994.

after eating shrimp. Blood was collected and saved from 34 shrimp-sensitive persons, who had positive skin tests, and from four volunteers who served as controls and showed no reaction to the shrimp extract. All skin tests were conducted at the NCRR-supported General Clinical Research Center (GCRC) at Tulane University Medical Center. "Skin testing of patients has to be performed under controlled conditions because it is possible to induce an anaphylactic reaction. The GCRC played a critical role in our studies," explains Dr. Lehrer.

Blood from hypersensitive persons who have been exposed to an allergy-producing substance contains a protein known as immunoglobulin E, or IgE. IgE is similar to the protective antibodies that are formed after immunization; it matches the specific allergy-producing substance just as these antibodies correspond to the disease-causing agent. However, when IgE reacts with a sensitizing substance, known as an allergen, it promotes release of chemical mediators such as histamine. These mediators are potent substances acting at many sites in the body to cause most allergic symptoms.

Shrimp-sensitive people have IgE that attaches specifically to an allergen in shrimp. This is the allergen Dr. Lehrer and his colleagues have isolated and identified.

In their study, the researchers separated individual proteins in the shrimp extract according to their molecular weights and tested them for reactivity against IgE from the 34 shrimp-sensitive people. The molecular weight and amino acid sequence of the main reactive protein indicated that it was identical to the shrimp muscle protein tropomyosin. Analyses performed at another NCRR-supported facility, the Resource Center for Biomedical Complex Carbohydrates at the University of Georgia in Athens, showed that the shrimp allergen also contained a small amount of carbohydrate.

People who are allergic to shrimp are often also allergic to other shellfish such as crawfish, lobster, and crab. Dr. Lehrer says this is because the areas of the tropomyosin molecule that induce allergy have similar structures in these crustaceans and therefore bind to the IgE from shrimp-sensitive people. In contrast, tropomyosin from mammalian species does not react.

"Why the shrimp tropomyosin is so allergenic compared to other tropomyosins such as beef, pork, chicken, and even human tropomyosin is not known, but it is an important issue that we need to study," notes Dr. Lehrer.

While scientists understand many details of how inhaled allergens interact with the body's immune system, much less is known about this interaction in the case of ingested allergens. Dr. Lehrer hopes that further studies of the shrimp allergen will help to clarify how immune tissue functions in the digestive tract. It might also be possible in the future to produce nonallergenic shrimp by genetic engineering techniques that could modify tropomyosin to reduce its allergenicity without affecting its functionality. Dr. Lehrer cautions, however that such alterations would require a fine touch.

"Any type of substantial modification or suppression of tropomyosin production would be fatal because shrimp is essentially one big muscle," he says.

—by Ole Henriksen, Ph.D.

This research was supported by the General Clinical Research Centers Program of the National Center for Research Resources, the Alton Ochsner Research Foundation, and the National Fisheries Institute.

Additional Reading

Daul, C.B., Slattery, M., Reese, G., and Lehrer, S.B., Identification of the major brown shrimp (Penaeus aztecus) allergen (Pen a1) as the muscle protein tropomyosin. *International Archives of Allergy and Immunology,* in press.

Shanti, K.N., Martin, B.M., Nagpal, S., et al., Identification of tropomyosin as the major shrimp allergen and characterization of its IgE-binding epitopes. *Journal of Immunology* 151:5354-5363, 1993.

Chapter 24

Cooking for People with Food Allergies

Many people have physical reactions after eating certain foods. Whether the reaction is called an allergy, a sensitivity, or an intolerance doesn't matter. After a doctor has diagnosed the allergy or intolerance, you must modify your diet, or your family's diet, to eliminate the offending substance. Some foods (tomatoes or nuts, for example) are easy to omit from the diet, but some foods are hard to avoid. Especially difficult are milk, eggs, corn, and wheat.

This chapter provides information to help in selecting and preparing foods that do not contain milk, eggs, corn, or wheat; tips to help recognize these ingredients in prepared foods; and recipes designed to help avoid them.

Food Allergies or Sensitivities

A true food allergy or sensitivity involves the body's immune system. Allergic reactions to foods may include asthma, hives, stomach cramps, diarrhea, vomiting, and other symptoms. Reactions may occur immediately, or hours after eating. A small amount of food may not always cause a response, while a large amount may cause a severe reaction.

People of all ages have allergic reactions to foods. Although food allergies sometimes seem to disappear after childhood, they may recur years later.

Department of Agriculture Home and Garden Bulletin No. 246, 1988.

Foods that often cause allergic reactions include cow's milk, egg white, corn, wheat, nuts, soybean products, finfish (flounder, trout, cod), and shellfish (shrimp, crab, lobster). Simple ingredients in foods, such as corn syrup, can also produce allergic responses.

When a food is found to cause an allergic reaction, all closely related foods should also be suspected. For example, someone allergic to chickpeas (garbanzo beans) may also be allergic to peanuts, since both foods are legumes. A doctor or dietitian who specializes in food allergies can provide information on related foods.

Food Intolerances

In contrast to a food allergy, a food intolerance is caused by an enzyme deficiency, a toxin, or a disease. Food intolerances can cause symptoms similar to food allergies—stomach cramping and diarrhea, for example. Lactose and gluten are two substances that many people do not tolerate well.

Lactose Intolerance. Lactose intolerance is caused by a lack of lactase, an intestinal enzyme that digests milk sugar (lactose). Those who do not tolerate milk as a beverage may be able to eat small amounts of yogurt or ice milk, especially as a part of a meal. Lactose-reduced milk is also available. You can purchase milk to which lactase has been added, or you can add the commercial lactase enzyme to your milk to break down the lactose. The enzyme can be purchased from a pharmacy without a prescription.

For severe intolerance, your doctor may advise avoiding all milk and milk products. If this is the case, a calcium supplement may be needed because milk is a major source of calcium in diets.

Gluten Intolerance. Gluten intolerance occurs when gluten, a combination of proteins found in wheat, rye, oats, barley, and buckwheat, irritates the lining of the small intestine. As a result, nutrients are inadequately absorbed from the intestine. Gluten intolerance can range from mild to severe. The proteins in corn, rice, soybean, and tapioca flours and potato, arrowroot, and corn starches contain no problem gluten.

Some people can tolerate the gluten in rye, oats, barley, and buckwheat but have an allergy to wheat. They generally need to omit only wheat flour, wheat starch, and combinations of flours that include wheat from their diets. Buckwheat is often confused with wheat, but it is a member of another plant family. However, some people are very sensitive to buckwheat.

Reading Food Labels

Be a label reader. Ingredients are listed on food labels in order by weight. The first ingredient is present in the greatest amount and the last in the least amount. The ingredients for a product may change, so you should make a practice of reading labels even on items you have used in the past.

Some basic food products, such as catsup and peanut butter, have a "Standard of Identity" approved by the U.S. Food and Drug Administration. Labels on these foods are not required to show a complete listing of all ingredients; only optional ingredients have to be listed. The processor or distributor named on the product's label can provide further information about its ingredients, especially for foods having a Standard of Identity.

Clues to Ingredient Names

Food ingredients made from milk, eggs, corn, or wheat are sometimes listed on the label only by their technical names. For example, did you know that caseinate comes from milk? When reading labels, look for words that are clues to the presence of milk, egg, corn, wheat, and gluten in a product. Here are names to look for:

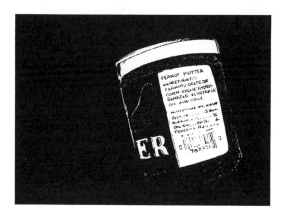

Table 24.1. *Technical names for milk, egg, and corn products*

Wheat	Gluten
Bran	All items listed
All-purpose flour	under wheat and
Wheat flour	the following:
Farina	Barley
Graham flour	Oats
Malt	Rye
Wheat germ	Buckwheat
Whole-wheat flour	
Wheat starch	

Table 24.2. Technical names for wheat and gluten products

The following foods may contain milk, eggs, corn, wheat, or gluten:

Milk may be found in—	Eggs may be found in—
Baked products	Baking mixes
Chocolate desserts and candies	Batter-fried foods
Yogurt, frozen yogurt	Baked products
Ice cream, sherbet, puddings	Breaded meats
Nondairy creamers	Custard, ice cream, sherbet
Nondairy whipped toppings	Coffee or root beer
Meatloaf, cold cuts, frankfurters	Meatloaf, croquettes, sausage
Margarine, cheese	Noodles
Sauces	No-cholesterol egg substitutes
Sour cream	Sauces, soups
Whipped potatoes	

Table 24.3. Foods containing milk or eggs

Corn may be found in—	Wheat or gluten may be found in—
Powdered sugar	Ale, beer, liquor
Baking powder	Baked products
Baking mixes	Cold cuts, frankfurters
Canned or frozen fruits or	Ice cream
juices	Hydrolyzed vegetable protein
Gum, mints, candy	Monosodium glutamate
Soft drinks	Ready-to-eat cereals
Sorbitol	Salad dressings
Sugar-cured ham or bacon	Sauces, soups

Table 24.4. Foods containing corn, wheat, or gluten

Nonwheat Flours and Starches

Nonwheat flours and starches differ from wheat flour, and from each other, in their characteristics and uses. Becoming familiar with these characteristics lets you choose the flour or starch that has the best qualities for individual recipes.

Characteristics and Uses

- Soy flour is generally milled from whole soybeans into one of three types of flour: full-fat, low-fat, or defatted. Full-fat soybean flour is the type usually available in stores for use in home baking. Soy flour is light yellow in color and has a strong nutty flavor. Because of its strong flavor, soy flour is best mixed with other nonwheat flours. Nuts, spices, or chocolate also help mask the soy flavor.

- Rice flour is milled from broken kernels of white or brown rice. It has a bland flavor with a slightly grainy texture. Since rice flour lacks a flavor of its own, it can be used in a variety of baked products.

- Corn flour is milled from white or yellow corn by the same process as cornmeal, but it is ground much finer. Corn flour is not available in all areas.

- Rye flour has a dark color, distinctive flavor, and a slight amount of gluten. Be sure to buy only 100 percent rye flour and not a rye-wheat combination flour. Most commercially baked rye breads contain wheat flour.

- Oat flour has a mild flavor. You can buy it ready to use, or you can make your own by grinding dry-rolled oats in a blender or food processor. One and one-half cups of regular or quick-cooking rolled oats makes 1 cup of oat flour. Commercially baked oatmeal breads and oatmeal cookies are usually made with some wheat flour.

- Cornstarch is a fine, white starch made from corn. It is the principal starch used in cooking in this country. Cornstarch is used to thicken gravies, sauces, and desserts.

- Arrowroot starch is a snow-white starch made from arrowroot, a tuberous root of a West Indian plant. Arrowroot starch thickens at a lower temperature than wheat flour or cornstarch, making it especially useful in egg sauces or other sauces that should not be boiled. Since arrowroot has no color or flavor, it's a good choice for thickening clear glazes and fruit sauces.

- Potato starch is a bland, white starch made from raw potatoes. It may be used in sauces or baked products. Potato starch works best in baked products that have eggs to provide needed structure, such as sponge cake.

- Quick-cooking tapioca is a granular product derived from the roots of the cassava plant. It can be used to thicken puddings.

Where to Buy Nonwheat Grains, Flours, Starches, and Other Products

Nonwheat flours, starches, and baked products are available in supermarkets, the food section of department stores, and specialty food stores. Oriental food stores have many rice-based foods that do not contain wheat. The various rice noodles, for instance, can be used in place of egg noodles or other pastas.

Food Preparation

Omitting a basic food or ingredient such as milk, eggs, corn, or wheat from meals can be a challenge. One or more of these foods are found in many baked products, salad dressings, soups, sauces, beverages, and mixed dishes. You may have to prepare foods that contain no milk, eggs, corn, or wheat at home in order to have varied meals and an adequate diet. Be willing to experiment.

Preparing some foods at home is almost the only way to have a varied diet while avoiding substances offensive to people with food allergies.

The following tips will make food preparation easier:

- Look for recipes that are quick and easy to prepare.

- Use convenience foods and mixes when possible. Check the label to be sure they contain only ingredients that are tolerated.

- Cook extra food so that some can be used the next day or frozen for future meals.

Quality of Baked Products

You will find that some foods made without milk, eggs, corn, or wheat will have a different taste, texture, and appearance.

Baking Without Eggs or Milk

Baked products made without eggs or milk:

- have less color and flavor,
- have crusts that brown less,
- are usually heavier in texture, and
- are more crumbly and dry out faster.

Eggs give structure and help to leaven or increase the volume of baked products. You can omit eggs from many cookies with little change in texture; cakes, however, tend to be more crumbly. To help avoid this problem, serve a cake made without eggs from the pan in

263

which it is baked, or bake it as cupcakes in paper liners. Try omitting eggs when preparing some one-layer cake mixes; however, be sure the other ingredients in the mix are those you can tolerate. Top with a tasty sauce, such as the Cherry Dessert Sauce from the following recipes, to add variety to a plain cake made without eggs. Milk is used in many baked products to add flavor or to increase nutritional value. If someone in your family is allergic to milk, try substituting one of the following ingredients: soy milk, fruit juice, liquid nondairy creamer (without milk or milk derivatives), or water. Fortified soy milk is nutritionally similar to milk.

Baking with Nonwheat Flours

When baking, you can use rice, soybean, oat, rye, or barley flour or potato starch instead of wheat flour. The strong gluten in wheat flour helps to form the structure of breads and cakes. Since nonwheat flours or starches contain weak gluten, or none, baked products made with these flours tend to be heavier and more crumbly than products made with wheat flour. Nonwheat flours work best in baked products when two or more flours are combined to make the most of the qualities of each.

Oat, rye, barley, and buckwheat flours contain small amounts of gluten; avoid them if you have a severe intolerance to gluten. In baking with nonwheat flours or starches, keep the following in mind:

- Stir flour or starch thoroughly before measuring. (Sifting is unnecessary).

- Expect the batters of nonwheat flours and starches to be of a different consistency than wheat-flour batters. Some flours make a thinner batter; others make a thicker batter. These variations are due to a lack of gluten and to the different thickening properties of the starches.

- Remember that baked products made with nonwheat flours and starches tend to be heavier, smaller in volume, and more crumbly than those made with wheat flour.

- Crumbling may be less of a problem with cookies or cupcakes than with layer or sheet cakes.

- Cover nonwheat baked products tightly and store at room temperature for a short time or freeze for longer storage. These baked products tend to become dry and pick up odors when stored in the refrigerator.

Thickening Foods with Nonwheat Flours and Starches

Nonwheat flours and starches can be used for thickening sauces, soups, puddings, and pie fillings. Because of differences in starch content, nonwheat flours and starches differ in their ability to thicken and in the clarity of the thickened food. Table 24.5 shows how much nonwheat flour or starch to use in place of wheat flour for thickening.

Foods thickened with most nonwheat flours or starches should not be cooked beyond the point at which they thicken. Be especially careful not to overbeat or overcook sauces thickened with arrowroot or potato starch, or else the sauce may become thinner. In addition, puddings, sauces, or other foods thickened with arrowroot or potato starch should be served the day they are made, as they tend to thin if held longer.

Rice flour is good for thickening foods because it does not affect color or taste. Oat, barley, rye, or soybean flour can also be used for thickening, but they have a stronger flavor and may change the color of the food.

Amounts of Flour or Starch to Substitute for Wheat Flour

The following tables show how much of other flours and starches to substitute for wheat flour. Combinations of flours tend to produce more acceptable baked products. For example, a mixture of 1 cup minus 2 tablespoons of rice flour and 1-1/4 cups of rye flour will substitute for 2 cups of wheat flour. The mild flavor of the rice flour minimizes the strong flavor of rye flour, while the rye flour minimizes the grainy texture produced by the rice flour.

Substitutes for 1 cup of wheat flour in baked products

Kind of flour	Amount
Barley flour	1-1/3 cups
Brown or white rice flour	1 cup minus 2 tablespoons
Corn flour	1 cup
Oat flour	1-1/3 cups
Potato starch	3/4 cup
Rye flour	1-1/4 cups
Soy flour	1-1/2 cups

Substitutes for 1 tablespoon of wheat flour to thicken sauces, gravies, and puddings

Kind of flour	Amount
Cornstarch	1/2 tablespoon
Potato starch	1/2 tablespoon
Arrowroot starch	1/2 tablespoon
Rice flour	1 tablespoon
Quick-cooking tapioca	2 teaspoons

Table 24.5. Substitutes for wheat.

Adapting Family Recipes

In most cases, your favorite recipes can be used with some changes in ingredients. Below are some suggestions for adapting recipes. The specific changes you make will depend on which foods you must avoid.

GENERAL GUIDES:

- Start with simple recipes so that substituting ingredients is easy.

- Replace forbidden ingredients with ingredients that do not cause reactions. See above for suggestions for replacing wheat flour and for milk substitutes.

TO AVOID WHEAT:

- Make cookies, pie crust, and the bottom layer of desserts with crushed breakfast cereal made from rice or corn. (See the recipe for Apricot-Pineapple Pie.)

- Substitute rolled oats for wheat flour in making fruit crisps.

- Use rice in place of wheat bread in poultry stuffing. (See the recipe for Rice Stuffing.)

- Make cornbread with all cornmeal and no wheat flour.

- Add fruits and vegetables to improve the eating quality of baked products made with nonwheat flours. Nuts and chocolate chips will also enhance flavor; however, they are higher in fat.

TO AVOID CHOCOLATE:

- Try replacing chocolate with carob. Carob is sold as a powder, flour, or chips. Carob chips and bars may contain milk products.

TO AVOID MILK:

- Use vegetable oil, shortening, or milk-free margarine in milk-free recipes. Kosher margarine contains no milk solids.

- Check the label to find chocolate chips made without milk.

TO AVOID CORN:

- Use margarines that do not contain corn oil.

- Use cereal-free baking powder in corn-free recipes—regular baking powders contain cornstarch. (Cereal-free baking powder can be purchased at specialty food stores.)

TO AVOID PEANUTS:

- Use sunflower or safflower oil rather than peanut oil.

Meal Planning

When possible, prepare foods that will be eaten by everyone in your family so that the family member with food allergies does not feel different. By creative planning and preparing ahead, you can omit certain foods or ingredients and still have tasty meals that follow Federal guidelines for health promotion. Such meals contain a variety of foods that provide needed nutrients and the food energy (calories) to maintain desirable weight. They also contain only moderate amounts of fat, cholesterol, sugar, and sodium. Keep a supply of suitable foods in your pantry, refrigerator, or freezer.

When eating at a new restaurant, call ahead to check the menu. Choose plain foods that you know contain no hidden ingredients.

Recipes

The Dietary Guidelines were considered in developing these recipes. In general, amounts of fat, saturated fat, cholesterol, sugar, and sodium they contain are limited to moderate levels. The fat, cholesterol, sodium, and total calories are given for each recipe. All of the recipes were tested in the Human Nutrition Information Service food laboratory and received a favorable rating for eating acceptability from trained taste panelists.

Dietary Guidelines

- Avoid too much sodium
- Avoid too much fat, saturated fat, and cholesterol
- Maintain a desirable weight
- Eat a variety of foods
- Eat foods with adequate starch and fiber
- Avoid too much sugar
- If you drink alcoholic beverages, do so in moderation

It's not easy to omit milk, eggs, corn, and wheat in cooking. Sometimes you will need special recipes. The following recipes for breads, main dishes, sauces, salad dressing, and desserts will get you started. Experiment with your own recipes. The results may not always measure up to products made with wheat flour, eggs, and milk, but their use will increase the variety in your daily menus.

Wheat is not an ingredient in any of these recipes. Some of the recipes are also free from milk, egg, corn, and/or gluten. In recipes that need baking powder, the cereal-free kind was used to avoid corn. Regular baking powder can be substituted for the cereal-free baking powder if corn is allowed.

The following symbols next to the name of the recipe indicate what ingredients are absent:

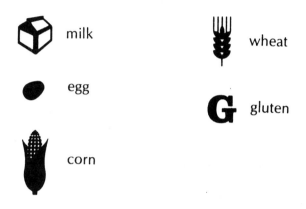

Table 24.6. *Ingredient omitted*

Yeast bread recipes are not included because the eating quality of yeast breads made from nonwheat flour is not generally acceptable unless gums or other special ingredients are used. Tasty and nutritious quick breads, such as those listed below, can be made without any special ingredients.

Some of these recipes can be adapted for a microwave oven or other cooking appliance. Refer to the cookbook that came with the appliance for similar recipes or contact your local county extension agent.

Cheese Pizza with Rice Crust

4 servings, 2 wedges each   NO: 🌾 🌽 **G**

Per serving:

Calories 255	Cholesterol .... 84 milligrams
Total fat .... 9 grams	Sodium .... 545 milligrams

Crust

Rice, cooked, unsalted .... 2-1/2 cups
Mozzarella cheese, lowfat, part skim milk, shredded . 1/4 cup
Egg, beaten.................................. 1
Onion, very finely chopped................... 2 tablespoons
Margarine, corn-free, melted................. 1 tablespoon

Topping

Tomato sauce............................... 8-ounce can
Oregano leaves .... 1/2 teaspoon
Basil leaves .... 1/4 teaspoon
Garlic powder .... 1/8 teaspoon
Green pepper, chopped .... 1/3 cup
Mozzarella cheese, lowfat, part skim milk, shredded . 3/4 cup

1. *Preheat oven to 425°F (hot).*
2. *Lightly grease 12-inch pizza pan.*
3. Mix ingredients for crust thoroughly. Spread evenly and press onto pizza pan.
4. Bake 20 minutes or until surface is lightly browned.
5. Mix tomato sauce and seasonings. Spread evenly over crust. Sprinkle with green pepper and cheese.
6. Bake 10 minutes or until sauce is bubbly and cheese melts.
7. Cut into eight wedges

Chicken-Rice Casserole

4 servings, about 1 cup each

NO: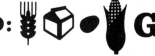

Per serving:

Calories	290	Cholesterol	44 milligrams
Total fat	10 grams	Sodium	495 milligrams

Mushroom stems and pieces	2-ounce can
Onion, chopped	1/2 cup
Margarine, milk- and corn-free	2 tablespoons
Rice flour	3 tablespoons
Chicken broth, unsalted	1-1/2 cups
Rice, cooked, unsalted	2 cups
Chicken, cooked, diced	1-1/2 cups
Pimiento, chopped	2 tablespoons
Salt	1/2 teaspoon
Pepper	1/8 teaspoon
Crisp rice cereal, crushed	1/4 cup

1. *Preheat oven to 350°F (moderate).*
2. Drain mushrooms; save liquid.
3. Cook mushrooms and onion in margarine until onion is tender, about 5 minutes. Stir in rice flour.
4. Gradually stir in mushroom liquid and chicken broth. Cook, stirring constantly, until thickened. Remove from heat.
5. Add remaining ingredients except cereal crumbs. Mix well.
6. Pour mixture into 1-1/2 quart casserole. Sprinkle crumbs over top.
7. Bake 25 minutes or until sauce is bubbly and top is lightly browned.

Variation

Fish-Rice Casserole

NO:

Per serving:

Calories	290	Cholesterol	44 milligrams
Total fat	9 grams	Sodium	535 milligrams

Use 1-1/2 cups milk in place of broth.
Use 1-1/2 cups cooked, unsalted, flaked fish in place of chicken.

Italian Ground Beef with Rice

4 servings, 1 cup each　　**NO:** 🌾 ▢ ● 🌽**G**

Per serving:

Calories 285	Cholesterol .... 62 milligrams
Total fat .... 8 grams	Sodium .... 447 milligrams

Lean ground beef.......................... 3/4 pound
Onion, chopped .... 1/2 cup
Green pepper, chopped .... 1/4 cup
Celery, chopped .... 1/4 cup
Tomatoes, crushed .... 8-ounce can
Tomato puree .... 10-3/4-ounce can
Oregano leaves .... 1 teaspoon
Basil leaves............................... 1 teaspoon
Rice, cooked, unsalted .... 2 cups

1. Cook beef, onion, green pepper, and celery in a large frypan until beef is lightly browned and onion is clear. Pour off fat.
2. Add tomatoes, tomato puree, and seasonings to meat mixture. Cover and simmer 15 minutes to blend flavors.
3. Stir in rice. Heat to serving temperature.

Meatloaf

4 servings, 2 slices each

NO:

Per serving:

Calories 305	Cholesterol .... 82 milligrams
Total fat .... 18 grams	Sodium .... 215 milligrams

Lean ground beef . . . . 1 pound
Quick-cooking rolled oats . . . . 1/2 cup
Apple juice . . . . 1/2 cup
Celery, chopped . . . . 1/4 cup
Onion, chopped . . . . 1/4 cup
Worcestershire sauce . . . . 3/4 teaspoon
Salt . . . . 1/4 teaspoon
Pepper . . . . 1/8 teaspoon
Ground nutmeg . . . . 1/8 teaspoon

1. *Preheat oven to 350°F (moderate).*
2. Mix all ingredients thoroughly.
3. Shape into a loaf in baking pan.
4. Bake 1-1/4 hours or until done.
5. Drain off excess fat.

NOTE: Mixture can also be packed lightly into a 9- by 5- by 3-inch loaf pan to bake.

Variation

Porcupine Meatballs

NO:  G

4 servings, 4 meatballs each

Per serving:

Calories 325	Cholesterol .... 82 milligrams
Total fat .... 18 grams	Sodium .... 216 milligrams

Omit rolled oats. Add 1/3 cup uncooked rice to meat mixture.
Shape into 16 meatballs.
Brown well on all sides in hot frypan. Pour off fat.
Add 1-1/2 cups hot water to meatballs in frypan. Heat to boiling, cover, reduce heat and simmer 50 minutes.
Remove from liquid and serve.

Rice Stuffing

4 cups
(sufficient stuffing for a 4-pound chicken)

NO: 🌾 📦 ● 🌽 **G**

Per 1/2 cup serving:

Made with broth	*Made with water*
Calories 125	Calories 115
Total fat . . . . . . 4 grams	Total fat . . . . . . 4 grams
Cholesterol . . . 0	Cholesterol . . . 0
Sodium . . . . . . 162 milligrams	Sodium . . . . . . 154 milligrams

Rice, uncooked, ...	1 cup
Celery, chopped	1 cup
Onion, chopped	1/2 cup
Oil, corn-free	2 tablespoons
Chicken broth, unsalted, or water	2 cups
Poultry seasoning	1 teaspoon
Salt	1/2 teaspoon

1. Cook rice, celery, and onion in oil in large frypan, stirring occasionally, until rice is lightly browned.
2. Stir in broth or water and seasonings. Heat to boiling. Reduce heat.
3. Simmer, covered, until rice is tender and liquid is absorbed, about 15 minutes.
4. Use to stuff a 4-pound chicken.

Rice Salad

4 servings, 3/4 cup each

NO: 🌾 📦 ● 🌽 **G**

Per serving:

Calories 160	Cholesterol 0
Total fat .... 5 grams	Sodium .... 235 milligrams

Rice, cooked, unsalted.........................	2 cups
Frozen green peas, cooked, unsalted, drained	1/2 cup
Celery, finely chopped.........................	1/2 cup
Pimiento, chopped	2 tablespoons
Onion, finely chopped.........................	1 tablespoon
Salad dressing, mayonnaise-type, egg-free	3 tablespoons
Vinegar	1 tablespoon
Prepared mustard............................	1 teaspoon
Salt	1/4 teaspoon
Garlic powder	Dash
Pepper	Dash
Salad greens	4 large leaves

1. Gently toss rice and vegetables.
2. Mix remaining ingredients except salad greens thoroughly. Lightly stir into rice mixture.
3. Chill.
4. Serve on salad greens.

Cooked Salad Dressing

1-1/4 cups dressing

NO: 🌾 ● 🌽 G

Per tablespoon:

Calories 15   Cholesterol .... 1 milligram
Total fat .... Trace   Sodium .... 65 milligrams

Sugar .... 2 tablespoons
Potato starch .... 1 tablespoon
Dry mustard .... 1 teaspoon
Salt .... 1/2 teaspoon
Paprika .... 1/8 teaspoon
Dried tarragon leaves, crumbled .... 1/8 teaspoon
Garlic powder .... 1/16 teaspoon
Lowfat milk .... 1 cup
Vinegar .... 3 tablespoons

1. Mix dry ingredients in saucepan. Gradually stir in milk.
2. Cook over low heat, stirring constantly, until thickened.
   Remove from heat. Cool completely.
3. Add vinegar; mix well.
4. Chill.

Date Bread

1 loaf, 18 slices

NO:

Per slice:

Calories 140	Cholesterol	16 milligrams
Total fat .... 3 grams	Sodium	137 milligrams

Boiling water	1/2 cups
Dates, chopped	1 cup
Rice flour	1 cup
Barley flour	1 cup
Baking powder, cereal-free	2 teaspoons
Baking soda	1/2 teaspoon
Salt	1/2 teaspoon
Sugar	3/4 cup
Vegetable shortening	1/4 cup
Egg	1
Lowfat milk	1/2 cup

1. *Preheat oven to 350°F (moderate).*
2. *Grease 9- by 5- by 3-inch loaf pan.*
3. Pour boiling water over dates. Let cool to lukewarm.
4. Mix dry ingredients except sugar thoroughly.
5. Beat sugar, shortening, and egg together until creamy.
6. Add milk to lukewarm date mixture.
7. Alternate adding dry ingredients and milk mixture to creamy mixture. Mix well after each addition.
8. Pour into baking pan.
9. Bake 45 minutes or until toothpick inserted in center of loaf comes out clean.
10. Cool on rack.
11. Remove from pan after 10 minutes.

Variation

Apricot Bread

NO:

Per slice:

Calories 135	Cholesterol	16 milligrams
Total fat .... 3 grams	Sodium	137 milligrams

Use 1 cup chopped dried apricots in place of dates.

Muffins

12 muffins **NO:**

Per muffin:

Calories 160	Cholesterol .... 24 milligrams
Total fat .... 5 grams	Sodium .... 210 milligrams

Potato starch . . . . 1 cup
Rice flour . . . . 1/2 cup
Oat flour . . . . 1/2 cup
Sugar . . . . 1/4 cup
Baking powder, cereal-free . . . . 1 tablespoon
Salt . . . . 1/2 teaspoon
Lowfat milk . . . . 1 cup
Egg, slightly beaten 1
Vegetable shortening, melted . . . . 1/4 cup

1. *Preheat oven to 400°F (hot).*
2. *Grease muffin tins.*
3. Mix dry ingredients thoroughly.
4. Mix milk, egg, and shortening. Add to dry ingredients and stir until dry ingredients are barely moistened.
5. Fill muffin tins about two-thirds full.
6. Bake 20 to 25 minutes or until lightly browned.

Variation

Blueberry Muffins **NO:**

Per muffin:

Calories 165	Cholesterol .... 24 milligrams
Total fat .... 6 grams	Sodium .... 211 milligrams

Stir 1 cup fresh or frozen, unsweetened blueberries into liquid mixture before adding to dry ingredients.

Rye Crackers

6 dozen crackers

NO: 🌾 ● 🌽

Per cracker:

Calories 30		Cholesterol	Trace
Total fat . . . . 2 grams		Sodium	63 milligrams

Rye flour . . . . 1-3/4 cups
Rice flour . . . . 1 cup
Salt . . . . 1-1/2 teaspoons
Baking soda . . . . 1 teaspoon
Vegetable shortening . . . . 1/2 cup
Buttermilk . . . . 3/4 cup

1. *Preheat oven to 375°F (moderate).*
2. Mix dry ingredients thoroughly.
3. Mix in shortening until mixture is crumbly.
4. Add buttermilk; mix well.
5. Divide dough in half.
6. Place half of dough on rye-floured board. Cover remaining half.
7. Roll very thin. Cut into pieces about 3 by 1-1/2 inches.
8. Place with sides touching on baking sheet.
9. Repeat steps 7 and 8 with other half of dough.
10. Bake 13 to 18 minutes or until lightly browned.
11. Remove from baking sheet; cook on rack.

Waffles

NO:

4 waffles, each about 7 inches in diameter

Per waffle:

Calories 325	Cholesterol .... 137 milligrams
Total fat .... 13 grams	Sodium .... 360 milligrams

Rice flour .... 1-1/2 cups
Baking powder, cereal-free .... 2 teaspoons
Sugar .... 2 teaspoons
Salt .... 1/4 teaspoon
Water .... 1 cup
Vegetable shortening, melted, or oil, corn-free ..... 3 tablespoons
Egg yolks, beaten 2
Egg whites, stiffly beaten 2

1. *Preheat waffle iron.*
2. Mix dry ingredients thoroughly.
3. Stir in water, shortening or oil, and egg yolks. Mix well.
4. Fold in beaten egg whites.
5. Bake in hot waffle iron, using 1/2 to 2/3 cup batter per waffle.

Apple Crisp

NO:

8 servings, about 1/3 cup each

Per serving:

Calories 175	Cholesterol 0
Total fat .... 6 grams	Sodium .... 4 milligrams

Apples, tart, pared, sliced .... 5 cups
Brown sugar, packed .... 1/2 cup
Oat flour .... 1/2 cup
Rolled oats, quick-cooking................... 1/2 cup
Ground cinnamon .... 1 teaspoon
Vegetable shortening .... 3 tablespoons

1. *Preheat oven to 350°F (moderate).*
2. *Grease 8- by 8- by 2-inch baking pan.*
3. Arrange apples in pan.
4. Mix dry ingredients thoroughly. Add shortening and mix until crumbly.
5. Sprinkle crumbly mixture evenly over apples.
6. Bake 40 minutes or until apples are tender and top is lightly browned.
7. Serve warm.

Applesauce Drop Cookies

5 dozen cookies

NO:

Per cookie:

Calories 35	Cholesterol 0
Total fat . . . . 1 gram	Sodium . . . . 17 milligrams

Oat flour	1-1/3 cups
Baking soda	1/2 teaspoon
Salt	1/4 teaspoon
Ground cinnamon	1/2 teaspoon
Ground nutmeg	1/4 teaspoon
Ground cloves	1/8 teaspoon
Vegetable shortening	1/3 cup
Sugar	2/3 cup
Applesauce, unsweetened	3/4 cup
Rolled oats, quick cooking	1-1/2 cups

1. *Preheat oven to 325°F (slow).*
2. *Grease baking sheet.*
3. Mix flour, baking soda, salt, and spices thoroughly.
4. Mix shortening and sugar until creamy. Stir in dry ingredients.
5. Add applesauce and rolled oats. Mix well.
6. Drop dough by teaspoonfuls onto baking sheet about 1 inch apart.
7. Bake about 15 minutes or until edges start to brown.
8. Remove from baking sheet while still warm.
9. Cool on rack.

Apricot-Pineapple Pie

8-inch pie, 8 servings

NO: 🌾 📦 ● 🌽 **G**

Per serving:

Calories 170	Cholesterol 0
Total fat .... 4 grams	Sodium .... 145 milligrams

Pie shell

Crisp rice cereal, crushed .... 1 cup
Margarine, milk- and corn-free, melted .... 3 tablespoons
Sugar .... 1 tablespoon

Filling

Apricot halves, juice pack .... 16-ounce can
Crushed pineapple, juice pack .... 15-1/4-ounce can
Sugar .... 1/4 cup
Quick-cooking tapioca .... 3 tablespoons
Ground cinnamon .... 1/2 teaspoon
Juice from pineapple and apricots .... 1 cup
Lemon juice .... 2 teaspoons

To make pie shell:

1. Preheat oven to 375°F (moderate).
2. Mix rice cereal, margarine, and 1 tablespoon sugar thoroughly. Save 1/4 cup of crumb mixture for top of pie.
3. Press remaining crumb mixture into 8-inch pie pan so the bottom and sides are completely covered.
4. Bake until crust is firm, about 8 minutes. Cool.

To make filling:

5. Drain apricots and pineapple; save 1 cup juice. Coarsely chop apricots.
6. Mix sugar, tapioca, and cinnamon in saucepan. Stir in fruit juice. Let stand 5 minutes.
7. Cook over low heat, stirring constantly, until thickened. Remove from heat.
8. Add apricots, pineapple, and lemon juice. Mix well.
9. Spoon filling into pie. Sprinkle crumbs over the top.
10. Chill until set.

Carrot-Raisin Cookies

4 dozen cookies

NO:

Per cookie:

Calories 50		Cholesterol 0	
Total fat .... 2 grams		Sodium .... 34 milligrams	

Barley flour..............................	2-1/2 cups
Baking soda	1/2 teaspoon
Salt	1/2 teaspoon
Vegetable shortening	1/2 cup
Sugar	3/4 cup
Vanilla	2 teaspoons
Carrots, finely shredded....................	1 cup
Raisins, chopped	1/2 cup
Water	1/4 cup

1. *Preheat oven to 350°F (moderate).*
2. *Grease baking sheet.*
3. Mix flour, baking soda, and salt.
4. Mix shortening, sugar, and vanilla until creamy.
5. Stir in carrots and raisins.
6. Alternate adding dry ingredients and water to carrot mixture. Mix well after each addition.
7. Drop dough by teaspoonfuls onto baking sheet, about 2 inches apart.
8. Bake 12 minutes or until cookies are set and lightly browned.
9. Remove from baking sheet while still warm.
10. Cool on rack.

Chiffon Cake

12 servings

NO: G

Per serving:

Calories 135	Cholesterol .... 68 milligrams
Total fat .... 6 grams	Sodium .... 117 milligrams

Rice flour .... 1 cup
Sugar .... 1/2 cup
Baking powder, cereal-free .... 1-1/2 teaspoons
Salt .... 1/4 teaspoon
Oil, corn-free .... 1/4 cup
Egg yolks, beaten 3
Water .... 1/4 cup
Lemon juice .... 1 tablespoon
Lemon rind, grated .... 1 teaspoon
Egg whites 3
Cream of tartar .... 1/4 teaspoon

1. *Preheat oven to 350°F (moderate).*
2. Mix flour, sugar, baking powder, and salt.
3. Add oil, egg yolks, water, lemon juice, and rind. Beat until smooth.
4. Beat egg whites with cream of tartar until stiff but not dry. Fold into egg yolk mixture.
5. Pour into ungreased 8- by 8- by 2-inch baking pan.
6. Bake 30 to 35 minutes or until firm to touch.
7. Invert in pan on rack to cool.

Variation

Peppermint Chiffon Cake

NO: G

Omit lemon juice and rind. Increase water to 1/3 cup.
Add 1/2 teaspoon peppermint flavoring.
Nutrients are the same as in the basic recipe.

Cranberry-Apple Sorbet

8 servings, about 1/2 cup each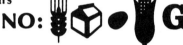

Per serving:

Calories. 85	Cholesterol 0
Total fat . . . . Trace	Sodium . . . . 22 milligrams

Sugar. . . . . 1/2 cup
Unflavored gelatin . . . . 1-1/2 teaspoons
(1/2 envelope)
Salt . . . . Dash
Cranberry juice cocktail . . . . 1 cup
Apple juice . . . . 1 cup
Lemon juice . . . . 3 tablespoons

1. Mix sugar, gelatin, and salt in saucepan.
2. Stir in cranberry juice cocktail.
3. Heat, stirring constantly, until gelatin is dissolved.
4. Remove from heat and add remaining ingredients. Mix well.
5. Pour into a 8- by 8- by 2-inch pan. Freeze until firm.
6. Remove from freezer and break into chunks. Place in chilled bowl. Beat with chilled beaters until smooth.
7. Return to pan, cover, and refreeze.

Cranberry-Apple Tapoica with Pears

4 servings, 1/2 cup each

Per serving:

Calories 100	Cholesterol 0
Total fat . . . . Trace	Sodium . . . . 44 milligrams

Quick-cooking tapioca . . . . 2 tablespoons
Sugar . . . . 1 tablespoon
Salt . . . . Dash
Ground cloves . . . . Dash
Cranberry juice cocktail . . . . 2/3 cup
Apple juice . . . . 2/3 cup
Canned pears, juice pack, drained, diced . . . . 1 cup

1. Mix tapioca, sugar, salt, and cloves in saucepan.
2. Add juices; stir until well blended. Let stand 5 minutes.
3. Cook over low heat, stirring constantly, until mixture thickens and just reaches boiling.
4. Cool, stirring occasionally.
5. Fold in pears.
6. Chill.

Grape Frappe

4 servings, about 3/4 cup each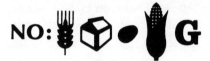

Per serving:

Calories 130	Cholesterol 0
Total fat .... Trace	Sodium .... 2 milligrams

Water .... 1-1/2 cups
Sugar .... 1/2 cup
Grape juice................................... 1 cup
Lemon juice .... 3 tablespoons

1. Mix water and sugar in saucepan. Bring to boiling, reduce heat, and cook gently for 5 minutes. Cool.
2. Add juices to cooled mixture.
3. Pour into 8- by 8- by 2-inch pan. Put in freezer until almost frozen.
4. Remove from pan into chilled mixing bowl. Beat with chilled beaters until fluffy and light in color.
5. Serve immediately or cover and return to freezer.

Lemon Pudding

4 servings, about 1/2 cup each **NO:** 🌾 📦 ● 🌽 **G**

Per serving:

Calories 110	Cholesterol 0
Total fat .... 2 grams	Sodium .... 103 milligrams

Sugar .... 1/3 cup
Potato starch .... 3 tablespoons
Salt .... 1/8 teaspoon
Water .... 1-3/4 cups
Margarine, milk- and corn-free .... 2 teaspoons
Lemon juice .... 1/4 cup
Lemon rind, grated .... 2 teaspoons

1. Mix sugar, potato starch, and salt in saucepan. Gradually stir in water. Mix well.
2. Cook over low heat, stirring constantly, until pudding thickens and just begins to boil.
3. Remove from heat; stir in remaining ingredients.
4. Chill.

Old-Fashioned Rice Pudding

4 servings, about 1/2 cup each

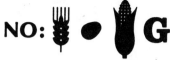

NO:

Per serving:

Calories 215	Cholesterol .... 12 milligrams
Total fat .... 3 grams	Sodium .... 227 milligrams

Rice, uncooked	1/2 cup
Sugar	1/4 cup
Salt	1/4 teaspoon
Ground cinnamon	1/4 teaspoon
Ground nutmeg	1/4 teaspoon
Lowfat milk................................	2-1/2 cups
Vanilla	1 teaspoon

1. Mix all ingredients except vanilla in saucepan.
2. Bring to a boil; reduce heat.
3. Cover and cook over very low heat, stirring occasionally, until rice is tender and milk is almost absorbed, about 50 minutes.
4. Remove from heat. Stir in vanilla.
5. Serve warm.

Variation

Apple Juice Rice Pudding   **NO:**

Per serving:

Calories 185	Cholesterol 0
Total fat .... Trace	Sodium .... 151 milligrams

Reduce sugar to 2 tablespoons. Omit nutmeg. Use 2-1/2 cups apple juice in place of milk.

Peanut Butter Bars

2 dozen bars

NO: ✻ ⬡ 🌽 **G**

Per bar:

Calories 105	Cholesterol . . . . 23 milligrams
Total fat . . . . 6 grams	Sodium . . . . 79 milligrams

Rice flour . . . . 1 cup
Baking powder, cereal-free . . . . 1 teaspoon
Salt . . . . 1/4 teaspoon
Brown sugar, packed . . . . 3/4 cup
Crunchy peanut butter . . . . 1/2 cup
Margarine, milk- and corn-free, softened . . . . 1/3 cup
Eggs 2
Vanilla . . . . 1/2 teaspoon

1. *Preheat oven to 350°F (moderate).*
2. *Grease 9- by 9- by 2-inch baking pan.*
3. Mix flour, baking powder, and salt thoroughly.
4. Mix sugar, peanut butter, and margarine until creamy.
5. Beat in eggs and vanilla. Add dry ingredients; mix well.
6. Spread batter into pan.
7. Bake about 25 minutes or until firm in the center.
8. Cool in pan on rack.
9. Cut into 24 bars while still warm.

Pineapple Upside-Down Cake

NO: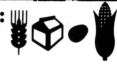

9 servings, about 2-1/2 × 2-1/2 inches each

Per serving:

Calories 315	Cholesterol 0
Total fat .... 12 grams	Sodium .... 240 milligrams

Vegetable shortening . . . . 3 tablespoons
Brown sugar, packed . . . . 1/3 cup
Canned pineapple slices, juice pack, drained 6
Vegetable shortening . . . . 1/3 cup
Brown sugar, packed . . . . 2/3 cup
Vanilla . . . . 1 teaspoon
Rye flour. . . . . 1 cup
Rice flour . . . . 1 cup
Baking powder, cereal-free . . . . 4 teaspoons
Salt . . . . 1/4 teaspoon
Pineapple liquid and water . . . . 1 cup

1. *Preheat oven to 375°F (moderate).*
2. Melt 3 tablespoons shortening together with 1/3 cup brown sugar in 8- by 8- by 2-inch baking pan in oven.
3. Arrange pineapple slices in sugar mixture.
4. Beat 1/3 cup shortening, 2/3 cup brown sugar, and vanilla until creamy.
5. Mix flours, baking powder, and salt.
6. Alternate adding dry ingredients and liquid to creamy mixture. Beat well after each addition.
7. Spread batter over pineapple slices.
8. Bake 40 minutes or until cake begins to leave sides of pan.
9. Cool a few minutes in pan on rack; loosen cake from sides of pan and invert on serving plate. Remove pan.

Plain Cake

Two 8-inch layers, 16 servings   **NO:**

Per serving:

Calories 190	Cholesterol .... 35 milligrams
Total fat .... 8 grams	Sodium .... 161 milligrams

Potato starch . . . . 3/4 cup
Rice flour . . . . 1/2 cup
Oat flour . . . . 1/2 cup
Baking powder, cereal-free . . . . 1 tablespoon
Salt . . . . 1/2 teaspoon
Vegetable shortening . . . . 1/2 cup
Sugar . . . . 1-1/4 cups
Egg yolks. 2
Vanilla . . . . 1-1/2 teaspoons
Lowfat milk. . . . . 1 cup
Egg whites, stiffly beaten 2

1. *Preheat oven to 375°F (moderate).*
2. *Grease two 8-inch layer pans. Use potato starch to coat pans.*
3. Mix dry ingredients except sugar thoroughly.
4. Beat shortening and sugar together until creamy.
5. Add egg yolks and vanilla; beat well.
6. Alternate adding dry ingredients and milk to creamy mixture, beating well after each addition.
7. Fold beaten egg whites into batter.
8. Pour batter into pans.
9. Bake 25 to 30 minutes or until cake surface springs back when touched lightly.
10. Cool cake in pans on rack for a few minutes. Remove cake from pans and complete cooling on rack.
11. Serve with slices of fruit or a fruit sauce.

Variation

Spice Cake   **NO:**

Add 1 teaspoon ground cinnamon, 1/2 teaspoon ground cloves, and 1/2 teaspoon ground nutmeg to dry ingredients. Mix thoroughly. Nutrients are the same as basic recipe.

Shortbread Cookies

24 cookies

NO: 🌾 📦 ● 🌽

Per cookie:

Calories 105	Cholesterol 0
Total fat . . . . 6 grams	Sodium . . . . 93 milligrams

Oat flour . . . . 1-1/3 cups
Potato starch . . . . 3/4 cup
Salt . . . . 1/4 teaspoon
Margarine, milk- and corn-free . . . . 3/4 cup
Sugar . . . . 1/2 cup
Vanilla . . . . 1 teaspoon

1. *Preheat oven to 350°F (moderate).*
2. Mix flour, potato starch, and salt thoroughly.
3. Beat margarine, sugar, and vanilla together until creamy. Add dry ingredients. Mix until smooth.
4. Spread mixture into ungreased 9- by 13- by 2-inch baking pan.
5. Bake 18 minutes or until lightly browned.
6. Cool in pan on rack.
7. Cut into 24 squares while still warm.

NOTE: 1/2 cup brown sugar, packed, may be used in place of granulated sugar.

Apricot Dessert Sauce

About 1-1/4 cups sauce

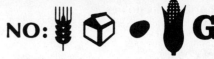

NO:

Per tablespoon:

Calories 10	Cholesterol 0
Total fat . . . . Trace	Sodium . . . . 1 milligram

Apricot nectar . . . . 1-1/4 cups
Potato starch . . . . 1 tablespoon

1. Mix apricot nectar and potato starch in saucepan.
2. Cook over low heat, stirring constantly, until sauce thickens and just begins to boil.
3. Serve warm over cake or other dessert.

Cherry Dessert Sauce

4 servings, 1/2 cup each

NO:

Per serving:

Calories 145	Cholesterol 0
Total fat . . . . 3 grams	Sodium . . . . 120 milligrams

Red sour pitted cherries, water pack . . . . 16-ounce can
Sugar . . . . 1/3 cup
Potato starch . . . . 1-1/2 tablespoons
Salt . . . . 1/8 teaspoon
Margarine, milk- and corn-free . . . . 1 tablespoon
Almond extract . . . . 1/8 teaspoon

1. Drain cherries; save liquid.
2. Mix sugar, potato starch, and salt in saucepan. Stir in cherry liquid until smooth.
3. Cook over low heat, stirring constantly, until mixture thickens and just begins to boil.
4. Remove from heat. Add cherries, margarine, and almond extract. Mix well.
5. Serve warm over cake or other dessert.

Lemon Dessert Sauce

About 1-1/3 cups sauce   **NO: 🌾 📦 ● 🌽 G**

Per tablespoon:

Calories 15	Cholesterol 0
Total fat .... Trace	Sodium .... 17 milligrams

Sugar . . . . 1/3 cup
Potato starch . . . . 1-1/2 tablespoons
Water . . . . 1 cup
Lemon juice . . . . 2 tablespoons
Lemon rind, grated . . . . 1 teaspoon
Salt . . . . 1/8 teaspoon
Margarine, milk- and corn-free . . . . 1 teaspoon

1. Mix sugar and potato starch in saucepan. Gradually stir in water.
2. Cook over low heat, stirring constantly, until sauce thickens and just begins to boil.
3. Remove from heat; stir in remaining ingredients.
4. Serve warm over cake or other dessert.

Medium White Sauce

1 cup sauce   **NO: 🌾 ● 🌽 G**

Per tablespoon:

Calories 15	Cholesterol .... 1 milligram
Total fat .... 1 gram	Sodium .... 53 milligrams

Margarine, corn-free . . . . 1 tablespoon
Potato starch . . . . 1 tablespoon
Salt . . . . 1/4 teaspoon
Lowfat milk . . . . 1 cup

1. Melt margarine in saucepan over low heat. Mix potato starch and salt until smooth.
2. Gradually stir in milk.
3. Cook, stirring constantly, until sauce thickens and just begins to boil.

Index to Recipes

Main Dishes

Cheese Pizza with Rice Crust 270
Chicken-Rice Casserole 271
Fish-Rice Casserole 271
Italian Ground Beef with Rice 272
Meatloaf 273
Porcupine Meatballs 273

Meat Accompaniments

Rice Stuffing 274

Salad, Salad Dressing

Rice Salad 275
Cooked Salad Dressing 276

Breads and Crackers

Apricot Bread 277
Blueberry Muffins 278
Date Bread 277
Muffins 278
Rye Crackers 279
Waffles 280

Desserts

Apple Crisp 280
Apple Juice Rice Pudding 287
Applesauce Drop Cookies 281
Apricot-Pineapple Pie 282
Carrot-Raisin Cookies 283
Chiffon Cake 284
Cranberry-Apple Sorbet 285
Cranberry-Apple Tapioca with Pears 285
Grape Frappe 286
Lemon Pudding 286

Desserts, continued

Old-Fashioned Rice Pudding 287
Peanut Butter Bars 288
Peppermint Chiffon Cake 284
Pineapple Upside-down Cake 289
Plain Cake 290
Shortbread Cookies 291
Spice Cake 290

Sauces

Apricot Dessert Sauce 292
Cherry Dessert Sauce 292
Lemon Dessert Sauce 293
Medium White Sauce 293

Chapter 25

The New Food Label: Better Information for Special Diets

This is the fifth and last in a series of articles which appeared in *FDA Consumer* telling how to use the new food label to meet specific dietary needs.

Articles cited in this chapter are among those included in the in depth and easy-to-understand *FDA Consumer* special report, *Focus on Food Labeling*. Copies cost $5 each at time of printing. To order, write to:

Superintendent of Documents,
P.O. Box 371954,
Pittsburgh, PA 15250-7954

Ask for stock number S/N 017-012-00360-5.

The right diet is important for everyone, but for Tony Robinson of Orlando, FL, it truly is his lifeblood.

Robinson has end-stage renal disease. Three times a week, he goes to a local medical center, where a dialysis machine does what his kidneys no longer can: purify his blood.

Between treatments, he's careful about what he eats because some nutrients can cause harmful—sometimes deadly—levels of substances to build up in his blood. He eats a diet low in protein, sodium and potassium to keep those dangerous substances minimal, and high in calories to maintain his weight.

FDA Consumer, January-February 1995.

Until recently, he and his wife, who does most of the cooking, kept mainly to foods listed in a brochure of "foods to eat" and "foods to avoid" for people with end-stage renal disease. But now they're using the new food label as another source of information.

"The new label adds to what we already know," Robinson said. "And mandatory nutrition labeling gives us the information we need to choose from a wider range of food products."

Label Benefits

Under the Nutrition Labeling and Education Act of 1990 and regulations from the Food and Drug Administration and the U.S. Department of Agriculture, virtually all food labels must now give information about a food's nutritional content.

That wasn't always the case. Until 1994, nutrition information was voluntary. Manufacturers had to provide it only when a food contained added nutrients or when nutrition claims appeared on the label. Nearly 40 percent of products didn't carry nutrition information.

"Just to have the information on the label is a big plus for consumers on therapeutic diets," said Camille Brewer, a registered dietitian and nutritionist in FDA's Office of Food Labeling.

Another group the regulations help is people with food sensitivities. Every product with two or more ingredients must now list the ingredients on the label. That includes standardized foods, such as peanut butter, and some baked goods. These foods previously were exempt from ingredient labeling because at one time, most Americans were familiar with the recipes since they were foods routinely prepared at home.

Also, the source of some ingredients (for example, hydrolyzed soy protein) must now be identified.

Get the Nutrition Facts

Consumers looking for nutrition information about a food should first look at "Nutrition Facts," usually on the side or back of the package.

For many people on special diets, the amount of the nutrient in grams or milligrams is most important because their diets are based on a set amount of one or more nutrients a day specific to their needs—for example, 60 grams (g) of protein or 2,000 milligrams (mg) of sodium a day. Special dieters can find the amount by weight of nutrients listed in the top part of the Nutrition Facts panel.

Some Important Points about the Nutrition Facts Panel

- The values listed for total carbohydrates include all carbohydrates, including dietary fiber and sugars listed below it.

- The sugars include naturally present sugars, such as lactose in milk and fructose in fruits, as well as those added to the food, such as table sugar, corn syrup, and dextrose. The label can claim "no sugar added" but still have naturally occurring sugar. An example is fruit juice.

- Also, potassium may be listed voluntarily with the nutrients listed on the top part of the panel, just below sodium. Its "% Daily Value" is based on a recommended intake of 3,500 mg a day.

- Other vitamins and minerals may be listed on the Nutrition Facts panel, along with vitamins A and C, iron, and calcium.

- Amounts of vitamins and minerals are only presented as percentages of the Daily Value.

- Calorie information appears at the top of the Nutrition Facts panel, following serving size information. This information is important for those needing to increase or decrease their calories.

Serving Size

The serving size information gives the amount of food to which all the other numbers on the Nutrition Facts panel apply.

Now serving sizes are more uniform among similar products and are designed to reflect the amounts people actually eat. Also, serving sizes must be about the same for the same types of products (for example, different brands of frozen yogurt) and for similar products within a food category (for example, ice cream, ice milk, and sherbet are within the category frozen dairy-type desserts).

Having more uniform serving sizes makes it easier to compare the nutritional values of related foods.

People who follow special diets should be aware that the serving size on the label may not be the same as that recommended for their specific needs. For example, the label serving size for cooked fish is 3 ounces (84 g). A person following a 60-gram protein diet may be allowed only 1 ounce (28 g) of fish at a meal. So, in this case, the nutrient values would have to be divided by 3 to determine the nutritional content of the 1-ounce portion eaten.

Ingredients

The ingredient list is a source of information especially useful for people with food sensitivities. (See Ingredient Labeling: What's in a Food?" in the April 1993 *FDA Consumer*.) Some new requirements that provide more information in the list are:

- **Listing protein hydrolysates by source:** Instead of "hydrolyzed vegetable protein," the list must state the type of vegetable (for example, "hydrolyzed corn protein").

- **Stating FDA food-certified color additives by name:** For example, "FD&C Blue No. 1" and "FD&C Yellow No. 6." Before, they could be listed simply as "colorings."

- **Declaring caseinate as a milk derivative:** The term "caseinate" often appeared on earlier labels even in foods that claimed to be non-dairy, such as coffee whiteners.

- **Voluntary listing of source of sweeteners:** On some labels, the ingredient list may state the source of sweeteners, although this is voluntary. For example, instead of "dextrose" or "dextrose monohydrate," the ingredient may be listed as "corn sugar monohydrate."

Nutrient Claims

Elsewhere on the label, consumers may find claims about the food's nutrient content. Often, these claims appear on the front of the package, where shoppers can readily see them. These claims signal that the food contains desirable levels of certain nutrients.

Some claims, such as "low-sodium,""high in calcium," or "good source of fiber," describe nutrient levels. (See "A Little 'Lite' Reading," in the June 1993 *FDA Consumer*.) Some, but not all, highlight foods containing beneficial amounts of nutrients for some people with special dietary needs. The same claim may warn other consumers, for whom the nutrient is detrimental, to avoid the product. For example, a product claiming to be an "excellent source of potassium" is not a wise buy for a person following a low-potassium diet. (See "Nutrient Claims Guide for Individual Foods" below.)

Health Claims

Health claims describe a relationship between a nutrient or food and a disease or health-related condition. FDA has authorized eight such claims; they are the only ones that can be used in a label. The claims may show a link between:

- calcium and a lower risk of osteoporosis;
- fat and a greater risk of cancer;
- saturated fat and cholesterol and a greater risk of coronary heart disease;
- fiber-containing grain products, fruits and vegetables and a reduced risk of cancer;
- fruits, vegetables and grain products that contain fiber and a reduced risk of coronary heart disease;
- sodium and a greater risk of high blood pressure;
- fruits and vegetables and a reduced risk of cancer;
- folic acid and a decreased risk of neural tube defect- affected pregnancy.

Nutrient and health claims can be used only under certain circumstances, such as when the food contains appropriate levels of the stated nutrients.

The intent of the new food label is not just to ensure that label information is truthful but to provide more complete and useful nutrition and ingredient information for consumers' use. People with special dietary needs will likely find the labeling changes a welcome bonus.

Special Diets

Label information can help individuals select foods appropriate for their special dietary needs, determined by a physician, registered dietitian, or nutritionist. Some medical conditions that require special attention to diet are:

- Kidney Disease
- Liver Disorders
- Food Sensitivities
- Celiac Disease
- Cancer
- Bowel Disease
- Osteoporosis

Kidney Disease

For many people whose kidneys have failed or are failing, protein, potassium and sodium are restricted. The nutrient phosphorus also may be restricted.

People undergoing dialysis may be encouraged to eat 20 to 25 grams (g) of fiber daily because fluid restrictions, lack of exercise, and some kidney medications can cause constipation. The Daily Value for fiber, which is based on a 2,000-calorie diet, is 25 g.

Daily Values are reference numbers based on recommended dietary intakes to help consumers use label information to plan a healthy diet. (See "'Daily Values' Encourage Healthy Diet" in the May 1993 *FDA Consumer*.)

Liver Disorders

People with hepatitis, cirrhosis, and other liver diseases often need a high-calorie, low-protein diet to help rejuvenate the damaged liver and maintain adequate nutrition. They also may need to increase their intake of vitamins—particularly folic acid, vitamin B12, and thiamin—and minerals.

Food Sensitivities

According to the Food Allergy Network (a national nonprofit organization), the most common food allergens are milk, eggs, wheat, peanuts and other nuts, and soy. The treatment: avoiding the food or foods containing them.

Celiac Disease

This is a genetic disorder in which the body cannot tolerate gliadin, the protein component of the gluten in wheat, barley, rye, and oats. So, people with celiac disease must avoid all products containing these grains—even foods that may contain only small amounts of the protein such as vinegar, bouillon, and alcohol-containing flavorings. The intolerance leads to malabsorption—not only of the offending food but virtually all nutrients.

Cancer

Because weight loss is common during cancer treatment, many cancer patients need to increase their calories and protein intake.

In the case of bowel obstruction—either from surgery, radiation or the tumor—cancer patients may need to eat less fiber. But, they may need more if they become constipated.

To help reduce their risk of developing cancer again, following treatment, patients may want to choose foods and nutrients whose role in reducing cancer risk has been borne out by significant scientific evidence. (See "Look for 'Legit' Health Claims on Foods" in the May 1993 *FDA Consumer*.)

Bowel Disease

Increased fiber is often recommended for people with chronic constipation, irritable bowel syndrome, and diverticulosis. Low-fiber diets may be called for during flare-ups of these and other bowel diseases, such as Crohn's disease and ulcerative colitis.

Osteoporosis

In osteoporosis, bone mass decreases, causing bones to become brittle and easily broken, especially in later life. A low-calcium intake throughout life is thought to be a major risk factor. The Daily Value for calcium, based on calcium needs for all ages, is 1,000 milligrams. Vitamin D also is important because it aids calcium absorption. The Daily Value for vitamin D is 400 International Units."

Nutrient Claims Guide for Individual Foods

Fiber

- **High-fiber:** 5 grams (g) or more per serving.

- **Good source of fiber:** at least 2.5 g per serving.

- **More or added fiber:** at least 2.5 g more per serving than the reference food. (Label will say 10 percent more of the Daily Value for fiber.)

Protein

- **High-protein:** 10 g or more of high-quality protein per serving.

- **Good source of protein:** at least 5 g of high-quality protein per serving.

- **More protein:** at least 5 g more of high quality protein per serving than reference food. (Label will say 10 percent more of the Daily Value for protein.)

Calcium

- **High-calcium:** 200 milligrams (mg) or more per serving.

- **Good source of calcium:** at least 100 mg per serving.

- **More calcium:** at least 100 mg more than reference food. (Label will say 10 percent more of the Daily Value for calcium.)

Vitamin D

- **High in vitamin D:** 80 International Units (IU) or more per serving.

- **Good source of vitamin D:** at least 40 IU per serving.

- **More or fortified with vitamin D:** at least 40 IU more than reference food. (Label will say 10 percent more of the Daily Value for vitamin D.)

—by Paula Kurtzweil

Paula Kurtzweil is a member of FDA's public affairs staff.

Part Four

Airborne Allergens

Chapter 26

Something in the Air: Pollen, Mold, and Dust Allergens

Cold or Allergy?

When is sneezing not a symptom of a cold? Very often, when it represents an allergic reaction to something in the air. It is estimated that 35 million Americans suffer from upper respiratory allergic reactions to airborne pollen. Pollen allergy, commonly called hay fever, is one of the most common chronic diseases in the United States. Worldwide, airborne dust causes the most problems for people with allergies. The respiratory symptoms of asthma, which affects approximately 15 million Americans, are often provoked by airborne allergens (substances that cause an allergic reaction).

Allergic diseases are among the major causes of illness and disability in the United States, affecting as many as 40 to 50 million Americans. The National Institute of Allergy and Infectious Diseases, a component of the National Institutes of Health, conducts and supports research on allergic diseases. The goals of this research are to provide a better understanding of the cause of allergy, to improve the methods for diagnosing and treating allergic reactions, and eventually to prevent allergies. This chapter summarizes what is known about the causes and symptoms of allergic reactions to airborne allergens, how these reactions are diagnosed and treated, and what medical researchers are doing to help people who suffer from these allergies.

NIH Publication No. 93-493 March 1993. National Institutes of Health & National Institute of Allergy and Infectious Diseases.

What is an Allergy?

An allergy is a specific immunologic reaction to a normally harmless substance, one that does not bother most people. Allergic people often are sensitive to more than one substance. Types of allergens that cause allergic reactions include food, dust particles, medicines, insect venom, mold spores, or pollen.

Why are Some People Allergic to these Substances while Others are not?

Scientists think that people inherit a tendency to be allergic, although not to any specific allergen. Children are much more likely to develop allergies if their parents have allergies. Even if only one parent is allergic, a child has a one in four chance of developing allergies. Exposure to allergens at certain times when the body's defenses are lowered or weakened, such as after a viral infection, during puberty, or during pregnancy, seems to contribute to the development of allergies.

What is an Allergic Reaction?

Normally, the immune system functions as the body's defense against invading agents such as bacteria and viruses. In most allergic reactions, however, the immune system is responding to a false alarm. When allergic persons first come into contact with an allergen, their immune systems treat the allergen as an invader and mobilize to attack. The immune system does this by generating large amounts of a type of antibody (a disease-fighting protein) called immunoglobulin E, or IgE. Only small amounts of IgE are produced in non-allergic people. Each IgE antibody is specific for one particular allergenic (allergy-producing) substance. In the case of pollen allergy, the antibody is specific for each type of pollen: one antibody may be produced to react against oak pollen and another against ragweed pollen, for example.

These IgE molecules attach themselves to the body's mast cells, which are tissue cells, and to basophils, which are blood cells. When the allergen next encounters the IgE, it attaches to the antibody like a key fitting into a lock, signalling the cell to which the IgE is attached to release (and in some cases to produce) powerful inflammatory chemicals like histamine, prostaglandins, and leukotrienes. These chemicals move into various parts of the body, such as the respiratory system, and cause the symptoms of allergy.

Some people with allergies develop asthma. The symptoms of asthma include coughing, wheezing, and shortness of breath due to a narrowing of the bronchial passages (airways) in the lungs and to excess mucus production. Asthma can be disabling and sometimes can be fatal. If wheezing and shortness of breath accompany allergy symptoms, it is a signal that the bronchial tubes also have become involved, indicating the need for medical attention.

Symptoms of Allergies to Airborne Substances

The signs and symptoms are familiar to many:

- Sneezing often accompanied by a runny or clogged nose
- Coughing and postnasal drip
- Itching eyes, nose, and throat
- Allergic shiners (dark circles under the eyes caused by increased blood flow near the sinuses)
- The "allergic salute" (in a child, persistent upward rubbing of the nose that causes a crease mark on the nose)
- Watering eyes
- Conjunctivitis (an inflammation of the membrane that lines the eyelids, causing red-rimmed, swollen eyes and crusting of the eyelids)

In people who are not allergic, the mucus in the nasal passages simply moves foreign particles to the throat, where they are swallowed or coughed out. But something different happens to a person who is sensitive to airborne allergens.

As soon as the allergen lands on the mucous membranes lining the inside of the nose, a chain reaction occurs that leads the mast cells in these tissues to release histamine. This powerful chemical enlarges the many small blood vessels in the nose. Fluids escape through these expanded vessel walls, which causes the nasal passages to swell, resulting in nasal congestion.

Histamine can also cause sneezing, itching, irritation, and excess mucus production, which can result in allergic rhinitis (runny nose). Other chemicals made and released by mast cells, including prostaglandins and leukotrienes, also contribute to allergic symptoms.

311

Pollen Allergy

Each spring, summer, and fall tiny particles are released from trees, weeds, and grasses. These particles, known as pollen, hitch rides on currents of air. Although their mission is to fertilize parts of other plants, many never reach their targets. Instead, they enter human noses and throats, triggering a type of seasonal allergic rhinitis called pollen allergy, which many people know as hay fever or rose fever (depending on the season in which the symptoms occur).

Of all the things that can cause an allergy, pollen is one of the most widespread. Many of the foods, drugs, or animals that cause allergies can be avoided to a great extent; even insects and household dust are escapable. Short of staying indoors when the pollen count is high—and even that may not help—there is no easy way to evade windborne pollen.

People with pollen allergies often develop sensitivities to other troublemakers that are present all year, such as dust. For these allergy sufferers, the "sneezin' season" has no limit. Year-round airborne allergens cause perennial allergic rhinitis, as distinguished from seasonal allergic rhinitis.

What is Pollen?

Plants produce microscopic round or oval pollen grains to reproduce. In some species, the plant uses the pollen from its own flowers to fertilize itself. Other types must be cross-pollinated; that is, in order for fertilization to take place and seeds to form, pollen must be transferred from the flower of one plant to that of another plant of the same species. Insects do this job for certain flowering plants, while other plants rely on wind transport.

The types of pollen that most commonly cause allergic reactions are produced by the plain-looking plants (trees, grasses, and weeds) that do not have showy flowers. These plants manufacture small, light, dry pollen granules that are custom-made for wind transport. Samples of ragweed pollen have been collected 400 miles out at sea and two miles high in the air. Because airborne pollen is carried for long distances, it does little good to rid an area of an offending plant; the pollen can drift in from many miles away. In addition, most allergenic pollen comes from plants that produce it in huge quantities. A single ragweed plant can generate a million grains of pollen a day.

The chemical makeup of pollen is the basic factor that determines whether it is likely to cause hay fever. For example, pine tree pollen is produced in large amounts by a common tree, which would make it a good candidate for causing allergy. The chemical composition of pine pollen, however, appears to make it less allergenic than other types. Because pine pollen is heavy, it tends to fall straight dow and does not scatter. Therefore, it rarely reaches human noses.

Among North American plants, weeds are the most prolific producers of allergenic pollen. Ragweed is the major culprit, but others of importance are sagebrush, redroot pigweed, lamb's quarters, Russian thistle (tumbleweed), and English plantain.

Grasses and trees, too, are important sources of allergenic pollens. Although more than 1,000 species of grass grow in North America, only a few produce highly allergenic pollen. These include timothy, Johnson, Bermuda, redtop, orchard, sweet vernal, and Kentucky bluegrass. Trees that produce allergenic pollen include oak, ash, elm, hickory, pecan, box elder, and mountain cedar.

It is common to hear people say that they are allergic to colorful or scented flowers like roses. In fact, only florists, gardeners, and others who have prolonged, close contact with flowers are likely to become sensitized to pollen from these plants. Most people have little contact with the large, heavy, waxy pollen grains of many flowering plants because this type of pollen is not carried by wind but by insects such as butterflies and bees.

When Do Plants Make Pollen?

One of the most obvious features of pollen allergy is its seasonal nature; people experience its symptoms only when the pollen grains to which they are allergic are in the air. Each plant has a pollinating period that is more or less the same from year to year. Exactly when a plant starts to pollinate seems to depend on the relative length of night and day, and therefore on geographical location, rather than on the weather. (On the other hand, weather conditions during pollination can affect the amount of pollen produced and distributed in a specific year.) Thus, the farther north you go, the later the pollinating period and the later the allergy season.

A pollen count, which is familiar to many people from local weather reports, is a measure of how much pollen is in the air. This count represents the concentration of all the pollen (or of one particular type, like ragweed) in the air in a certain area at a specific time. It is expressed in grains of pollen per square meter of air collected over 24 hours. Pollen counts tend to be highest early in the morning on warm, dry, breezy days and lowest during chilly, wet periods. Although a pollen count is an approximate and fluctuating measure, it is useful as a general guide for when it is advisable to stay indoors and avoid contact with the pollen.

Mold Allergy

Along with pollens from trees, grasses, and weeds, molds are an important cause of seasonal allergic rhinitis. People allergic to molds may have symptoms from spring to late fall. The mold season often peaks from July to late summer. Unlike pollens, molds may persist after the first killing frost. Some can grow at subfreezing temperatures, but most become dormant. Snow cover lowers the outdoor mold count drastically but does not kill molds. After the spring thaw, molds thrive on the vegetation that has been killed by the winter cold.

In the warmest areas of the United States, however, molds thrive all year and can cause year-round (perennial) allergic problems. In addition, molds growing indoors can cause perennial allergic rhinitis even in the coldest climates.

What is Mold?

There are thousands of types of molds and yeast, the two groups of plants in the fungus family. Yeasts are single cells that divide to form clusters. Molds consist of many cells that grow as branching threads called *hyphae*. Although both groups can probably cause allergic reactions, only a small number of molds are widely recognized offenders.

The seeds or reproductive particles of fungi are called spores. They differ in size, shape, and color among species. Each spore that germinates can give rise to new mold growth, which in turn can produce millions of spores.

What is Mold Allergy?

When inhaled, microscopic fungal spores or, sometimes, fragments of fungi may cause allergic rhinitis. Because they are so small, mold spores may evade the protective mechanisms of the nose and upper respiratory tract to reach the lungs and bring on asthma symptoms.

Build-up of mucus, wheezing, and difficulty in breathing are the result. Less frequently, exposure to spores or fragments may lead to a lung disease known as hypersensitivity pneumonitis, which will be discussed later.

In a small number of people, symptoms of mold allergy may be brought on or worsened by eating certain foods, such as cheeses, processed with fungi. Occasionally, mushrooms, dried fruits, and foods containing yeast, soy sauce, or vinegar will produce allergic symptoms. There is no known relationship, however, between a respiratory allergy to the mold *Penicillium* and an allergy to the drug penicillin, made from the mold.

Where do Molds Grow?

Molds can be found wherever there is moisture, oxygen, and a source of the few other chemicals they need. In the fall they grow on rotting logs and fallen leaves, especially in moist, shady areas. In gardens, they can be found in compost piles and on certain grasses and weeds. Some molds attach to grains such as wheat, oats, barley, and corn, making farms, grain bins, and silos likely places to find mold.

Hot spots of mold growth in the home include damp basements and closets, bathrooms (especially shower stalls), places where fresh food is stored, refrigerator drip trays, house plants, air conditioners, humidifiers, garbage pails, mattresses, upholstered furniture, and old foam rubber pillows.

Bakeries, breweries, barns, dairies, and greenhouses are favorite places for molds to grow. Loggers, mill workers, carpenters, furniture repairers, and upholsterers often work in moldy environments.

Which Molds Are Allergenic?

Like pollens, mold spores are important airborne allergens only if they are abundant, easily carried by air currents, and allergenic in their chemical makeup. Found almost everywhere, mold spores in some areas are so numerous they often outnumber the pollens in the air. Fortunately, however, only a few dozen different types are significant allergens.

In general, *Alternaria* and *Cladosporium (Hormodendrum)* are the molds most commonly found both indoors and outdoors throughout the United States. *Aspergillus, Penicillium, Helminthosporium,*

Epicoccum, Fusarium, Mucor, Rhizopus, and *Aureobasidium (Pullul-aria)* are also common.

Are Mold Counts Helpful?

Similar to pollen counts, mold counts may suggest the types and relative quantities of fungi present at a certain time and place. For several reasons, however, these counts probably cannot be used as a constant guide for daily activities. One reason is that the number and types of spores actually present in the mold count may have changed considerably in 24 hours because weather and spore dispersal are directly related. Many of the common allergenic molds are of the dry spore type; they release their spores during dry, windy weather. Other fungi need high humidity, fog, or dew to release their spores. Although rain washes many larger spores out of the air, it also causes some smaller spores to be shot into the air.

In addition to the effect of day-to-day weather changes on mold counts, spore populations may also differ between day and night. Day favors dispersal by dry spore types and night favors wet spore types.

Are There Other Mold-related Disorders?

Fungi or micro-organisms related to them may cause other health problems similar to allergy. Some kinds of *Aspergillus* especially may cause several different illnesses, including both infections and allergy. These fungi may lodge in the airways or a distant part of the lung and grow until they form a compact sphere known as a "fungus ball." In people with lung damage or serious underlying illnesses, *Aspergillus* may grasp the opportunity to invade and actually infect the lungs or the whole body.

In some individuals, exposure to these fungi can also lead to asthma or to an illness known as *"allergic bronchopulmonary aspergillosis."* This latter condition, which occurs occasionally in people with asthma, is characterized by wheezing, low-grade fever, and coughing up of brown-flecked masses or mucous plugs. Skin testing, blood tests, x-rays, and examination of the sputum for fungi can help establish the diagnosis. Corticosteroid drugs are usually effective in treating this reaction; immunotherapy (allergy shots) is not helpful. The occurrence of allergic aspergillosis suggests that other fungi might cause similar respiratory conditions.

Inhalation of spores from fungus-like bacteria, called actino-mycetes, and from molds can cause a lung disease called hypersensi-tivity pneumonitis. This condition is often associated with specific occupations. For example, farmer's lung disease results from inhal-ing spores growing in moldy hay and grains in silos. Occasionally, hypersensitivity pneumonitis develops in people who live or work where an air conditioning or a humidifying unit is contaminated with and emits these spores.

The symptoms of hypersensitivity pneumonitis may resemble those of a bacterial or viral infection such as the flu. Bouts of chills, fever, weakness, muscle pains, cough, and shortness of breath develop four to eight hours after exposure to the offending organism. The symp-toms gradually disappear when the source of exposure is removed. If this is not possible, such as in occupational settings, it may be neces-sary to increase the ventilation of the workplace, wear a mask with a filter capable of removing spores, or change jobs. If hypersensitivity pneumonitis is allowed to progress, it can lead to serious heart and lung problems.

Dust Allergy

An allergy to dust found in houses is perhaps the most common cause of perennial allergic rhinitis. House dust allergy usually pro-duces symptoms similar to pollen allergy.

What is House Dust?

Rather than a single substance, house dust is a varied mixture of potentially allergenic materials. It may contain fibers from different types of fabrics: cotton, lint, feathers, and other stuffing materials; bacteria; mold and fungus spores (especially in damp areas); food particles; bits of plants and insects; and other allergens peculiar to an individual home.

Dust also may contain microscopic mites. These mites, which also live in bedding, upholstered furniture, and carpets, thrive in summer and die in winter. However, in a warm, humid house, they continue to thrive even in the coldest months. The particles seen floating in a shaft of sunlight are dead dust mites and their waste-products. These waste-products, which are proteins, actually provoke the allergic re-action. House dust mite allergy is the major year-round allergy in the world, though ragweed allergy is more prevalent in the United States.

Waste-products of cockroaches are also an important cause of allergy symptoms from household allergens, particularly in some urban areas of the United States.

Animal Allergy

Household pets are the main culprits in causing allergic reactions to animals. It was once thought that pet allergy was provoked by dander or fur from cats and dogs. Now, however, the allergen is known to be proteins in the saliva that is present on the dander or fur. Cats win the prize for causing the most allergic reactions. One reason may be that cats preen themselves more than other furry pets. This preening coats the hairs with saliva containing allergens, which become airborne when the saliva dries. Also, it may be because cats are held more and often spend more time in the house, close to humans, than do dogs.

Some rodents, such as guinea pigs and gerbils, have become increasingly popular as household pets. They, too, can cause allergic reactions in some people. Urine is the major source of allergens from these animals.

Allergies to animals can take two years or more to develop and may not subside until six months or more after ending contact with the animal. Carpet and furniture are a reservoir for pet allergens, and the allergens can remain in them for four to six weeks. In addition, these allergens can stay in household air for months after the animal has been removed. Therefore, it is wise for people with an animal allergy to check with the landlord or previous owner to find out if furry pets had lived previously on the premises.

Chemical Sensitivity

Allergic to the twentieth century is a phrase that has been used to describe people who seem to react to everything in their environment, indoors and outdoors. These allergy-like reactions can result from exposure to man-made substances, such as those found in paints or carpeting, or to natural substances, such as odors emitted by plants and flowers. Although the symptoms may resemble some of the manifestations of true allergies, sensitivity to chemicals does not represent a true allergic reaction.

Diagnosing Allergic Diseases

People with allergy symptoms, such as allergic rhinitis, may at first suspect they have a cold, but the "cold" lingers on. It is important to see a doctor about any respiratory illness that lasts longer than a week or two. When it appears that the symptoms are caused by an allergy, the patient should see a physician who understands the diagnosis and treatment of allergies. If the patient's medical history indicates that the symptoms recur at the same time each year, the physician will work under the theory that a seasonal allergen (like pollen) is involved. Properly trained specialists recognize the patterns of the local seasons and the association between these patterns and symptoms. The medical history suggests which allergens are the likely culprits. The doctor will also examine the mucous membranes, which often appear swollen and pale or bluish in persons with allergic conditions.

Skin Tests

To confirm which allergen is responsible, skin testing may be recommended using extracts from allergens such as dust, pollens, or molds commonly found in the local area. A diluted extract of each kind of allergen is injected under the patient's skin or is applied to a scratch or puncture made on the patient's arm or back.

With a positive reaction, a small, raised, reddened area with a surrounding flush (called a wheal and flare) will appear at the test site. The size of the wheal can provide the physician with an important diagnostic clue, but a positive reaction does not prove that a particular pollen is the cause of a patient's symptoms. Although such a reaction indicates that IgE antibody to a specific allergen is present in the skin, respiratory symptoms do not necessarily result.

Blood Tests

Skin testing is not advisable in some people such as those with widespread skin conditions like eczema. Diagnostic tests can be done using a blood sample from the patient to detect levels of IgE antibody to a particular allergen. One such blood test is called the RAST (radioallergosorbent test), which can be performed when eczema is present or if a patient has taken medications that interfere with skin testing.

It is expensive to perform, takes several weeks to yield results, and is somewhat less sensitive than skin testing. Overall, skin testing is the most sensitive and least costly diagnostic tool.

Treating Allergic Diseases

There are three general approaches to the treatment of these allergies:

- avoidance of the allergen,
- medication to relieve symptoms, and
- allergy shots.

Although no cure for allergies has yet been found, one of these strategies or a combination of them can provide varying degrees of relief from allergy symptoms.

Avoidance

Complete avoidance of allergenic pollen or mold means moving to a place where the offending substance does not grow and where it is not present in the air. But even this extreme solution may offer only temporary relief since a person who is sensitive to a specific pollen or mold may subsequently develop allergies to new allergens after repeated exposure. For example, people allergic to ragweed may leave their ragweed-ridden communities and relocate to areas where ragweed does not grow, only to develop allergies to other weeds or even to grasses or trees in their new surroundings. Because relocating is not a reliable solution, allergy specialists do not encourage this approach.

There are other ways to evade the offending pollen:

- Remain indoors in the morning, for example, when the outdoor pollen levels are highest. Sunny, windy days can be especially troublesome.

- If persons with pollen allergy must work outdoors, they can wear face masks designed to filter pollen out of the air and keep it from reaching their nasal passages.

- As another approach, some people take their vacations at the height of the expected pollinating period and choose a location where such exposure would be minimal. The seashore, for example, may be an effective retreat for many with pollen allergies.

Mold allergens can be difficult to avoid, but some steps can be taken to at least reduce exposure to them. First, the allergy sufferer should avoid those hot spots mentioned earlier where molds tend to be concentrated. The lawn should be mowed and leaves should be raked up, but someone other than the allergic person should do these chores. If such work cannot be delegated, wearing a tightly fitting dust mask can greatly reduce exposure and resulting symptoms. Travel in the country, especially on dry, windy days or while crops are being harvested, should be avoided as should walks through tall vegetation. A summer cabin closed up all winter is probably full of molds and should be aired out and cleaned before a mold-sensitive person stays there.

Around the home, a dehumidifier will help dry out the basement, but the water extracted from the air must be removed frequently to prevent mold growth in the machine.

Those with dust allergy should pay careful attention to dust-proofing their bedroom. The worst things to have in the bedroom are wall-to-wall carpets, venetian blinds, down-filled blankets, feather pillows, heating vents with forced hot air, dogs, cats, and closets full of clothing. Shades are preferred over venetian blinds because they do not trap dust. Curtains can be used if they are washed periodically in hot water to kill the dust mites. Bedding should be encased in a zippered, plastic, airtight, and dust-proof cover.

Although shag carpets are the worst type for the dust-sensitive person, all carpets trap dust and make dust control impossible. In addition, vacuuming can contribute to the amount of dust, unless the vacuum is equipped with a special high-efficiency particulate air (HEPA) filter. Wall-to-wall carpets should be replaced with washable throw rugs over hardwood, tile, or linoleum floors. Reducing the amount of dust in a home may require new cleaning techniques as well as some changes in furnishings to eliminate dust collectors. Water is often the secret to effective dust removal. Washable items should be washed often using water hotter than 130 degrees Fahrenheit. Dusting with a damp cloth or oiled mop should be done frequently.

The best way for a person allergic to pets, especially cats, to avoid allergic reactions is to find another home for the animal. There are, however, some suggestions that help keep cat allergens out of the air:

- Bathe the cat weekly and brush it more frequently.
- Remove carpets and soft furnishings.
- Use a vacuum cleaner with a high-efficiency filter and a room air cleaner (see section below).
- Wear a face mask while house and cat cleaning.
- Keep the cat out of the bedroom are other methods that allow many people to live more happily with their pets.

Irritants such as chemicals can worsen airborne allergy symptoms and should be avoided as much as possible. For example, during periods of high pollen levels, people with pollen allergy should try to avoid unnecessary exposure to irritants such as dust, insect sprays, tobacco smoke, air pollution, and fresh tar or paint.

Air Conditioners and Filters

Use of air conditioners inside the home or in a car can help prevent pollen and mold allergens from entering. Various types of air-filtering devices made with fiberglass or electrically charged plates may help reduce allergens produced in the home. These can be added to the heating and cooling systems. In addition, portable devices that can be used in individual rooms are especially helpful in reducing animal allergens.

An allergy specialist can suggest which kind of filter is best for the home of a particular patient. Before buying a filtering device it is wise to rent one and use it in a closed room (the bedroom, for instance) for a month or two to see whether allergy symptoms diminish. The airflow should be sufficient to exchange the air in the room five or six times per hour; therefore, the size and efficiency of the filtering device should be determined in part by the size of the room.

Persons with allergies should be wary of exaggerated claims for appliances that cannot really clean the air. Very small air cleaners cannot remove dust and pollen, and no air purifier can prevent viral or bacterial diseases such as influenza, pneumonia, or tuberculosis. Buyers of electrostatic precipitators should compare the machine's ozone output with Federal standards. Ozone can irritate the nose and airways of persons with allergies, especially those with asthma, and can increase the allergy symptoms. Other kinds of air filters such as HEPA filters do not release ozone into the air.

Medication

For people who find they cannot adequately avoid the allergens, the symptoms often can be controlled with medications. Effective medications that can be prescribed by a physician include antihistamines, topical nasal steroids, and cromolyn sodium, any of which can be used alone or in combination. Many effective antihistamines and decongestants also are available without a prescription.

Antihistamines. As the name indicates, an antihistamine counters the effects of histamine, which is released by the mast cells in the body's tissues and contributes to allergy symptoms. For many years, antihistamines have proven useful in relieving sneezing and itching in the nose, throat and eyes and in reducing nasal swelling and drainage.

Many people who take antihistamines experience some distressing side effects: drowsiness and loss of alertness and coordination. In children, such reactions can be misinterpreted as behavior problems. During the last few years, however, antihistamines that cause fewer of these side effects have become available by prescription. These new non-sedating antihistamines are as effective as other antihistamines in preventing histamine-induced symptoms, but do so without causing sleepiness.

Topical nasal steroids. This medication should not be confused with anabolic steroids that have serious side effects. Topical nasal steroids are anti-inflammatory drugs that stop the allergic reaction. In addition to other beneficial actions, they reduce the number of mast cells in the nose and reduce mucus secretion and nasal swelling. The combination of antihistamines and nasal steroids is a very effective way to treat allergic rhinitis.

Cromolyn Sodium. Cromolyn sodium stops allergic reactions from starting. It is administered as a nasal spray, and it can prevent the release of chemicals like histamine from the mast cell.

Immunotherapy

Immunotherapy, or a series of allergy shots, is the only available treatment that has a chance of reducing the allergy symptoms over the long haul. Patients receive injections of increasing concentrations of the allergen(s) to which they are sensitive. These injections reduce the amount of IgE antibodies in the blood and cause the body to make a protective antibody called IgG. About 85 percent of patients with allergic rhinitis will have a significant reduction in their hay fever symptoms and in their need for medication within 24 months of starting immunotherapy. Many patients are able to stop the injections with good, long-term results. As better allergens for immunotherapy are produced, this technique will become an even more effective treatment.

Allergy Research

The National Institute of Allergy and Infectious Diseases (NIAID) conducts and supports research on allergies focused on understanding what happens to the body during the allergic process: the sequence of events leading to the allergic response and the factors responsible for allergic diseases. This understanding will lead to better methods of preventing and treating allergies.

NIAID supports a network of Asthma, Allergic and Immunologic Diseases Cooperative Research Centers throughout the United States. The centers encourage close coordination among scientists studying the immune system, genes, biochemistry, and pharmacology. This interdisciplinary approach helps move research knowledge as quickly as possible from research scientists to physicians and their allergy patients.

Educating patients and health care workers is an important tool in controlling allergic diseases. All of these research centers conduct and evaluate educational programs focused on methods to control allergic diseases.

NIAID's National Cooperative Inner-City Asthma Study Centers are examining ways to prevent asthma in minority children in inner-city environments. Asthma, a major cause of illness and death among these children, is provoked by a number of possible factors, including allergies to airborne substances.

Although several factors provoke allergic responses, scientists know that heredity is a major influence on who will develop an allergy. Therefore, researchers are trying to identify and describe the genes that make a person susceptible to allergic diseases. Other studies are aimed at seeking better ways to diagnose and treat people with allergic diseases and to better understand the factors that regulate IgE production in order to reduce the allergic response in patients. Several research institutions are focusing on ways to influence the cells that participate in the allergic response.

These studies offer the promise of improving treatment and control of allergic diseases and the hope that one day allergic diseases will be preventable as well.

Information Resources

American Academy of Allergy and Immunology
611 East Wells Street
Milwaukee, WI 53202
1-800-822-ASMA

Asthma and Allergy Foundation of America
1125 15th Street, NW, Suite 502
Washington, DC 20005
1-800-7-ASTHMA

Allergy and Asthma Network
3554 Chain Bridge Road, Suite 200
Fairfax, VA 22030
1-800-878-4403

U.S. Department of Health and Human Services
Public Health Service National Institutes of Health
Bethesda, MD 20892

For Information on Air-cleaning Devices

Environmental Protection Agency
Public Information Service
401 M Street, SW
Washington, DC 20460
1-800-438-4318

Chapter 27

Indoor Allergens

One of five Americans will experience allergy-related illness at some point during his/her life, and indoor allergens will be responsible for a substantial number of those cases, according to a recent report from the Institute of Medicine, *Indoor Allergens: Assessing and Controlling Adverse Health Effects.*

The report describes allergy, generally speaking, as "the state of immune hypersensitivity that exists in an individual who has been exposed to an allergen and has responded with an over-production of certain immune system components such as immunoglobulin E (IgE) antibodies. About 40 percent of the population have IgE antibodies against environmental allergens, 20 percent have clinical allergic disease, and 10 percent have significant or severe allergic disease."

The report lists major sources of indoor allergens in the United States as house dust mites, fungi and other micro-organisms, domestic pets (usually cats and dogs), and cockroaches. The most common allergic diseases related to these allergens are allergic rhinitis, asthma, and allergic skin diseases.

Allergy plays a key but sometimes unrecognized role in triggering asthma, a disease that deserves special attention because of its prevalence, cost, and potential severity. In 1988, 4,580 people died of asthma in the United States, and the mortality rate is rising, particularly in Blacks. Depending on age, Blacks are three to five times more likely than Whites to die from asthma. In 1987 (the most recent available

EPA Journal, 19:4, October/November 1993.

data), asthma was the first-listed diagnosis for more than 450,000 hospitalizations in the United States.

Allergy to house dust mites and cats increases the risk of childhood asthma fourfold to sixfold. In addition, indoor allergens are thought to be responsible for much of the acute asthma in adults under the age of 50 years.

The total annual cost associated with asthma in the United States has been estimated at more than $6.2 billion. This estimate includes direct and indirect costs and is a 30-percent increase over the estimated cost of the disease in 1985.

For most allergenic agents, exposure clearly creates a risk of allergic sensitization, but insufficient data are available to identify thresholds or risk levels. The report indicates, however, that a positive relationship has been found between cumulative exposure to dust mite allergen and the risk of sensitization. This finding has long been suspected, but never demonstrated.

Avoiding specific allergens can lessen the probability of initial sensitization and can improve dramatically the condition of people with a known sensitivity by reducing the cascade of symptoms that result from exposure. Because of the amount of time people spend sleeping, the bedroom is one area where steps to reduce exposure to allergens can be especially beneficial. For example, covering mattresses and pillows with impermeable materials is an effective way to limit exposure to dust mite allergens.

Wall-to-wall Carpeting Is a Good Reservoir

Wall-to-wall carpeting in homes, schools, hospitals, and offices is a good reservoir for both dust mite and mold allergens if the premises are damp; vacuum cleaning is probably not an effective intervention. In fact, vacuum cleaning disperses and suspends allergens and other particles in the air. (Removing carpet might work better in such circumstances.)

A thorough understanding of how building systems and structures operate and perform is essential for assessing and controlling indoor air quality problems. The reduction and/or elimination of human exposure is probably best achieved by simultaneously controlling allergen sources and improving building ventilation—that is, the design, operation, and maintenance of heating, ventilation, and air-conditioning systems.

—by Andrew M. Pope

Dr. Pope is Study Director, Division of Health Promotion and Disease Prevention, Institute of Medicine.

Indoor Allergens is the work of a multidisciplinary committee on the Health Effects of Indoor Allergens (Roy Patterson, M.D., Chair, and Harriet Burge, Ph.D., Vice-Chair). The report is available from the National Academy Press; call (202) 334-3313 or 800-624-6242.

Chapter 28

How to Create a Dust-Free Bedroom

Dust-sensitive individuals, especially those with allergies and asthma, can reduce some of their misery by creating a "dust-free" bedroom. Dust may contain dander, molds, and fibers as well as tiny mites. These mites, which also live in bedding, upholstered furniture, and carpets, thrive in the summer and die in the winter. The particles seen floating in a shaft of sunlight are dead dust mites and their waste products; the waste products actually provoke the allergic reaction.

Most people cannot control the dust conditions under which they work or spend their daylight hours. But everyone can, to a large extent, eliminate dust from the bedroom. To create a dust-free bedroom, reduce the number of surfaces on which dust can collect. Dr. Michael Kaliner, head of the Allergic Diseases Section, National Institute of Allergy and Infectious Diseases, suggests the following guidelines:

- Steam or hot water heat is preferable to hot air heat. If there is a hot air furnace outlet in the room, install a dust filter made of several layers of cheesecloth or some other adequate material (old nylon hose); change the filter frequently. Seal holes or cracks in the floor around heating or other pipes with adhesive tape, although for some cracks transparent tape is adequate. In addition, change or clean furnace and air-conditioning filters every two to four weeks.

NIH Publication "How to Create a Dust-Free Bedroom," January 1991.

- Completely empty the room, just as if one were moving. Empty and clean all closets and, if possible, store contents elsewhere and seal closets. If this is not possible, keep clothing in zippered plastic bags and shoes in boxes off the floor. Give the woodwork and floors a thorough cleaning and scrubbing to remove all traces of dust. Wipe wood, tile, or linoleum floors with water, wax, or oil. If linoleum is used, cement it to the floor.

- Keep only one bed in the bedroom. Encase box springs and mattress in a dust-proof cover (zippered plastic). Scrub bed springs outside the room. If a second bed must be in the room, prepare it in the same manner.

- Carpeting makes dust control impossible. Although shag carpets are the worst type for the dust-sensitive person, all carpets trap dust. Therefore, hardwood, tile, or linoleum floors are preferred. Washable throw rugs may be used.

- Use a *Dacron* mattress pad and pillow. Avoid fuzzy wool blankets or feather- or wool-stuffed comforters; use only washable materials on the bed. Launder sheets and blankets frequently.

- Keep furniture and furnishings to a minimum. Avoid upholstered furniture and venetian blinds. A wooden or metal chair that can be scrubbed may be used in the bedroom. If desired, hang plain, lightweight curtains on the windows. Wash the curtains once a week.

- Clean the room daily. Do a thorough and complete cleaning once a week: clean the floors, furniture, tops of doors, window frames, sills, etc., with a damp cloth or oil mop; air the room thoroughly; then close the doors and windows until the dust-sensitive person is ready to occupy the room.

- Keep the doors and windows of the bedroom closed as much as possible, especially when not using the room. Use this room for sleeping only. Dress and undress and keep clothing in another room, if possible.

- If the dust-sensitive person is a child, do not keep toys that will accumulate dust in the room. Do not use stuffed toys at all: use only washable toys of wood, rubber, metal, or plastic, and store them in a closed toy box or chest.

- Keep all animals with fur or feathers out of the room.

- Try using room air cleaners fitted with high efficiency particulate activating (HEPA) filters to help control the dust.

While these steps may seem difficult at first, experience plus habit will make them easier. The results—better breathing, fewer medications, and greater freedom from allergy and asthma attacks—will be well worth the effort.

—by Laurie K. Doepel

Laurie K. Doepel, Office of Communications, National Institute of Allergy and Infectious Diseases, National Institutes of Health, Bethesda, MD 20892.

Chapter 29

Allergies to Dogs and Cats: Man's Best Friends?

Pets That Make You Sneeze, Wheeze, and Scratch

A dog may be man's best friend, but only if that man doesn't suffer from allergies. Surveys have found that 15 to 30 percent of allergic persons have allergic reactions to cats and dogs. Cat allergies are about twice as common as dog allergies. One of the reasons that animals commonly cause allergic disease is that humans insist on close contact with them. Over half of the homes in the United States have at least one cat or dog. The total pet population is over a hundred million (about 40 percent as many pets as people). Cat and dog allergens have been found in household dust from almost every home sampled, even when there wasn't a resident pet.

Allergy reactions to cats and dogs range from ordinary skin inflammation, nasal congestion and inflamed eyes to severe life-threatening asthma. Reddened areas on the skin are usually caused by a scratch or a lick. Sometimes an intense rash appears on the face, neck and upper trunk associated with respiratory symptoms. In most cases, respiratory systems occur 15 to 30 minutes following exposure. However, under circumstances where allergen levels are low or where the person's sensitivity is minor, symptoms may not appear until after several days of exposure.

Cat and dog allergens have now been identified as small proteins which are generally contained in animal secretions, including saliva and oil glands in the skin. In the cat, the major allergen is produced in both saliva and skin glands. The dog has its own major allergen, but its saliva contains several other important allergens, as well. In general, allergic patients are allergic to all breeds of dogs, but because some dog allergens are present only in some breeds, some people may be able to tolerate some dogs better than others.

Animal allergens, contained in secretions, dry on fur or bedding. They become airborne only with disturbances such as petting, grooming, or sitting on a common couch. Airborne animal particles are capable of staying suspended in the air for long periods of time. This is quite different from larger pollen particles that settle quickly. In addition, animal particles appear to be sticky and adhere to walls, clothing and other surfaces. As a consequence, cat and dog allergens are virtually everywhere, even in homes which have only been briefly occupied with these animals.

The diagnosis of animal allergy in most people can be accomplished with a careful history and laboratory tests. However, in spite of positive tests, some people will deny that a pet is causing their symptoms. In these cases, a trial of avoidance in which the patient is separated from the animal while the symptoms are closely monitored is commonly recommended. The separation could occur on an extended vacation. It is critical that the person be removed from the environment containing the animal rather than removing the animal. If the person remains in the environment, the allergen will likely persist for months after the removal of the animal.

Avoidance is clearly the most effective treatment and may provide substantial relief without the use of medications or immunotherapy. Unfortunately, the patient or family may refuse to give up the offending pet. If the symptoms are mild and the pet is especially important, this may be a reasonable decision. If this choice is made, it may be helpful to take some preventive measures to at least limit exposure, such as confining the animal to one room or using aggressive cleaning measures. Since animal allergens are sticky, aggressive cleaning measures must include removal of the animal's favorite furniture, removal of wall-to-wall carpet and scrubbing the walls and woodwork. An intriguing study has shown that airborne allergen concentrations were reduced by washing the pet every week or two. Electrostatic filters are effective in removing particles the size of animal allergens, but it is not clear that these devices can have a true impact on patient symptoms.

When avoidance is not possible or only partially possible, medication may be needed to alleviate the allergic symptoms. Antihistamines can be used for irritated nasal passages and eyes. Cromolyn or steroid ointments may help skin irritation. Cromolyn, beta-agonists, corticosteroids, and/or theophylline may be needed to control asthmatic symptoms. Generally, immunotherapy is not very helpful for patients who are continuously exposed to pet allergens, but should be reserved for highly sensitive individuals who have occasional unavoidable animal contact.

This information should not be used as a substitute for responsible professional care.

—*by Peyton A. Eggleston, MD. and Robert A. Wood, MD.*

Dr. Peyton A. Eggleston and Dr. Robert A. Wood are Professors of Pediatrics at Johns Hopkins University in Baltimore, Maryland.

Cat-Induced Asthma

Over 31 percent of American households are shared by humans and felines and since 1984, according to the Humane Society of the United States, cat ownership has climbed while that of dogs has diminished somewhat. Yet, for families containing one or more individuals with asthma, the presence of cats can be a frequent trigger of potentially severe illness.

Causes of Cat-Induced Asthma

Symptoms of cat-induced asthma are caused by allergic reactions to cat allergens, the most important of which is called Fel d 1. The allergen is produced by the salivary glands and by the skin sebaceous glands of the animal, and is applied to the fur and dander when the cat licks himself and the sebaceous glands secrete. Cat hair and dander carrying the Fel d 1 are shed continually. Two cats have been shown to shed between .01 and .33 grams of hair and dander per day. Moreover, the Fel d 1 allergen in cat hair and dander is quite stable. Under standard room conditions, no loss of potency has been detected during one month of observation, as reported in the scientific literature.

Most airborne particles of cat hair and dander in a typical cat environment can easily contact exposed surfaces of the eyes, nasal airways, and the skin of humans sharing that environment. Many particles are small enough (under 10 micrometers in size) to penetrate the peripheral lung. In susceptible individuals, exposure to cat allergens causes the immune system to make specific antibodies known as anti-cat IgE. These antibodies attach to and sensitize mast cells in the airways and skin. When inhaled, these allergens combine with the anti-cat IgE and stimulate the mast cell to release various chemical mediators, such as histamine and leukotriene, which produce the typical reactions of asthma within a few minutes.

Other cells attracted by mediators induce inflammation. They include neutrophils, eosinophils and mononuclear cells. They produce other chemical mediators in turn that induce, after several hours, a more dangerous and prolonged late-phase response that promotes chronic asthma. Manifestations of this late-phase response are more debilitating and more difficult to treat than those of the immediate response.

The Prevalence and Symptoms of Cat Induced Asthma

Studies from various parts of the world have shown that 20 to 30 percent of patients with asthma evidence reaction to cat allergen. Patients have typical symptoms and signs of asthma, such as coughing, wheezing and shortness of breath. They also often display itching and tearing eyes, sneezing, nasal discharge and obstruction, and itching skin. Symptoms such as these are debilitating and, when severe, can be devastating.

Diagnosis of cat-induced asthma is based on demonstrating the coexistence of two pieces of evidence: the typical asthma symptoms that occur upon exposure to cat or cat allergen, and reaction to a skin test or to a blood test called RAST (radioallergosorbent test). Because many patients with positive skin or RAST tests to cat do not have asthma following exposure, it is important in patients with positive test results to also demonstrate cat-induced symptoms and signs of asthma. Therefore, the physician carefully observes, on several occasions, the effects of exposure to cat and of separation from cat. In situations where asthma occurs consistently and promptly after multiple exposures to an environment containing cat allergens, cat-induced asthma can then be presumed to exist. On the other hand, when multiple observations indicate that no symptoms of asthma are induced by cat exposure, cat-induced asthma can be excluded with considerable confidence.

Prevention, Control and Treatment

Avoidance. Although the saying, "no cat, no cat-induced asthma" remains true, strict elimination of contact with cats and their hair and dander is quite difficult to achieve. The affinity for these household pets in our society is great. Many, for whom separation from cats would mean better health, have such strong attachments to their pets that they seem unable or unwilling to consider such a choice. But living with feline pets is not the only threat to those with cat-allergic symptoms. Significant quantities of cat allergen have been found in dust from houses where cats were not kept or, at least, were alleged to be absent. Consequently, inadvertent casual exposure to cat is virtually inevitable for most cat-allergic patients, even those who allow no cats in their own homes.

Under circumstances of continuing exposure, the more dangerous and difficult-to-treat symptoms of late-phase allergic response are likely to occur. Contact with cats within a specific dwelling can be reduced by confining the pets to a single area. This area should be isolated from cat-free ones. Circulation of the air (and thus the airborne cat allergen) into the rest of the house must be prevented by weather stripping all entrances, and by use of a separate ventilation system. The area of the house that is to be kept free of cat allergen must be carefully cleaned to remove residual cat allergen from floors, carpets, and furniture because such residential allergen is stable and will continue to have the power to provoke symptoms until removed.

Frequently, cat exposure is blamed for manifestations of asthma that are provoked by factors unrelated to cat allergy. These include other allergens (such as pollens, molds, dust mite), respiratory tract irritants (such as tobacco smoke), respiratory tract infections, exercise, climatic factors, and/or emotional tension. One or more of these non-cat factors are almost always important in patients who have proven to have cat-induced asthma. What is required is a thorough general allergy workup for all patients with cat-induced asthma, except for those whose symptoms are promptly and completely controlled by cat avoidance.

Medications. Bronchodilators, such as inhaled adrenergic drugs and oral theophylline, are often needed to control cat-induced asthma.

Prednisone may be required for more severe symptoms. In situations where significant asthma has been deliberately induced by briefly exposing individuals to a cat for two hours or less, it has been shown that asthma symptoms can be completely relieved within 5 to 30 minutes by immediate termination of the exposure, followed within 5 minutes by two inhalations from an albuterol inhaler. It is important to emphasize that the exposure to cat allergen should be terminated at the time such bronchodilator therapy is begun. Using a bronchodilator to permit continuing cat exposure can be a dangerous practice, because continuing exposure may result in severe asthma that is very difficult to relieve. Oral bronchodilators can be useful, such as sustained release theophylline preparations or oral adrenergic drugs. Severe chronic asthma is usually associated with considerable inflammation of the lower airway, presumably induced by the effects of the late-phase allergic response (discussed above). In such circumstances, the patient should receive anti-inflammatory medication such as corticosteroid and/or inhaled cromolyn products, in addition to the use of bronchodilators.

Immunotherapy. Regular injections of cat extract have been shown in controlled trials to decrease bronchial sensitivity to inhaled cat allergen sufficiently to provide protection against limited exposure for brief periods. However, high enough levels of exposure will induce asthma symptoms which then require medication. Consequently, an adequate immunotherapy program requires that injections be combined with cat avoidance and medication.

This information should not substitute for seeking responsible, professional medical care.

—by Thomas E. Van Metre, Jr., M.D.

Dr. Thomas E. Van Metre, Jr. is associate professor of medicine at the Johns Hopkins Medical School, a practicing allergist in Baltimore, and a former president of the American Academy of Allergy and Immunology.

Chapter 30

Populations at Risk from Particulate Air Pollution— United States, 1992

Despite improvements in air quality since the 1970s, air pollution remains an important environmental risk to human health. A national health objective for the year 2000 is to reduce exposure to air pollutants so that at least 85 percent of persons live in counties that meet U.S. Environmental Protection Agency (EPA) standards (objective 11.5)(1). This report provides estimates from the American Lung Association (ALA) of populations potentially at risk from exposure to particulate air pollution in the United States during 1992.

The National Ambient Air Quality Standard for particulate matter <10 μm in diameter (PM_{10}) is 150 μg/m^3, averaged over 24 hours (2). The federal standard is met if this value is not exceeded more than once per calendar year, and the annual arithmetic mean is less than or equal to 50 μg/m^3. Information in this report is based on the second highest maximum 24-hour PM_{10} concentrations recorded by at least one monitor in 1992 (EPA, unpublished data, 1993). Both the federal "exceedance" definition (greater than or equal to 155 μg/m^3) and a similar approach applied to the California standard (greater than or equal to 55 μg/m^3) were used as cutoff values. California's particulate matter air quality standard of 50 μg/m^3 averaged over 24 hours (3) is the most stringent standard in the United States. Estimates of the numbers of persons potentially exposed to levels of PM_{10} above these cutoff values were derived from 1991 census figures for each county (U.S. Bureau of the Census, unpublished data, 1992).

Mortality and Morbidity Weekly Report, April 29, 1994.

For this report, a population at risk was defined as persons who have a "significantly higher probability of developing a condition, illness, or other abnormal status," as described by EPA (4). Five at-risk populations were included: preadolescent children (aged less than or equal to 13 years), the elderly (aged greater than or equal to 65 years), persons aged less than 18 years with asthma, adults (aged greater than or equal to 18 years) with asthma, and persons with chronic obstructive pulmonary disease (COPD) (e.g., chronic bronchitis and emphysema). Age-specific county populations for 1991 were estimated by applying the population age distribution of each state (U.S. Bureau of the Census, unpublished data, 1992) to the counties within that state. The number of persons with asthma or COPD in each county was estimated by applying age-specific prevalences from CDC's National Health Interview Survey (5) to age-specific population estimates for each county. Although PM_{10} levels are presented on a county basis, they do not indicate that all areas of the county were subject to that level or that all persons in the county were exposed to the recorded concentration.

During 1992, PM_{10} levels were greater than or equal to 155 μg/m^3 in 16 counties; an estimated 23 million persons (9.1 percent of the total U.S. population) resided in these counties (Table 30.1). Approximately 92 million additional persons (36 percent of the U.S. population) resided in counties in which PM_{10} levels were 55 μg/m^3-154 μg/m^3. Overall, an estimated 115 million persons (45 percent of the U.S. population) resided in counties with PM_{10} levels greater than or equal to 55 μg/m^3 (Table 30.1). In the United States during 1992, 46 percent of persons with asthma lived in communities with levels of particulate air pollution higher than the California standard.

Reported by: P Vigliarolo, Communications Div; S Rappaport, MPH, K Lieber, MPH, A Gorman Epidemiology and Statistics Div; R White, MST; National Programs Div, American Lung Association, New York. Air Pollution and Respirstory Health Br, Div of Environmental Hazards and Health Effects, National Center for Environmental Health, CDC.

Table 30.1. Estimated number and percentage of the total population and at-risk* subgroups residing in counties with particulate air pollution with a diameter of less than 10 μm (PM_{10}) at levels greater than or equal to 155 μg/m³ and greater than or equal to 55 μ/m³†—United States, 1992§

Population at risk	PM_{10} level≥155μg/m³ No.	% ¶	PM_{10} levels≥55μg/m³ No.	% ¶
Total population	**22,894,856**	**(9.1)**	**114,671,632**	**(45.5)**
Preadolescent children (aged ≤13 yrs)	4,931,408	(9.5)	23,794,139	(46.0)
Elderly (aged ≥65yrs)	2,649,477	(8.3)	14,010,297	(44.1)
Persons (aged <18 yrs) with asthma	387,220	(9.5)	1,878,848	(45.9)
Persons (aged ≥18 yrs) with asthma	697,444	(9.1)	3,528,475	(46.2)
Persons with chronic obstructive pulmonary disease**	1,243,407	(9.1)	6,263,409	(46.0)

*Population-at-risk estimates should not be added to form totals. These categories are not mutually exclusive.
†PM_{10} greater than or equal to 155 μg/m³ is the federal "exceedance" definition; PM_{10} greater than or equal to 55 μg/m³ is the California "exceedance" standard.
§The PM_{10} level of the county does not imply responsibility for the disease status of its population.
¶Of the total population in the category, the proportion of each population subgroup potentially exposed.
**Includes chronic bronchitis and emphysema.

MMWR Editorial Note: Particulate matter (e.g., dust, dirt, and smoke) is a complex and varying mixture of substances. Sources include motor-vehicle emissions, factory and utility smokestacks, residential wood burning, construction activity, mining, agricultural tilling, open burning, wind-blown dust, and fire. Some particles are formed in the atmosphere through the condensation or transformation of other chemical substances. Particles with diameters less than 10 µm pose a greater health risk than larger particles because particles of this size are easily inhaled deep into the lungs.

Increased risks for illness and death have been associated with particulate air pollution at levels comparable to those presented in this report (6-8). Acute effects on the respiratory system are well established and include exacerbations of chronic respiratory disease, restrictions in activity, and increases in emergency department visits and hospitalizations for respiratory illness (8). Persons with asthma are particularly sensitive to the effects of particulate air pollution (8). A national health objective for the year 2000 is to reduce asthma morbidity, measured by a reduction in asthma hospitalizations, from 188 per 100,000 in 1987 to no more than 160 per 100,000 (objective 11.1) (1).

The estimates presented in this report underscore the potential public health importance of particulate air pollution. Although levels of airborne particulate pollution declined substantially from 1988 to 1992 (emissions of PM_{10} decreased 8 percent and air concentrations of PM_{10} decreased 17 percent) (9), continued efforts are required to reduce health risks associated with particulate air pollution. EPA is reviewing technical and scientific information to determine whether the federal ambient air quality standard for particulate matter, established in 1987, should be revised.

The American Lung Association recently issued *The Perils of Particulates* (10), which includes national and county estimates of populations at potential risk for exposure to particulate air pollution. Copies are available from local offices of the ALA—telephone (800) 586-4872.

References

1. Public Health Service. *Healthy People 2000: national health promotion and disease prevention objectives.* Washington, DC: US Department of Health and Human Services, Public Health Service, 1991; DHHS publication no. (PHS)91-50213.

2. US Environmental Protection Agency. Revisions to the National Ambient Air Quality Standard for particulate matter: final rule. *Federal Register* 1987;52:24634.

3. Air Resources Board. *California ambient air quality standard for particulate matter (PM_{10})*. Sacramento, California: State of California, Air Resources Board, Research Division, December 1982.

4. US Environmental Protection Agency. *Air quality criteria document for lead*. Washington, DC: US Environmental Protection Agency, 1977.

5. NCHS. *Current estimates from the National Health Interview Survey, 1991*. Hyattsville, Maryland: US Department of Health and Human Services, Public Health Service, CDC, 1992; DHHS publication no. (PHS)92-1509. Vital and health statistics; series 10, no. 1841.

6. Ostro B. The association of air pollution and mortality: examining the case for inference. *Arch Environ Health* 1993;48:336-42.

7. Schwartz J. Air pollution and daily mortality: a review and meta analysis. *Environ Res* 1994;64:36-52.

8. Dockery DW, Pope CA. Acute respiratory effects of particulate air pollution. *Annual Revue Public Health* 1994,15:107-32.

9. Curran T, Faoro R, Fitz-Simons T, et al. *National air quality and emissions trends report*. Research Triangle Park, North Carolina: US Environmental Protection Agency, Office of Air Quality Planning and Standards, October 1993; publication no. EPA-454/R-93/031.

10. American Lung Association. *The perils of particulates: an estimation of populations at risk of adverse health consequences from particulate matter in areas with particulate matter levels above the National Ambient Air Quality Standards (NAAQS) of the Clean Air Act and the state of California's air quality standard*. New York: American Lung Association, 1994.

Part Five

Contact and Proximity Allergens

Chapter 31

Insect Allergies

As early as 2621 B.C., hieroglyphics on the walls of King Menes' tomb in Egypt recorded his death from a hornet or wasp sting. No one knows for sure how common insect sting allergy may be today, but it is estimated that at least 4 of every 1,000 people are affected. It is known that every year 50 to 100 people in this country die from reactions to stings. The number may be even higher because many summer deaths attributed to heart attacks or drownings, for example, may actually be due to an allergic reaction to an insect sting. In fact, more people are killed in this country each year by a group of insects classified as Hymenoptera—bees, wasps, hornets, yellow jackets, and fire ants—than by any other venomous creatures, even rattlesnakes.

What is an Allergy?

Some people are sensitive and their bodies overreact to a substance that has little or no effect on most people. For sensitive persons, that substance is an allergen, and they are said to have an "allergy." Many substances can cause an allergic reaction. Foods, pollens, house dust, animal hairs, molds, medicines, cosmetics, and insects are the most common allergens. Symptoms may be mild, such as stuffiness in the nose or itching of the eyes, or they may be more severe, such as obstruction of the airways. In some people, the reactions can be serious, even life-threatening.

NIH Publication No. 82-1046.

It is possible for allergens to be inhaled, injected, rubbed on the skin, or taken by mouth. In insect allergy, all of these routes are used although the usual exposure is by a sting or bite, during which the allergen is injected into the victim by the offending insect. An estimated 35 to 50 million Americans have allergies. No one knows exactly why some people have allergies while others do not, but evidence shows that heredity is an important factor in their development. When an allergy-prone individual is first exposed to a particular allergen, he or she produces a protein called IgE antibody, a specific kind of antibody responsible for allergies. (Other antibodies protect the body by helping to fight off and destroy foreign invaders, such as bacteria and viruses.) The IgE antibodies attach to the surfaces of two types of cells known as mast cells and basophils. Mast cells are found primarily in the respiratory and digestive tracts and the skin. Basophils are found in the blood.

When an allergic person again encounters the allergen, it binds to the IgE antibodies that are already sitting on the cell's surface. However, each antibody will react only with the specific allergen against which it was made. The combining of the allergen with its antibody is a signal to these cells to release irritating chemicals that cause the various allergic symptoms, such as wheezing, sneezing, hives, and abdominal pain. One of these chemicals, histamine, causes blood vessels to expand and to leak fluids. This leads to swelling and, if leakage is not checked, to a drop in blood pressure and to shock. Sudden, severe allergic reactions are called anaphylaxis.

What is an Insect Allergy?

Insect allergy simply means that exposure to an insect brings about an overreaction of the immune system in a sensitive person. Most often, exposure involves a sting or bite. In most cases, insect allergy might be called more correctly insect sting allergy or insect venom allergy, since the allergic reaction is usually not caused by the whole insect but by the venom that it injects.

The Committee on Insect Allergy of the American Academy of Allergy has described some of the characteristics of people with insect allergy:

- First, allergy to insects is present as often in people who have no other allergies as in those who do.

- Second, severe reactions occur most often after the age of 30, although they have been found in people of all ages.

350

- Third, a person's previous reaction to an insect sting may be a warning of a future severe reaction. However, about one-half the victims of stings may have an entirely normal response on one occasion but suffer a serious allergic reaction to the next sting.

Insect sting reactions are most common during the summer months when insects are abundant and most active. Also, during those months people are out-of-doors and thus encounter insects more often.

Which Insects Cause Allergy?

The salivary secretions of biting insects (such as mosquitoes, flies, lice, and fleas) or the irritating substances left on the skin by some crawling insects may lead to sensitivity, but it is the stinging insects that are generally the most dangerous.

The Hymenoptera or "membrane winged" insects are the only insects that sting, and only a few of the stinging Hymenoptera—honey bees, wasps, hornets, yellow jackets, and ants—cause serious allergic reactions in man. Of those five, reactions to the yellow jacket and the bee are the most common.

In the Hymenoptera the stinger, a modified egg depositor, works like a hypodermic needle. Found only in the female, the stinger has small venom-filled sacs located at its base. The venom is injected through a hollow tube in the center of the stinger.

Most stinging Hymenoptera can remove the stinger and use it again and again, but the stinger of the honey bee is barbed. When the honey bee tries to remove its stinger from human skin, both stinger and venom sacs are torn off and left in the victim as the injured bee flies away and dies.

Some Hymenoptera stingers may be contaminated with bacteria and occasionally cause infections in man. Curiously, infections occur less commonly with honey bee stings, even though the honey bee leaves its stinger in the victim's skin.

The venoms of different stinging Hymenoptera vary in their make-up, although some components are the same. Toxic components cause the irritating local reactions experienced by most people. In addition, the venoms contain chemicals, such as histamine, that are similar to those released by the body during an allergic reaction. The venom also contains certain proteins known as allergens, which are the agents responsible for allergic reactions. Honey bee venom has been studied the most, and four allergens have been identified thus far.

351

What is the Behavior of Stinging Insects?

Bees feed their young (larvae) honey and pollen, so they sting only to protect themselves or their hives. Yellow jackets, wasps, and hornets, however, sting in order to kill smaller insects that are used as food for their young, and thus they tend to be more aggressive than bees.

There are two behavioral types of bees:

* solitary and
* social.

Solitary bees. The carpenter, miner, mason, and cuckoo do not form colonies, and their stings are usually quite mild.

Social Bees. Of the two kinds of social bees—the bumblebee and the honey bee—the bumblebee is less vicious and less organized, and it nests in the ground. Large colonies of honey bees may be either wild or domesticated. All members of a colony depend on one another. The queen lays the eggs, the males or drones fertilize the queen, and the workers gather food and care for the young. Honey bees not only produce honey but also fertilize crops.

Wasps. Wasps may also be solitary or social. The most common wasp threats to man—hornets, yellow jackets, and the *Polistes wasps* (also known as "paper wasps")—fall in the social group and are very protective of their nests. Usually dark blue, yellow, or reddish brown, wasps can be identified by their narrow "waists" (the "wasp waist"). Although these three types of wasps prefer to feed on other insects, they are also attracted to nectars and overripe fruit. Some wasps nest underground, but others build their nests in the open, in trees (hornets) or under eaves (paper wasps).

Ants. Colonies of hardworking ants with their highly structured societies are found almost everywhere, but only two kinds are believed to cause allergic reactions in man. These are harvester, or agricultural, ants and fire ants. The aggressive harvester ant lives in warm, dry, sandy areas and builds mounds that are easily recognized and avoided. The **fire ant,** especially the **imported fire ant,** is becoming common in the southeastern United States. It also constructs large mounds, but these are harder to avoid since they are low and sometimes naturally camouflaged.

The ant's stinger is much like that of the bee, but it does not have barbs. Ants seem to sting because of what they see or hear and sometimes what they smell. The fire ant attaches itself to its victim by biting the skin before it stings, but probably only the sting—when venom is released—is significant for allergy sufferers.

Do Other Insects Cause Allergy?

Some biting insects cause allergic reactions, but fewer people seem to be bothered by these insects than by stinging insects, and reactions are generally less severe.

Mosquitoes. Mosquitoes, for example, bite humans to obtain blood for food. Usually, the allergic reaction to their bites consists of hives or an eczema-like rash with red, itchy lesions that become moist and then encrusted when scratched. This allergy is diagnosed by the location of the reaction, medical history, and the circumstances surrounding the bites. Avoiding exposure to mosquitoes is the best way to prevent these reactions.

Flies. Some flies, but not the house fly, bite and may cause allergic reactions. These include black flies, biting midges, deer flies, and stable flies. Bites from these cause pain, swelling, severe itching, and on rare occasions, anaphylactic shock. Local reactions can be treated by antihistamines given by mouth or by steroid creams applied to the area of skin affected. Systemic (throughout the body) reactions should be treated like those resulting from Hymenoptera stings.

Fleas. Fleas usually cause only a local rash consisting of grouped, itchy, raised lesions. Antihistamines and applied medications will relieve itching due to flea bites. The best prevention is to treat the environment and household pets with appropriate insecticides.

Kissing Bugs. Kissing bugs bite at night and cause a full range of reactions from local itching to extensive swelling and shock. Antihistamines, injections of epinephrine, or corticosteroids are the proper treatment, depending on the type and severity of the symptoms. Desensitization shots (immunotherapy) may be used in selected cases.

Caterpillars. Some caterpillars (the worm-like larvae of moths and butterflies) are covered for their protection by tiny hairs that contain an irritating substance. If one of these larvae crawls on the skin of a sensitive person, the resulting symptoms may range from a local rash to a severe systemic reaction. These reactions may also occur if the hairs are swallowed or inhaled. The **puss caterpillar** is the worst offender. Diagnosis is relatively simple because the rash follows the grid-like track of the insect on the skin. If a sticky tape is applied to the skin as soon as possible, some of the hairs can be removed. Ice packs and antihistamines given by mouth are used to treat local reactions.

Smaller Insects. Some insects cause allergic reactions when they are inhaled or accidentally swallowed. For example, small insects like the **mayfly** and **caddis fly** are abundant near bodies of water in late spring and summer. There they can easily be inhaled. Also insect parts, such as scales, wings, bits of the hard outer body covering, and dried secretions, may be blown around by the wind. Such materials, along with the minute **house-dust mite** (an arachnid, not an insect) and the **cockroach,** can be components of house dust allergy.

These creatures cause symptoms resembling those of hay fever (allergic rhinitis) or asthma, and when no other cause can be found for seasonal respiratory allergy, insects might be suspected. Skin testing can give positive indication of this allergy.

Food Pests. Regardless of the precautions taken, insects are common wherever there is food, especially grains or cereals. The insect may come from the field where the food is grown, enter at any step in the food processing, or appear after the food is brought into the home. Such pests most commonly found are the **cockroach, weevil, moth, beetle, mite,** and **silverfish.** There is some reason to suspect that insects contaminating food may actually cause some cases of "food" allergy.

What are the Symptoms?

Insect stings can cause a variety of reactions, depending on the type of insect, the amount of venom injected, the presence or absence of a specific type of allergy in the person attacked, and the site of the sting. In general, reactions fall into three main groups.

Normal reactions. Normal reactions to stings involve pain, redness, swelling, itching, and warmth at the site of the sting. These symptoms, lasting for a few hours, may be quite severe, but as long as they are confined to the area of the sting, they are considered normal inflammatory responses and pose no danger. They are the result of direct action on body tissues by toxins or irritating chemicals in the venom.

Toxic reactions. Toxic reactions are the result of multiple stings. Five hundred stings within a short time are considered enough to kill because of the effects of extremely large amounts of venom injected into one person. Fewer stings, but usually at least ten, closely spaced over time, can cause serious illness and discomfort. Muscle cramps, headache, fever, and drowsiness are the most common symptoms of a toxic reaction.

Allergic reactions. Allergic reactions, the third type, produce some of the same symptoms as those of toxic reactions, but allergic reactions differ in that they can be triggered by only one sting or a minute amount of venom. Any reaction to a single sting involving extensive swelling of a large area beyond the site of the sting probably should be considered allergic until proved otherwise.

Allergic reactions to insect stings have been classified by the American Academy of Allergy as local or systemic, and both of these types may vary in severity. Local allergic reactions involve swelling at the site of the sting, accompanied by severe itching and sometimes a few hives near the sting. Any amount of swelling, even if it involves the entire limb, is considered local if it is continuous with the sting area and if no additional symptoms are apparent in other parts of the body. Systemic allergic reactions are those which affect any part of the body in addition to the portion that is stung. A slight systemic reaction involves the spread of hives to areas of the skin distant from the sting in addition to itching and a feeling of being "under par" and filled with anxiety. A victim with a moderate systemic reaction has the symptoms described above plus at least two of the following complaints: edema (swelling) of areas distant from the sting site, sneezing, chest constriction, abdominal pain, dizziness, and nausea. A severe systemic reaction may be recognized by the above symptoms plus two of the following:

- difficulty in swallowing,
- labored breathing,
- hoarseness and thickened speech,

- weakness,
- confusion, and
- feelings of impending disaster.

The most serious reaction to a sting is closing of the airways or shock (anaphylaxis), in which the patient suffers not only from the above symptoms but also turns blue (cyanosis) or shows evidence of a drop in blood pressure, collapse, or unconsciousness. These reactions may develop within minutes or hours after a sting, and the patient may die if treatment is not given promptly.

The onset of allergic reactions can be immediate or delayed. In most cases, the shorter the time between the sting and the start of symptoms, the more severe the reaction will probably be. Most systemic allergic reactions begin 10 to 20 minutes after the sting.

A delayed reaction, occurring several hours to two weeks after a sting, is similar to a drug reaction known as serum sickness. In this situation painful joints, fever, hives or other skin rashes, and swollen lymph glands may develop. Both immediate and delayed reactions can occur in the same person following a sting, although immediate reactions are more common in the allergic person.

Most ant stings cause very little pain or itching. Stings of the imported fire ant, however, can produce severe local or systemic allergic reactions. In the local reaction, pain and a small raised area at the site of the sting are followed in a few hours by several fluid-filled blisters that eventually break or dry up. After the first day, the sting site itself becomes red and filled with pus. Days later, this spot crusts over and scar tissue forms. A systemic allergic reaction involves progressively larger local reactions, and future stings may even cause symptoms of anaphylactic shock.

Are Diagnostic Tests Available?

Most people who have a local reaction to a single sting do not feel the need to consult a physician. However, when stings lead to more severe reactions, expert help should be sought.

A complete medical history and exact identification of the insect are the doctor's best tools for diagnosing a possible insect allergy. Careful questioning may reveal other less severe allergic reactions to previous stings. If the insect is not available, the doctor may be able to identify the culprit by asking about its appearance, its ability to fly or crawl, and the circumstances of the sting or bite (for example, the time of day and the place where the attack occurred).

The sting or bite may provide other clues to the insect's identity. Some insects leave mouthparts or a stinger at the site, and others produce characteristic symptoms or patterns of multiple bites. The location of the bite on the body may suggest a certain insect. Identification of the insect, whenever possible, is important for the doctor to be able to make a diagnosis and determine the required treatment.

Many allergies—such as those to pollen—can be diagnosed by a skin test. In this procedure a small, diluted, specially treated amount of the substance believed to be responsible for the allergy is applied to a scratch or prick on the skin (scratch or prick test) or injected into the top layer of skin (intracutaneous test). If a small area of redness and swelling develops at the site of the test within about 20 minutes, the person is suspected of being allergic to that substance. For many years skin tests have been used to diagnose insect allergy. The arm is often used for insect allergy tests because a tourniquet can be applied to impede absorption if the person reacts too strongly to the test material. Also, in suspected severe insect allergy, the scratch or prick test is often tried first because it is less likely to cause an allergic reaction than the intracutaneous method. However, it is a less sensitive technique, and the results are not always clear-cut.

Medical scientists working in the field of allergy have developed improved testing procedures based upon evidence that what most people are allergic to is the insect's venom, not its body, and that testing with venom alone will provide more accurate test results. These tests with venom can be performed by the skin test methods described above or by a blood test called the RAST (radioallergosorbent test). In this method, a blood sample from the person is exposed to specially prepared venom from the suspected insect. The RAST reveals whether the victim is producing IgE antibody in response to the venom.

Until recently, both the RAST and the use of venom were considered experimental procedures. Now venoms from honey bees, yellow jackets, hornets, and wasps are commercially available and can be used routinely for skin testing.

Because the skin will often not respond to test materials until perhaps 2 weeks after a sting, diagnostic studies should be delayed for at least that long. The skin needs time to replenish its supply of skin-sensitizing antibodies (IgE) used up during the allergic reaction.

People who have had an allergic reaction to insect parts that they have inhaled are presumably allergic to a component of the insect body. Such allergies can be diagnosed by the technique of skin testing with extract of the insect's whole body.

How are Non-Allergic Reactions Treated?

Following any insect sting, the stinger with the attached venom sac, if left behind, should be removed immediately by gently flicking it up and out with a fingernail or tweezers. The honey bee's venom sac continues to contract for some time after being torn from the insect, so prompt removal may prevent additional venom from being injected. Care must be taken not to squeeze or press on the venom sac when removing the stinger. The affected area should be washed thoroughly after the stinger has been taken out.

In a normal reaction, ice (not heat) applied to the spot may help to lessen the pain and swelling. Antihistamines taken by mouth and a calamine solution applied to the skin may help to control the itching, and aspirin or codeine (by prescription) may lessen pain.

A toxic reaction to an insect sting is treated in this same manner, but other medication may be needed to combat symptoms. Antibiotics to control secondary infections may also be necessary. A tetanus toxoid booster is advisable if one is due.

How are Allergic Reactions Treated?

When a person is presumed to be allergic to an insect sting, three general approaches may be considered:

1. avoidance of the causative substance,

2. treatment and medication to lessen the symptoms of the allergic reaction, and

3. measures to reduce the person's sensitivity to the allergenic substance.

Avoidance. Keeping away from the allergen, a major approach to treating any allergy, is vital in the prevention of allergic reactions to insect stings, and steps can be taken to reduce the chances of being stung.

Some people seem to attract insects more than others, but there are ways to make oneself less appealing and vulnerable. Close-fitting clothes will prevent the insect from getting between the material and the skin. Dark-colored clothing such as brown or black may provoke an attack; white or light khaki color is least attractive to bees. A flowered print may cause bees to come near to investigate but will not incite them to sting.

Scented soaps, perfumes, suntan lotions, and other cosmetics should be avoided, as should shiny buckles or jewelry. The amount of skin exposed out-of-doors should be minimized by wearing long-sleeved shirts, slacks, hats, socks, and shoes (not sandals). Some Hymenoptera nest in the ground, and others are attracted to low-growing plants; such insects may attack unprotected feet. Honey bees are often found close to the ground in grass and clover and are provoked to sting when trapped in sandals or loose clothing. Wasps are attracted to food and drink, and people are frequently stung at picnics and swimming pools. There are no effective repellents for the stinging Hymenoptera.

In the out-of-doors, any article that someone with an insect allergy may touch should be checked first for the presence of the insect. The feeding areas of Hymenoptera—flower beds, clover fields, garbage cans, and ripe fruit—must be avoided. As much as possible, car windows should be kept closed. An insecticide spray carried in the glove compartment can be helpful if an insect does get into the car. A piece of gauze or cheesecloth kept in the car can be used to catch the intruder.

In and around the house, screens or windows and doors should be checked for holes. Garbage cans should be kept clean, sprayed with an insecticide if necessary, and closed tightly. Nests under eaves, in trees, or in the ground should be removed by a professional exterminator. Pamphlets giving advice on this subject are available from the U.S. Department of Agriculture.

Weather can affect the temperament of Hymenoptera. For example, a rain may wash pollen from the flowers and thus anger bees. At such times an allergic person must take care to avoid attack. If that is impossible, he should move away slowly or lie on the ground, always protecting the face with the arms. Wild motion of the arms or frantic running will only anger and further provoke an insect to attack.

Preventing attack by ants involves taking special care to keep food stored properly, covering arms and legs, and locating and eliminating any nests indoors (between the floor and subfloor, under cracked basement floors, or in decaying wood). Entrances to the home as well as suspicious areas in the yard can be treated with appropriate chemicals—dimpylate, lindane, malathion, and propoxur.

Treatment and Medication. Allergic sting reactions may require special attention. When stung, an allergic person should try to keep the amount of venom in the blood low by carefully removing any stinger as soon as possible and by placing a tourniquet above the sting site if it is on an arm or leg. The tourniquet should be loosened every 10 minutes so that circulation is not impaired. If possible, a cold pack should be applied.

A serious allergic reaction to a sting should be treated as an emergency. Epinephrine (adrenalin) is given by injection as soon as possible, and such an injection may have to be repeated if symptoms do not improve. Antihistamines given by injection or by mouth reduce later appearing symptoms but are not an effective emergency treatment.

Adrenal steroids (cortisones), which act more slowly than epinephrine or even antihistamines, may be given for persistent symptoms such as severe itching, swelling, and hives. Intravenous fluids, oxygen, and a tracheotomy (which provides an opening in the trachea, or windpipe, to maintain breathing) may also be necessary in acute shock or airway closure.

Antihistamines and steroids given by mouth are administered for several days for a delayed allergic reaction to a sting.

Prompt treatment is vital for any person with a history of allergic reactions to insect stings. Unfortunately, most stings occur at some distance from a doctor's office or a hospital—in parks at the beach, on the golf course, or at the swimming pool. Therefore, anyone who has had an allergic reaction to a sting should take two steps:

- First, wear a Medic Alert Identification bracelet or tag and/or carry information on a card which states that s/he is allergic to specific insects and needs definitive treatment. Such knowledge can be lifesaving if the wearer should faint and is unable to explain what is wrong.

- Second, s/he should always have emergency insect sting treatment at hand, such as epinephrine in a syringe ready for injection or a kit containing epinephrine in a syringe, antihistamine tablets, a tourniquet, and alcohol swabs for cleansing the injection site.

Such kits are available only with a doctor's prescription. When a doctor prescribes one, he will also instruct the allergic person on techniques for self-injection. The instructions in the kit are simple and easy to follow. The fluid in the syringe should be checked periodically, and if it has turned brown the fluid is ineffective and should be replaced.

This kit should be carried at all times. The emergency treatment will provide the precious time needed to get the allergic person to a physician or a hospital for complete professional care. The kit is not intended to replace medical help.

A consensus development conference on the emergency treatment of insect sting allergy was held at the National Institutes of Health in September 1978. The experts in this field agreed that, to the maximum extent allowed by law, permission and encouragement should be given to all those who are properly trained to administer emergency treatment for stings at the site of the emergency. Such persons would include lifeguards, forest rangers, scout leaders, and school nurses.

Measures To Reduce Sensitivity. Traditionally, allergy "shots"—injection treatments known as immunotherapy or desensitization—have been used to reduce or prevent future symptoms of allergy. In this procedure, injections of small diluted amounts of the allergen are given once or twice a week. As the person's tolerance builds up, the injections are given less often and contain increasing amounts of the allergen. Usually the shots are given by a doctor or by a nurse under the doctor's direction, and the patient remains in the office for 15 to 30 minutes to make sure that no side effect of treatment occurs.

This form of immunotherapy is believed to increase the body's supply of protective or blocking antibody, called immunoglobulin G (IgG). This is thought to combine with the allergen before it can attach to IgE, the allergy antibody on the cell's surface. Thus IgE is not stimulated to trigger the chain of events that result in the allergic reaction.

What About the Future?

Altering our environment is usually not a practical solution to an allergic problem. Pollens, molds, and insects are all vital to the ecology of this planet. Thus allergies to these things must be controlled in the individual, rather than by attempts—probably futile, in any case—to eradicate a particular allergen.

In the past, insect allergy has been one of the less successfully treated allergies. However, NIAID-supported research has recently made venom therapy available to doctors. The increasingly active field of immunology is providing hope that people may be able to live free of their fear of insects and enjoy nature and the environment during all seasons.

361

Chapter 32

Insect Sting Allergy and Venom Immunotherapy

The warm weather brings with it great enjoyment for most people, but also brings the threat of insect stings from bees, yellow jackets, hornets, and wasps.

Occurrence

We are not sure about the true prevalence of insect sting allergy. One survey of boys attending a scout summer camp estimated the prevalence of systemic sting reactions (involving parts of the body in addition to the immediate site of the sting) at from 0.4 to 0.8 percent. A study among adult industrial employees found the prevalence to be 3.3 percent. That study suggested, in addition, that 30 to 40 percent of those who had been recently stung became sensitized, but just half among those stung over three years prior to the testing remained so. The longer one goes without being re-stung, the less one seems to be sensitized.

Each year, about 40 to 50 deaths are reported in the U.S. from insect sting allergy. However, we believe that this estimate is probably quite low, since many cases of anaphylaxis (a life threatening allergic reaction marked by lowered blood pressure and shock) may be reported as *myocardial infarction* or a "cerebrovascular accident."

The History of Venom Immunotherapy

The idea of injecting people who are diagnosed as sensitive to insect venom with minute quantities of the venom, in order to reduce allergic reactions when they are re-exposed to it, first came to the attention of physicians in the years after World War I. It was first reported in a case of a patient in South Africa who had developed symptoms of anaphylaxis after being stung by honeybees and was helped by injecting her with a then novel preparation made by grounding up the bodies of bees and then extracting the venom (whole body extract). Although her symptoms lessened during the course of immunotherapy, harsh side effects brought her treatment to an early end.

A few years later, a scientific report in the first edition of the *Journal of Allergy* described a beekeeper with respiratory symptoms and anaphylaxis. From their testing, the authors concluded there was a sort of universal bee allergen distributed through the bees' bodies that seemed to be responsible for both the respiratory and systemic reactions. A professional following developed for the use of whole body extracts to desensitize patients, although treatment failures using unstandardized extracts from whole insect bodies were reported. A well-respected American allergist, Dr. Mary Loveless, treated her insect-allergic patients with injections of freshly extracted venom or by allowing one or more specimens of the suspected insects to sting her patients.

Still uncertain whether insect sting reactions were toxic (poisonous) or allergic (the latter involving the multiplication of IgE, the allergy antibody, and the overproduction of inflammation-causing chemicals), researchers at Johns Hopkins in the early 1970s were able to show that insect-allergic patients released histamine, a characteristic of IgE-mediated reactions, when they were exposed to low, nontoxic concentrations of venom. This finding led to the use of venoms for skin testing, and then to immunotherapy.

Soon afterwards, the Hopkins researchers began a controlled trial of immunotherapy for insect-sting allergy that compared venom, whole insect body extracts, and a placebo (the last, a medically harmless substance) in 60 sensitive adults. In addition to demonstrating the superiority of venom specific to the type of insect that caused the patient's diagnosed sensitivity, the researchers were able to observe that:

- The patient usually reacts in a predictable way each time an insect sting creates a reaction.

• The risk of a system-wide reaction in unimmunized people with previous histories of reactions to insect stings is about 60 percent, not 100 percent as earlier thought.

In a later study, unimmunized, insect-allergic children whose earlier reactions only involved skin symptoms, just 10 to 20 percent were at risk of any future sting reaction. Also, it was shown that in any case, future reactions would almost never be worse than the original reaction.

Modern Diagnostic and Treatment Approaches

Proving the Diagnosis. In looking for the most reliable proof as to whether a patient has an allergic response to insect venom, researchers discovered that the level of blocking (protective) IgG, another immune system antibody, would rise to about twice its previous level when insect-sensitive patients were immunized with insect venom.

Who Should Receive Immunotherapy? Today, there is general agreement among experts that venom immunotherapy should be offered to any child or adult who has a history of a previous systemic sting reaction that is potentially life-threatening, and also to adults with sting-caused skin reactions. We know that non-threatening reactions can be expected in unimmunized children with histories of previous reactions limited to the skin, but we still lack similar data for adults.

Starting Venom Immunotherapy. The decision to start therapy is a clinical one. That is, it depends on the results of skin tests or RAST (radioallergosorbent test), and other health-related factors. For example, older patients with cardiovascular complications, and patients who take beta-blockers can risk more severe reactions if they occur. Certain occupational and leisure interests—such as beekeeping and golf—must also be considered.

Ending Venom Immunotherapy. In recent years, studies with adult and child patients at Johns Hopkins have established that stopping venom therapy after five uninterrupted years of treatment can produce lasting resistance to future insect stings in 90 percent of patients. This appears to be so even though the patients may continue to show elevated quantities of IgE or antibodies in their blood sera and be reactive to venom in skin testing. We do not fully understand these contradictions.

Taking Precautions. It is certainly preferable to avoid sting reactions, but exposure to stinging insects is practically inevitable. This is so despite a variety of common sense precautions, such as not eating or drinking where insects are plentiful, and not walking barefoot when out doors.

Mild systemic reactions confined to the skin are easily treated with oral antihistamines. More severe reactions that cause nasal symptoms, bronchospasm or mild decreases in blood pressure usually require injected epinephrine. Kits for self-treatment are available from pharmacies with a doctor's prescription. Their tradenames are *Epi-Pen* and *Epi-Pen Jr.*, and *Ana-Kit* or *Ana-Guard*.

This information should not substitute for seeking responsible, professional medical care.

—by Martin D. Valentine, M.D.

Dr. Martin Valentine is an allergist and professor of medicine at the Johns Hopkins School of Medicine in Baltimore.

Chapter 33

Poison Ivy, Poison Oak, and Poison Sumac: They're Still Out There

Those nasty weeds—poison ivy, poison oak and poison sumac—grow practically everywhere in the United States, except Hawaii, Alaska and some desert areas of Nevada. They are the most common causes of allergic reactions in the United States and will affect 10 to 50 million Americans every year.

Poison Ivy. In the East, Midwest, and South, it grows as a vine. In the Northern states, Canada and around the Great Lakes, it grows as a shrub.

Poison Oak. In the East it grows as a shrub. In the West it may grow as a vine as well as a shrub. Hair is found on the fruit, trunk and leaves.

Poison Sumac. Grows in standing water in peat bogs in the North and in swampy areas in parts of the South. Each leaf has 7-13 leaflets.

For the sake of convenience, "poison ivy" in this chapter will refer not only to ivy but to sumac and oak as well.

For a more detailed description of the various forms of poison ivy, oak, and sumac, see the following chapter.

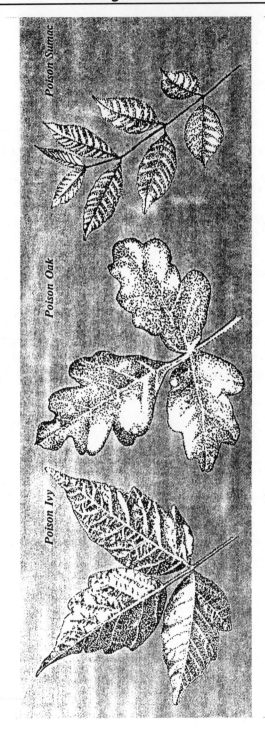

Figure 33.1. Leave these "three-leaflets" be

Poison Ivy Rash

Poison ivy rash is really an allergic contact dermatitis caused by a substance called *urushiol,* (you-ROO-shee-ol), found in the sap of poison ivy, poison oak and poison sumac.

Urushiol is a colorless or slightly yellow oil that oozes from any cut, or crushed part of the plant, including the stem and the leaves.

You may develop a rash without ever coming into contact with poison ivy, because the *urushiol* is so easily spread. Sticky, and virtually invisible, it can be carried on the fur of animals, on garden tools, or sports equipment, or on any objects that have come into contact with a crushed or broken plant. After exposure to air, *urushiol* turns brownish-black, making it easier to spot. It can be neutralized to an inactive state by water.

Once it touches the skin, the *urushiol* begins to penetrate in a matter of minutes. In those who are sensitive, a reaction will appear in the form of a line or streak of rash (sometimes resembling insect bites) within 12 to 48 hours. Redness and swelling will be followed by blisters and severe itching. In a few days, the blisters become crusted and begin to scale. The rash will usually take about ten days to heal, sometimes leaving small spots, especially noticeable in dark skin.

The rash can affect almost any part of the body, especially areas where the skin is thin; the soles of the feet and palms of the hands are thicker and less susceptible.

Who's Sensitive, Who's Not

Sensitivity to poison ivy is not something we are born with. It develops only after several encounters with the plants, and sometimes over many years. Studies have shown that approximately 85 percent of the population will develop an allergic reaction if exposed to poison ivy. This sensitivity varies from person to person. Although they are not sure why, scientists believe that an individual's sensitivity to poison ivy changes with time and tends to decline with age.

The first bout of poison ivy usually occurs in children between the ages of 8 and 16, and can be quite severe. If there is no repeated exposure to poison ivy, or urushiol, sensitivity will probably decrease by half by the time these individuals reach their thirties.

Investigators have found that people who reach adulthood without becoming sensitized have only a 50 percent chance of developing an allergy to poison ivy. Those who were once allergic may lose their sensitivity later in life. However, dermatologists say you should not assume that you are one of the few people who are not sensitive; only 10 to 15 percent of the population is believed to be resistant. That same percentage (25 to 40 million people) is thought to be very susceptible to poison ivy. These people will develop a rash and extreme swelling on the face, arms and genitals. In such severe cases, treatment by a dermatologist will be required.

Recognizing Poison Ivy

Identifying the plant is the first step toward avoiding poison ivy. The popular saying "leaves of three, let them be," is a good rule of thumb, but it's only partially correct. Poison oak or poison ivy will take on a different appearance depending on the environment. The leaves may vary from groups of three, to groups of five, seven, or even nine.

Poison oak is found in the West and Southwest, poison ivy usually grows east of the Rockies, and poison sumac east of the Mississippi River. The plants grow near streams and lakes, and wherever there are warm, humid summers.

Poison ivy grows as a low shrub, vine or climbing vine. It has yellow-green flowers and white berries. Poison oak is a low shrub or small tree with clusters of yellow berries and the oak-like leaves. Poison sumac grows to a tall, rangy shrub producing 7 to 13 smooth-edged leaves, and cream-colored berries. These weeds are most dangerous in the spring and summer. That's when there is plenty of sap, the *urushiol* content is high, and the plants are easily bruised. Although poison ivy is usually a summer complaint, cases are sometimes reported in winter, when the sticks may be used for firewood, and the vines for Christmas wreaths. The best way to avoid these toxic plants is to know what they look like in your area and where you work, and to learn to recognize them in all seasons.

For a more detailed description of the various forms of poison ivy, oak, and sumac, see the following chapter.

What To Do About Poison Ivy

Prevention is the best cure. The best way to avoid the misery of poison ivy is to be on the look-out for the plant whenever you are out-of-doors. Know what you are looking for, and stay away from it. The weeds can be destroyed with herbicides in your own back yard, but this is not a practical solution for forest preserves and other natural areas. If you are going to be in areas where you know poison oak or ivy is likely to grow, wear long pants and long sleeves, and, whenever possible, gloves and boots. Remember that the plant's virtually invisible, oily resin— urushiol—sticks to almost all surfaces, and can even be carried in the wind if it is burned in a fire. Studies have shown that a sensitive person may develop an internal inflammation from inhaling *urushiol*. In addition, don't let pets run through wooded areas since *urushiol* may be carried home on their fur.

Barrier creams offer little hope against poison oak and ivy, although new products may offer some protection. These may soon be marketed throughout the United States. Dermatologists are also working on a skin treatment to prevent *urushiol* from penetrating the skin. Ask your physician about new treatments available that might help to protect you.

Treatment: A Poison Ivy Primer

If you think you've had a brush with poison ivy, poison oak or poison sumac, follow this simple procedure:

- Wash all exposed areas with cold running water as soon as you can reach a stream, lake or garden hose. If you can do this within five minutes, the water will neutralize or deactivate the *urushiol* in the plant's sap and keep it from spreading to other parts of the body. Soap is not necessary, and may even spread the oil.

- When you return home, wash all clothing outside, with a garden hose, before bringing it into the house, where resin could be transferred to rugs or to furniture. Handle the clothing as little as possible until it is soaked. Since *urushiol* can remain active for months, it's important to wash all camping, sporting, fishing or hunting gear that may also be carrying the resin.

- If you do develop a rash, avoid scratching the blisters. Although the fluid in the blisters will not spread the rash, fingernails may carry germs that could cause an infection.

Cool showers will help ease the itching and over-the-counter preparations, like calamine lotion or Burow's solution, will relieve mild

371

rashes. Soaking in a lukewarm bath with an oatmeal or baking soda solution is often recommended to dry oozing blisters and offer some comfort. Over-the-counter hydrocortisone creams will not help. Dermatologists say they aren't strong enough to have any effect on poison ivy rashes.

In severe cases, prescription corticosteroid drugs can halt the reaction if taken soon enough. If you know you've been exposed and have developed severe reactions in the past, be sure to consult your dermatologist. He or she may prescribe steroids, or other medications, which can prevent blisters from forming.

Immunization

Investigators have found that most people could be immunized against poison ivy through prescription pills. These pills contain gradually increasing amounts of active extract from the plants. However, this procedure can take four months to achieve a reasonable degree of "hyposensitization." In addition, the medication must be continued over a long period of time and it can often cause uncomfortable side effects. This procedure is recommended only if the doses are given before contact with the plant, and only for individuals, such as fire-fighters, who must live or work in areas where they come into constant contact with poison ivy. Consult your dermatologist for his or her advice on whether you should consider immunization.

Common Myths About Poison Ivy

- **Scratching poison ivy blisters will spread the rash.** This is not true. The rash is spread by *urushiol* on the hands—scratching the nose, for instance, or wiping the forehead—before blisters have formed.

- **Poison ivy is "catching."** It's not. The rash cannot be passed from person to person; only *urushiol* can be spread by contact.

- **Once allergic, always allergic.** False. A person's sensitivity changes over time, even from season to season. People who were particularly sensitive to poison ivy as children may not be allergic as adults.

- **"Leaves of three, let them be."** This is usually true, but not always.

- **Dead poison ivy plants are no longer toxic.** This is not true. *Urushiol* remains active for up to several years. Never risk handling dead plants.

- **There's no immunization against poison ivy.** There is, but it's not recommended; the procedure is tedious, and carries unwelcome side effects.

- **Hydrocortisone creams will relieve poison ivy itches.** They may help with very mild rashes, but, in most cases, these over-the-counter remedies are far too weak to combat the itch of poison ivy.

Not Just a Summer Hazard

If you think that summer's end means no more poison ivy precautions, think again. A physician at the National Institutes of Health in Bethesda, MD, is determined to weed out some major myths surrounding this fearsome flora.

"One myth is that poison ivy is strictly a summer hazard," says Dr. Laurence H. Miller, Special Advisor for Skin Diseases at the National Institute of Arthritis and Musculoskeletal and Skin Diseases. "You can get just as bad a case of poison ivy in the fall, winter, or spring."

Myth number two concerns the spread of poison ivy. Dr. Miller explains that the allergic reaction the skin undergoes results from contact with *urushiol*, the active oily ingredient in the resin of the plant. Before you bathe or shower, you can unknowingly spread this invisible substance from one part of your body to another. *Urushiol* also can cling to clothing, shoes, the fur of a pet, or the surface of garden tools and gloves, where it can remain active for weeks to months.

Prompt bathing with soap and laundering contaminated clothes will reduce the possibility of *urushiol* spreading and affecting anyone else.

Source for "Not Just a Summer Hazard": NIH Healthline September 1989.

Perhaps the greatest misunderstanding concerning the spread of poison ivy involves the blisters that break out within 24 hours in areas of maximum exposure (less exposed areas break out several days later). Although scratching blisters is not a good idea, the clear serum that is released will not spread the rash to other parts of your body or to another person.

Prevention and Treatment

- **Learn how to recognize poison ivy.** It is a vine (or sometimes a bush) with three shiny green leaves at the tip of the same stem which turn reddish brown in the early fall. In late fall, winter, and early spring, the plant has greenish white berries. It tends to grow around the base of trees, near fences, and up through bushes such as azaleas.

- **Save weeding for the last chore of the day.** Protect yourself with gloves, long sleeves, and slacks. If you do become contaminated and shower immediately, you probably will not break out in a rash, or at least not as severely.

- **When the rash is in its initial stage of bumps and no blisters, an over-the-counter cortisone cream will lessen itching.** Once blisters form, drying preparations such as calamine lotion and hydrogen peroxide will help. Applying ice is soothing and taking antihistamine, Benadryl, will reduce itching.

- **For severe rashes, a physician can prescribe cortisone in pill or injection form.** In either case, marked improvement occurs quickly. If you take cortisone orally, complete the dosage; otherwise the rash may return.

— by Mary Gamboa

Chapter 34

Poison Ivy, Poison Oak, and Poison Sumac: Identification, Precautions, Eradication

Many people are accidentally poisoned each year from contact with plants that they did not know were harmful. If they had known how to recognize these poisonous plants, they could have escaped the painful experience of severe skin inflammation and water blisters. Many people do not recognize these plants, although they occur in almost every part of the United States in one or more of their various forms (Figure 34.1).

Few persons have sufficient immunity to protect themselves from poisonous plants. However, poisoning is largely preventable. You can easily learn to identify plants in their various forms by studying pictures and general descriptions; then train yourself by diligent practice in observing the plants in your locality. Children should be taught to recognize the plants and to become poison ivy conscious.

Poison Ivy and Poison Oak

Poison ivy and poison oak are neither ivy nor oak species. Rather, they belong to the cashew family and are known by a number of local names; actually, several different kinds of plants are called by these names. Poison ivy and poison oak plants vary greatly throughout the United States. They grow in the form of:

1. woody vines attached to trees or objects for support,

United States Department of Agriculture. Farmers' Bulletin No. 1972. GPO Stock #001-000-03883-4.

2. trailing shrubs mostly on the ground, or
3. erect woody shrubs entirely without support.

They may flourish in the deep woods, where soil moisture is plentiful, or in very dry soil on the most exposed hillsides. Plants are most frequently abundant along old fence rows and edges of paths and roadways. Plants ramble over rock walls and climb posts or trees to considerable height. Often they grow with other shrubs or vines in such ways as to escape notice.

Leaf forms among plants, or even on the same plant, are as variable as the habit of growth; however, the leaves almost always consist of three leaflets. The old saying, "Leaflets three, let it be," is a reminder of this consistent leaf character but may lead to undue suspicion of some harmless plant. Only one three-part leaf leads off from each node on the twig. Leaves never occur in pairs along the stem.

Flowers and fruit are always in clusters on slender stems that originate in the axils, or angles, between the leaves and woody twigs. Berry-like fruits usually have a white, waxy appearance and ordinarily are not hairy, but may be so in some forms. The plants do not always flower and bear fruit. The white or cream-colored clusters of fruit, when they occur, are significant identifying characters, especially after the leaves have fallen. For convenience, these plants are discussed under three divisions:

- common poison ivy,
- poison oak, and
- Pacific poison oak.

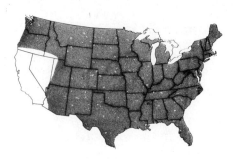

Figure 34.1. *The shaded part shows the extensive area where some form of common poison ivy may grow.*

Common Poison Ivy (**Rhus radicans**)

The plant is known by various local names: poison ivy, three-leaved ivy, poison creeper, climbing sumac, poison oak, markweed, picry, and mercury. Common poison ivy may be considered as a vine in its most typical growth habit.

Vines often grow for many years, becoming several inches in diameter and quite woody. Slender vines may run along the ground, grow with shrubbery, or take support from a tree. A plant growing along the edge of a lawn and into the shrubbery may be inconspicuous compared with a vine climbing on a tree. The vine develops roots readily when in contact with the ground or with any object that will support it. When vines grow on trees, these aerial roots attach the vine securely. A rank growth of these roots often causes the vines on trees to have the general appearance of a fuzzy rope.

The vines and roots apparently do not cause injury to the tree except where growth may cover the supporting plant and exclude sunlight. The vining nature of the plant makes it well adapted to climbing over stone walls or on brick and stone houses.

Poison ivy may be mixed in with ornamental shrubbery and vines. Sometimes people do not recognize the plant and cultivate it as an ornamental vine. An ivy plant growing on a house may be prized by an unsuspecting owner. The vine is attractive and sometimes turns a brilliant color in the fall. This use as an ornamental can result in cases of accidental poisoning, and these plants may serve as propagating stock for more poison ivy in the vicinity.

Poison ivy, mixed in with other vines, may be difficult to detect, unless you are trained in recognizing the plant. Virginia creeper and some forms of Boston ivy often are confused with it. You can recognize Virginia creeper by its five leaflets radiating from one point of attachment. Boston ivy with three leaflets is sometimes difficult to detect. Study a large number of Boston ivy leaves and you will usually find some that have only one deeply lobed blade or leaflet. Poison ivy has the three leaflets. A number of other plants are easily confused with poison ivy. Learn to know poison ivy on sight through practiced observation, then make sure by looking at all parts of the suspected plant.

Common poison ivy when in full sunlight grows more like a shrub than like a vine along fence rows or in open fields. In some localities, the common form is a low-growing shrub that is 6 to 30 inches tall. Both forms usually have rather extensive horizontal systems of rootstocks or stems at or just below the ground level. Under some conditions, the vining form later becomes a shrub. Plants of this type may start as a vine supported on a fence and later extend upright stems that are shrub-like. In some localities, the growth form over a wide range is consistently either vine or shrub type. In other areas, common poison ivy apparently may produce either vines or shrubs.

Leaves of common poison ivy are extremely variable, but the three leaflets are a constant character. The great range of variation in the shape or lobing of the leaflets is impossible to describe. The five leaves shown in Figure 34.2 give a fair range of patterns. Other forms may be found. One plant may have a large variety of leaf forms, or it may have all leaves of about the same general character. The most common type of leaf having leaflets with even margins is shown in Figure 34.2:A. Other forms in Figure 34.2 are not quite so widespread but may be the usual type throughout some areas.

Most vines or shrubs of poison ivy produce some rather inconspicuous flowers (Figure 34.2:A) that are always in quite distinct clusters arising on the side of the stem immediately above a leaf. Frequently, the flowers do not develop or are abortive and no fruit is produced. Poison ivy fruits are white and waxy in appearance and have rather distinct lines marking the outer surface, looking like the segments in a peeled orange.

In some forms of poison ivy, the fruit is covered with fine hair, giving it a downy appearance; however, in the more common form, fruits are entirely smooth. The fruit is especially helpful in identifying plants in late fall, winter, and early spring when the leaves are not present.

Poison Oak (**Rhus toxicodendron**)

Poison oak is more distinctive than some other types. Some people call it oakleaf ivy while others call it oakleaf poison ivy.

Poison oak usually does not climb as a vine but occurs as a low-growing shrub. Stems generally grow upright. The shrubs have rather slender branches, often covered with fine hairs that give the plant a kind of downy appearance. Leaflets occur in threes, as in other ivy, but are lobed, somewhat as the leaves of some kinds of oak. The middle leaflet usually is lobed alike on both margins and resembles a small oak leaf, while the two lateral leaflets are often irregularly lobed. The lighter color on the underside of one of the leaves is caused by the pubescence, or fine hairs, on the surface. The range in size of leaves varies considerably, even on the same plant.

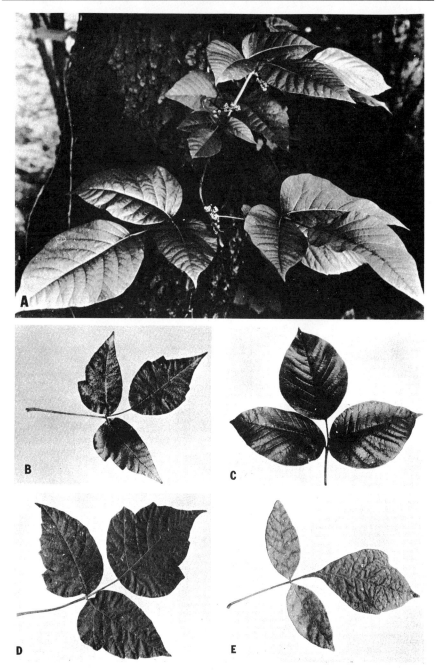

Figure 34.2:A. Common poison ivy vine with clusters of flowers in the axil of each leaf. **B,C,D,E,** less-common leaf forms that may occur on the same or different plants of common poison ivy.

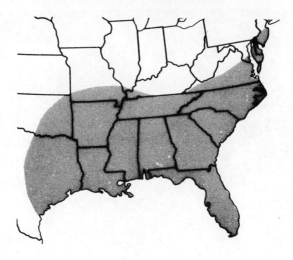

Figure 34.3. *Region where poison oak is likely to occur. Other forms also may be in the same region.*

Pacific Poison Oak (Rhus diversiloba)

Pacific poison oak of the Pacific Coast States, usually known as poison oak, occasionally is referred to as poison ivy or yeara. This species is in no way related to the oak but is related to poison ivy.

The most common growth habit of this western poison oak is as a rank upright shrub that has many small woody stems rising from the ground. It frequently grows in great abundance along roadsides and in uncultivated fields or on abandoned land.

Pacific poison oak sometimes attaches itself to upright objects for support and takes more or less the form of a vine. The tendency is for individual branches to continue an upright growth rather than to become entirely dependent on other objects for support. In some woodland areas, 70 to 80 percent of the trees support vines extending 25 to 30 feet in height.

In open pasture fields, Pacific poison oak usually grows in spreading clumps from a few feet to several feet tall. Extensive growth greatly reduces the area for grazing. It is a serious menace to most people who frequent such areas or tend cattle that come in contact with the plants while grazing.

Low-growing plants, especially those exposed to full sunlight, often are quite woody and show no tendency for vining. These plants are common in pasture areas or along roadsides. Livestock, in grazing, do not invade the poison ivy shrub. As a rule, these plants spread both by rootstock and seed.

As in other poison ivy, leaves consist of three leaflets with much irregularity in the manner of lobing, especially of the two lateral leaflets. Sometimes lobes occur on both sides of a leaflet, giving it somewhat the semblance of an oak leaf. The middle, or terminal, leaflet is more likely to be lobed on both sides, and resembles an oak leaf more than the other two. Some plants may have leaflets with an even margin and no lobing whatsoever. The surface of the leaves is usually glossy and uneven, giving the leaves a thick leathery appearance.

Flowers are borne in clusters on slender stems diverging from the axis of the leaf. Individual flowers are greenish white and are about one-fourth inch across. The cluster of flowers matures into greenish or creamy white berry-like fruits about mid-October. These are about the size of small currants and look much like other poison ivy fruits. Many plants bear no fruit although others produce it in abundance.

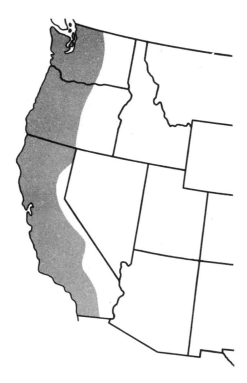

Figure 34.4. The region where Pacific poison oak is likely to occur. Other forms may also be in the same region.

Fruits sometimes have a somewhat flattened appearance. They remain on plants throughout fall and winter and help identify poison oak after leaves have fallen.

Poison Sumac (Rhus vernix)

Poison sumac grows as a coarse woody shrub or small tree and never in the vine-like form of its poison ivy relatives. This plant is known also as swamp sumac, poison elder, poison ash, poison dogwood, and thunderwood. It does not have variable forms, such as occur in poison oak or poison ivy. This shrub is usually associated with swamps and bogs. It grows most commonly along the margin of an area of wet acid soil.

Mature plants range in height from 5 or 6 feet to small trees that may reach 25 feet. Poison sumac shrubs usually do not have a symmetrical upright tree-like appearance. Usually, they lean and have branched stems with about the same diameter from ground level to middle height.

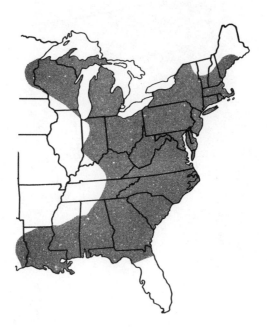

Figure 34.5. *The region where poison sumac is likely to occur; isolated plants are sometimes found in dry soil.*

Isolated plants occasionally are found outside swampy regions. These plants apparently start from seed distributed by birds. Plants in dry soil are seldom more than a few feet tall, but may poison unsuspecting individuals because single isolated plants are not readily recognized outside their usual swamp habitat.

Leaves of poison sumac consist of 7 to 13 leaflets, arranged in pairs with a single leaflet at the end of the midrib.

The leaflets are elongated oval without marginal teeth or serrations. They are 3 to 4 inches long, 1 to 2 inches wide, and have a smooth velvet-like texture. In early spring, their color is bright orange. Later, they become dark green and glossy on the upper surface, and pale green on the lower, and have scarlet midribs. In the early fall, leaves turn to a brilliant red-orange or russet shade.

The small yellowish-green flowers are borne in clusters on slender stems arising from the axis of leaves along the smaller branches. Flowers mature into ivory-white or green-colored fruits resembling those of poison oak or poison ivy, but they usually are less compact and hang in loose clusters that may be 10 to 12 inches in length.

Because of the same general appearance of several common species of sumac and poison sumac, there is often considerable confusion as to which one is poisonous. Throughout most of the range where poison sumac grows, three nonpoisonous species are the only ones

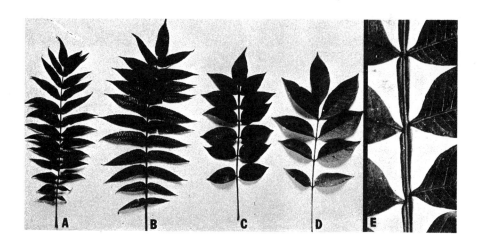

Figure 34.6. *Leaves of species of sumac that are often confused:* **A:** *Smooth Sumac;* **B:** *staghorn sumac;* **C:** *dwarf sumac;* **D:** *poison sumac;* **E:** *enlarged portion of dwarf sumac leaf from* **C***, showing the wing margin of the midrib. Poision sumac does not have the winged midrib.*

likely to confuse. These are the smooth sumac (*Rhus glabra*), staghorn sumac (*Rhus typhina*), and dwarf sumac (*Rhus copallina*), all of which have red fruits that together form a distinctive terminal seed head. These are easily distinguished from the slender handing clusters of white fruit of the poison sumac. Sometimes more than one species of harmless sumac grow together.

When seed heads or flower heads occur on plants, it is easy to distinguish poisonous from harmless plants; however, in many clumps of either kind, flowers or fruit may not develop. The leaves have some rather distinct characteristics.

Leaves of the smooth sumac and of staghorn sumac have many leaflets, which are slender and lance shaped and have a toothed margin. These species usually have more than 13 leaflets. Leaves of dwarf sumac and poison sumac have fewer leaflets; these are more oval shaped and have smooth or even margins. The dwarf sumac is readily distinguished from poison sumac by a winged midrib. Poison sumac never has the wing margin on the midrib.

Introduced Poisonous Sumac and Related Species

The small Japanese lacquer-tree (*Rhus verniciflua*), uncommon in the United States, is related to native poison sumac. Native to Japan and China, it may be a source of Japanese black lacquer. Poisoning has followed contact with lacquered articles. Never plant this tree.

A native shrub or small tree (*Metopium toxiferum*) called poisonwood, doctor gum, Metopium, Florida poison tree, or coral sumac is commonly found in the pinelands and hummocks of extreme southern Florida, the Keys, and the West Indies. It is much like, and closely related to, poison sumac. The shrub or small tree has the same general appearance as poison sumac. However, the leaves have only three to seven, more-rounded leaflets. Fruits are borne in clusters in the same manner as those of poison sumac, but they are orange colored and each fruit is two to three times as large. All parts of the plant are poisonous and cause the same kind of skin irritation as poison-ivy or poison sumac.

Poisoning

Many people know through experience that they are susceptible to poisoning by poison ivy, poison oak, or poison sumac. Others, however, either have escaped contamination or have a certain degree of immunity. The extent of immunity appears to be only relative. After repeated contact with the plants, persons who have shown a degree of immunity may develop poisoning.

The skin irritant of poison ivy, poison oak, and poison sumac is a nonvolatile phenolic substance called urushiol, found in all parts of the plant. The danger of poisoning is greatest in spring and summer and least in late fall or winter.

Poisoning usually is caused by contact with some part of the bruised plant, as actual contact with the poison is necessary to produce dermatitis. A very small amount of the poisonous substance can produce severe inflammation of the skin. The poison is easily transferred from one object to another. Clothing may become contaminated and is often a source of prolonged infection. Dogs and cats frequently contact the plants and carry the poison to children or other unsuspecting persons. The poison may remain on the fur of animals for a considerable period after they have walked or run through poison ivy plants.

Smoke from burning plants carries the toxin and can cause severe cases of poisoning.

Children who have eaten the fruit have been poisoned although the fruit when fully ripe is reported as nonpoisonous. A local belief that eating a few leaves of the plant will develop immunity in the individual is unfounded. Never taste or eat any part of the plant.

Cattle, horses sheep, hogs, and other livestock apparently do not get the skin irritation caused by these plants, although they graze on the foliage occasionally. Bees collect nectar from the flowers, but no ill effects from use of the honey have been reported.

The time between contamination of the skin and first symptoms varies greatly with individuals and probably with conditions. The first symptoms of itching or burning sensation may develop in a few hours or even after 7 days or more. The delay in development of symptoms is often confusing when an attempt is made to determine the time or location when contamination occurred. The itching sensation and subsequent inflammation that usually develops into water blisters under the skin may continue for several days from a single contamination. Persistence of symptoms over a long period is most likely caused by new contacts with plants or by contact with previously contaminated clothing or animals.

Severe infection may produce more serious symptoms, which result in much pain through abscesses, enlarged glands, fever, or other complications.

If it is necessary to work among poisonous plants, some measure of prevention can be gained by wearing protective clothing. It is necessary, however, to remember that the active poison can be easily transferred. Some protection also may be obtained by using protective creams or lotions. They prevent the poison from contact with the skin, make it easily removable by washing with soap and water, or neutralize it to a certain degree.

All measures to get rid of the poison must be taken within a few minutes after contact. A 10-percent water solution of potassium permanganate, obtainable in any drugstore, usually is effective if applied within 5 to 10 minutes after exposure.

Many ointments and lotions are sold for prevention of poisoning by chemical or mechanical means. Their use should always be followed by repeated washings with soap and water to remove the contaminant.

Contaminated clothing and tools often are difficult to handle without causing further poisoning. Automobile door handles or steering wheels may, after trips to the woods, cause prolonged cases of poisoning among persons who have not been near the plants. Decontaminate such articles by thorough washing in several changes of strong soap and water. Do not wear contaminated clothing until it is thoroughly washed. Do not wash it with other clothes. Take care to rinse thoroughly any implements used in washing. Dry cleaning processes will probably remove any contaminant; but there is always danger that clothing sent to commercial cleaners may poison unsuspecting employees.

Dogs and cats can be decontaminated by washing; take care, however, to avoid poisoning while washing the animal.

There seems to be no absolute, quick cure for all individuals, even though many studies have been made to find effective remedies. Remedies may be helpful in removing the poison or rendering it inactive, and for giving some relief from the irritation. Mild poisoning usually subsides within a few days, but if the inflammation is severe or extensive, consult a physician.

Control by Mechanical Means

Poison ivy and poison oak can be grubbed out by hand quite readily early in spring and late in fall, only if a few plants are involved. Roots are most easily removed when soil is thoroughly wet. Grubbing when soil is dry and hard is almost futile because the roots break off in the ground, leaving large pieces that later sprout vigorously. Grubbing is effective if well done.

Poison ivy vines climbing on trees should be severed at the base, and as much of the vine as possible should be pulled away from the tree. Often the roots of the tree and weed are so intertwined that grubbing is impossible without injury to the tree. Bury or destroy roots and stems removed in grubbing because the dry material is almost as poisonous as the fresh.

Smoke from burning poison ivy plants or contaminated articles may carry the poison in a dispersed form. Take extreme caution to avoid inhalation or contact of smoke with the skin or clothing.

Old plants of poison ivy produce an abundance of seeds, and these are freely disseminated, especially by birds. A poison ivy seedling 2 months old usually has a root that one mowing will not kill. Seedling plants at the end of the first year have well established underground runners that only grubbing or herbicides will kill. Seedlings are a threat as long as old poison ivy is in the neighborhood.

Plowing is of little value in combating poison ivy and poison oak.

Mowing with a scythe or sickle is not an efficient means of controlling poison ivy and poison oak. It has little effect on the roots unless frequently repeated.

Weed burners are also inefficient in controlling poison ivy and poison oak.

Control by Herbicides

Poison ivy and poison oak can be destroyed with herbicides without endangering the operator. One usually may stand at a distance from the plants and apply the herbicide without touching them. Most herbicides are applied as a spray solution by sprayers equipped with nozzles on extensions 2 feet or more in length. The greatest danger of poisoning occurs in careless handling of gloves, shoes, and clothing after the work is finished.

Any field or garden sprayer, or even a sprinkling can, can be used for applying the spray liquid, but a common compressed-air sprayer holding 2 to 3 gallons is convenient and does not waste the spray.

Use moderate pressure giving relatively large spray droplets, rather than high pressure giving a driving mist, because the object is to wet the leaves of the poison ivy and poison oak and avoid wetting the leaves of desirable plants. High pressures cause formation of many fine droplets that may drift to desirable plants.

Follow the manufacturer's recommendations shown on the container label in preparing the spray solution. Cover all foliage, stems, shoots, and bark of poison plants with herbicide spray. Although best results normally are obtained soon after maximum foliage development in the spring, applications may be made up to 3 weeks before fall frost is normally expected under good growing conditions in the humid areas.

Many herbicides used on poison ivy and poison oak will injure most broad-leaved plants. Apply them with caution if the surrounding vegetation is valuable. During the early part of the growing season, the leaves of poisonous plants usually tend to stand conspicuously apart from those of adjacent plants, and they can be treated separately if sprayed with care. Later the leaves become intermingled, and injury to adjacent species is unavoidable. Chemicals other than oil are not injurious to the thick bark of an old tree, and poison ivy clinging to the trunk safely can be sprayed with them. However, cutting the vine at the base of the tree and spraying regrowth may be more practical.

Apply sprays when there is little or no air movement. Early morning or late afternoon, when the air is cool and moist, usually is a favorable time.

No method of herbicidal eradication can be depended on to kill all plants in a stand of poison ivy and poison oak with one application. Retreatments made as soon as the new leaves are fully expanded are almost always necessary to destroy plants missed the first time, to treat new growth, and to destroy seedlings. Plants believed dead sometimes revive after many months. An area under treatment must be watched closely for at least a year and retreated where necessary.

Dead foliage and stems remaining after the plants have been killed with herbicides are slightly poisonous. Cut off dead stems and bury or burn them, taking care to keep out of the smoke.

Use of Pesticides

Pesticides are registered by the Environmental Protection Agency (EPA) for country-wide use unless otherwise indicated on the label.

The use of pesticides is governed by the provisions of the Federal Insecticide, Fungicide, and Rodenticide Act, as amended. This act is administered by EPA. According to the provisions of the act, "It shall be unlawful for any person to use any registered pesticide in a manner inconsistent with its labeling" (Section 12(a)(2)(G)).

EPA has interpreted this Section of the Act to require that the intended use of the pesticide must be on the label of the pesticide being used or covered by a Pesticide Enforcement Policy Statement (PEPS) issued by EPA.

The optimum use of pesticides, both as to rate and frequency, may vary in different sections of the country. Users of this publication may also wish to consult their Cooperative Extension Service, State agricultural experiment stations, or county extension agents for information applicable to their localities.

The user is cautioned to read and follow all directions and precautions given on the label of the pesticide formulation being used.

Federal and State regulations require registration numbers. Use only pesticides that carry one of these registration numbers.

—by Donald M. Crooks (retired),
and Dayton L. Klingman,
Sea agronomist,
Weed Science Laboratory,
Beltsville Agricultural Research Center West,
Beltsville, Md. 20705

Chapter 35

Chemical and Other Environmental Sensitivities

A variety of often vague, hard-to-pinpoint "asthma and allergy-like" symptoms and syndromes are experienced by an undetermined but possibly sizeable number of adults and children. We don't yet know a great deal about what are referred to as chemical sensitivities; but they are being talked of as a growing problem, and the variety of adverse health effects can easily confuse the public as well as their health care providers.

Why Are Chemical Sensitivities Gaining So Much Interest?

There are several reasons, among which are:

- the natural environment around us being disturbed to a greater degree than in earlier times by complex chemical compounds (polymers);

- less indoor air exchange in more energy-efficient houses and buildings;

- more diverse media reaching us with news and opinions about chemical sensitivities and their possible effects on our health.

©Asthma and Allergy Foundation. Reprinted with permission.

391

Some physicians who refer to themselves as "ecologically oriented" have proposed diagnoses such as the "twentieth century disease," "chemical AIDS," "multiple chemical sensitivities," or "Candida hypersensitivity." Intriguing as these labels may be to some whose symptoms seem to frustrate the attempts of a medical diagnosis and treatment, no single, widely accepted test of physiologic function has yet to clearly identify the causes of these symptoms. Nevertheless, physicians have been advised to be more sensitive to patients with vague complaints, and to satisfy them and keep them from fleeing in desperation to seek care and "cures" that either totally lack a medical-scientific basis or require much more study before anyone can say anything certain about them.

Attempting To Classify Chemical Sensitivity

There are four general ways that we can classify chemical sensitivity:

- **Annoyance reactions.** These are due to a heightened sensitivity to unpleasant odors, called olfactory awareness, in some susceptible individuals. Your ability to cope with offensive, but mostly nonirritating, odors has a lot to do with genetic or acquired factors, among which are infection and inflammation of the mucous membranes or polyps (growths of the nasal or sinus membranes), and abuse of tobacco and nasal decongestants.

- **Irritational syndromes.** Caused by significant exposure to irritating chemicals that are more likely than others to penetrate the mucous membranes, these types of reactions can affect certain nerve endings and cause burning sensations in the nose, eyes, and throat. They usually come and go, and can be reversed.

- **Immune hypersensitivity.** At present, only a relatively few chemicals are known to have the capability of provoking a true immune system response. Among them are certain industrial chemicals, particularly acid anhydrides and isocyanates, that are able to bind to human proteins.

- **Intoxication syndrome.** In some cases, long-term exposure to noxious chemicals may cause serious illness, or even death. Permanent damage to health may be the outcome of such reactions, which are dependent on the nature and extent of the chemical exposure.

Pollutants

The most common complaints of people who believe they have symptoms due to chemical sensitivity concern exposure to pollution, either out-of-doors or indoor. The atmosphere is made up of a complex mixture of volatile and particle substances. Out-of-doors pollution may result from natural causes (the eruption of volcanoes, dust storms, forest fires), or man-made causes (vehicle exhaust, fossil fuel combustion, petroleum refining).

Sulfur Dioxide

We do have substantial scientific evidence linking specific air pollutants to increased respiratory illness and decreased pulmonary function, especially in children. People prone to allergy, especially those with allergic asthma, can be very sensitive to inhaled sulfur dioxide, for example. Symptoms can include bronchospasm, hives, gastrointestinal disorders, and inflammation of the walls of the blood vessels (vasculitis-related disorder).

Ozone and Nitrogen Dioxide

Temporary or perhaps permanent bronchial hypersensitivity has been connected to inhaling ozone and nitrogen dioxide. Long-term exposure to nitrogen dioxide has been associated with the increased occurrence of respiratory illness.

The greatest exposures to airborne pollution occur inside homes, offices, and non-industrial buildings. These settings have not received nearly the attention by pollution control agencies that they deserve.

Cigarette Smoke

One of the most disagreeable and potentially dangerous indoor pollutants is cigarette smoke. It is made up of a complex mixture of gases and particles that contain a variety of chemicals. Indoor tobacco smoking substantially increases levels of carbon monoxide, formaldehyde, nitrogen dioxide, acrolein, polycyclic aromatic hydrocarbons, hydrogen cyanide, and many other substances and inhaled particles found in the air.

Building Products

Toxic pollutants are given off by a number of building products, such as furniture, cleaning fluids, pesticides, and paints.

- **Woodburning stoves.** There are over 11 million woodburning units in U.S. homes today. Wood burning usually occurs in cold, oxygen-poor conditions that heighten the emission of carbon monoxide and other inhaled chemicals and particles. Increased use of wood as a heating fuel has raised concern due to its ability to contaminate a home. Poorly ventilated stoves give off increased levels of carbon monoxide, nitrogen and sulfur oxides, formaldehyde, and benzopyrene.

- **Formaldehyde.** While the greatest source of formaldehyde outdoors is gasoline and diesel fuel combustion, its primary indoor source is cigarette smoke. Data indicates that formaldehyde is capable of acting as a respiratory irritant. Also, it is known to cause skin sensitivity. However, there is no convincing evidence that this pollutant is able to sensitize the respiratory system.

- **Building-related illness.** Poor air quality in tightly-built homes and other buildings has been associated with a variety of syndromes, or group of symptoms. The term "building-related illness" is applied to an office building in which one or more occupants develop a generally accepted, well-defined syndrome for which a specific cause related to the building is found. A variety of illnesses broadly known as *hypersensitivity pneumonitis*—in which one or more organic dusts can create complex immune system reactions and symptoms including mucous membrane irritation, coughing, chest tightness, headache, and fatigue—may be diagnosed. While building occupants with these symptoms have been identified as having "multiple chemical sensitivities" or other forms of environmental illness, one study showed that the majority of nonspecific complaints by office workers had developed before they began working in the building suspected of causing their symptoms. A collaboration between physician, industrial hygienist, and building engineer may be necessary to clearly establish a cause-and-effect relationship between any indoor air quality level and disease.

Issues in Diagnosing Chemical Sensitivity

Chemical sensitivity can be an issue in considering workers' compensation claims or in legal action that involves product liability. Since the stakes are significant, we believe that there is a basic plan in evaluating patients who are believed to be at risk. Several major "pitfalls" can sidetrack the diagnosis:

- Failure to recognize a pre-existing medical disorder.

- Failure to diagnose an underlying medical condition that is masquerading as chemical sensitivity.

Diagnosing Suspected Chemical Sensitivity

The Most Productive Strategies in Diagnosing Suspected Chemical Sensitivity

Our experience has convinced us that there are strategies that can produce reliable diagnoses with relatively low cost, reliable diagnoses at significant cost, or questionable diagnoses at great expense. Obviously, the first alternative is most often preferable. It includes:

- A careful patient medical history that includes a review of all previous medical records and, when symptoms may be related to potentially hazardous substances in the workplace, reviewing a **Materials Safety Data Sheet** supplied by the employer.

- Upper respiratory tract and selective skin tests, and a neurologic examination.

- Routine laboratory studies, including nasal smear

- Lung function measurements (spirometry and peak flow monitoring).

If these diagnostic procedures do not produce a definite diagnosis, more expensive, but worthwhile, evaluations may help. They include an industrial hygiene evaluation of the workplace, an evaluation of the home environment, and psychiatric evaluations.

Unproductive Strategies

Diagnostic approaches we believe to be expensive and not very effective in explaining suggested chemical sensitivity include RAST testing, blood work for Epstein-Barr and autoimmune disease, food allergy testing, and evaluations for airborne molds and bacteria.

This information should not substitute for seeking responsible, professional medical care.

—by Emil J. Bardana, Jr., M.D.

Dr. Bardana is professor and vice chairman of the Department of Medicine and head of the Division of Allergy and Clinical Immunology at the Oregon Health Sciences University in Portland.

Chapter 36

Contact Dermatitis: Solutions to Rash Mysteries

When it comes to solving mysteries, a super sleuth like Sherlock Holmes has nothing on a good dermatologist.

Consider the case of the woman whose 21-year-long bout of eczema of the right palm was traced by her dermatologist to a carving knife she received as a wedding present 21 years before. The knife's wooden handle was the culprit causing her allergic rash.

Or the lady who had eczema of the palms for six years. The dermatologist deduced that the guilty party was the car she had bought six years earlier. The steering wheel contained a compound to which she was allergic.

Or the recent widower who suddenly developed an itchy rash on his hands. His dermatologist determined that it was not a psychosomatic disorder brought on by grief, but a sensitivity to oils in the skin of oranges, which he was squeezing for himself for the first time.

Allergies

The red, raw hands that tormented these people resulted from the skin's reaction to a substance (allergen) to which they had become sensitized, or allergic. This type of eczema, or superficial skin inflammation, is called allergic contact dermatitis. Normally, the skin doesn't react the first time it meets up with an allergen. Sometimes it occurs with the second exposure. But in other cases, it takes years

DHHS Publication No. (FDA) 91-1166. Reprint of *FDA Consumer*, May 1990.

and many exposures for hypersensitivity to a particular substance to develop. Once sensitized, the skin will usually become inflamed within hours or days after contact.

Irritants

Unlike allergic contact dermatitis, irritant contact dermatitis—a more common type—is a nonallergic inflammatory skin reaction caused by exposure to irritating substances that actually damage the skin. Not everyone develops allergies, but everybody's skin can become irritated if abused. Contact with strong irritants, such as acid or lye, can result in blisters, erosion and ulcers within minutes or hours. For weaker irritants, such as soaps or detergents, exposure over days or weeks may be necessary before eczema develops. Any substance can act as an irritant if it is concentrated enough and if the skin is exposed to it long enough.

The eczema usually starts with a red, itchy rash and progresses to tiny blisters that ooze.

Doctors can usually distinguish contact dermatitis from other types of dermatitis by its unusual pattern. The eruption often appears with clear-cut margins, acute angles, and geometric outlines, although poison ivy and other poison plants cause lines or groups of blisters.

Though the configuration of the rash aids in diagnosis, it's not so easy to determine whether an allergy or irritant is involved. The skin reaction produced by either, especially when mild, frequently looks the same. Redness or an itchy rash may be the first sign. However, blisters that weep or form a crust, along with swelling, are more likely to appear in allergic dermatitis, such as poison ivy. As the inflammation lessens, the skin may scale and become temporarily thickened. When the dermatitis becomes chronic, the skin becomes dry, thickened and cracking.

Sometimes, if the inflammation with mild irritants continues for a long time, the original irritation disappears because the skin becomes hardened.

Finding the Source

A person may know what caused the inflammation—for example, recent hand contact with a corrosive, such as an oven cleaner—or may not have a clue. The patient's hobbies, diet, occupation, sports activities, clothing and cosmetics, as well as medications that are taken internally—all come under suspicion.

An irritant or allergen at home or at work may be responsible. In one particularly puzzling case, Walter B. Shelley, M.D., professor of dermatology, Medical College of Ohio in Toledo, decided to visit the home of a patient who had been hospitalized twice for severe contact dermatitis. All tests had been negative, but after seeing her stainless steel kitchen, the cause of the dermatitis was apparent: the stainless steel polish she used to keep her kitchen shiny.

The location of the rash will sometimes tell the tale, except for hands, which are into everything. Anything on the scalp, face and neck suggests cosmetics such as hair sprays, shampoos, makeup, sunscreens, perfumes, shaving cream, acne medications—the list is endless. Eyelid dermatitis is often traced to nail polish, which can cause an allergic reaction if nails touch the eye area before the polish dries completely, a two-hour process. Lips can become sensitive to ingredients in lipsticks, toothpastes or chapped lip medications. Armpits can become allergic to or irritated by ingredients in deodorants or antiperspirants.

Dyes, elastic materials, fabric finishes such as sizing and permanent press, laundry detergents, and fabric softeners can cause dermatitis on the torso and arms and legs. "Some of those anti-static laundry products are really mean," says Shelley. "They can cause terrible problems. They set off itching, and people scratch, of course, which only makes things worse. It takes a lot of laundering to get that stuff out of the clothes."

The feet can be affected by dyes, rubber compounds, and leather-tanning products in shoes, or elastic fibers in hosiery. Nickel used in jewelry, bra fasteners, eyelash curlers, metallic eyeglass frames, and many other products can produce inflammation wherever it touches the body. People may become sensitized to nickel from ear-piercing instruments and from nickel-plated earrings inserted after piercing.

Fragrances in cosmetics are frequent offenders. Redness under the ears may be caused by perfume dermatitis. Some components of fragrances may interact with sunlight or other sources of ultraviolet light to produce dermatitis by a process called photosensitization. When dermatitis occurs on the left side of a man's face and neck—the side exposed to the sun while driving a car—photosensitization caused by aftershave lotion fragrances should be suspected.

Betrayed by Medications

And the unkindest cut of all—people can become sensitized to the very medications that they're using to relieve a skin problem, such as acne. If a skin product does not seem to be working, if things are getting worse instead of better, there's a chance that an allergy to some ingredient in the medication has developed, especially if puffiness, redness and itching appear.

Dermatitis may be caused by topical (externally applied) medications, such as anesthetics containing benzocaine, dibucaine and other chemicals that end in "caine," topical antibiotics such as neomycin and streptomycin, topical antihistamines such as diphenhydramine and promethazine, and topical mercury compounds such as mercurochrome and merthiolate.

Some drugs delivered to the individual by skin patches (transdermal therapeutic systems) such as scopolamine for motion sickness, and clonidine and nitroglycerin for treatment of cardiovascular disease can cause either irritant or allergic dermatitis, due either to the drug itself, a patch component, or the adhesive.

In addition, people who've been contact-sensitized by certain topical drugs may develop fever, feel unwell, or have excessive thirst when they take the drug orally as a tablet or capsule, or by injection.

Even inhaling the vapor can cause problems. One example of inhalation-related dermatitis is the "baboon syndrome" (named after the red-bottomed baboon), a curious type of red, spreading rash that develops on the buttocks and upper thighs. Japanese doctors have reported a number of cases in which mercury-allergic people, previously sensitized by the use of mercurochrome on the skin, developed the syndrome after inhaling the vapor from crushed thermometers. This ailment points out the importance of never allowing mercury to touch the skin. Alexander Fisher, M.D.. One of the world's leading dermatologists, advises in *Current Dermatologic Therapy* (ed. Stuart Maddin, M.D.) that if a thermometer breaks, a "shiny copper object, such as a penny," should be used to pick up the mercury.

Allergy Testing

If the physician suspects an allergy, patch testing may identify the responsible agent. However, to prevent the condition from worsening, these tests are not done until the inflammation has subsided. The dermatologist uses groups of medicines, metals, preservatives, rubber compounds, and various chemicals that go by the name **North American Contact Dermatitis Group Standard Patch Test Series.** A small amount of the suspected allergen(s) is applied to the patient's back, covered with a nonabsorbent adhesive patch, and left on for 48 hours. (The patch is removed if itching or burning develops before that time.) If redness, some hardness, or blistering occurs, the test is considered positive, indicating probable allergy to the substance. Since some reactions do not occur until after the patches are removed, the doctor will take another look at the patch sites in 72 hours. Other patch test series are available if the tests are negative.

Occupational Contact

Sometimes, the offending allergen can't be easily identified. But dermatologists don't like to give up.

"When the allergen is not found, you just keep looking. So many of these cases are due to occupational contact," says Shelley. "While you're looking, treatment is directed at relieving the inflammation. It's rare that you can't do something for the patient."

Industrial statistics show that contact dermatitis accounts for more than 50 percent of all occupational illness, excluding injury, and results in about a fourth of the time lost from work. About one in every thousand workers in the United States suffers from contact dermatitis, costing millions of dollars each year.

Occupational dermatitis is common among hairdressers, workers who handle animal intestines in slaughterhouses, shrimp peelers, furniture makers working with woods like teak and African mahogany, bakers in contact with cinnamon, and many others. People with hay fever and asthma or other allergies are well advised to stay away from occupations in which they would be exposed to chemicals, water and soil, because their skin is more susceptible to dermatitis. In the workplace, about 70 percent of contact dermatitis cases are irritant and 30 percent are allergic.

A Lifelong Problem

Contact dermatitis can make its appearance as early as infancy. Acute skin problems account for one-third of visits to the pediatrician, with irritant dermatitis the most frequent type in children. A baby's thin delicate skin can become irritated from urine and bowel movements, or it can become allergic to a chemical in the diaper or medicines used to treat diaper rash. Dermatitis of the cheeks and around the mouth can occur as a result of irritation by drooling, water, juices, food, and dry air. A rash all over the body and in the folds of a baby's skin may result from contact with detergents, soaps, fabric softeners, and bleach.

Problems can continue throughout adulthood. The problem of "dishpan" hands is common in those whose hands are constantly in contact with water, soaps or detergents. Sun lovers may develop an itchy rash following too much of a good thing, especially after the first exposure in the spring or summer. Ski enthusiasts are familiar with dermatitis and chapped skin from exposure to cold, dry air.

Frictional irritant dermatitis can result from improperly fitted shoes. Handling golf clubs and tennis rackets may produce inflamed skin, blisters and calluses. Tattooing has its dangers: people who've been sensitized to mercury, chromium, cobalt, and cadmium can develop rashes and roughened skin when tattooed with the salts of these metals.

Neither do the elderly escape. Topical medications should be used with care by older people, because changes in the skin make it more susceptible to dermatitis, and it generally takes longer to clear up than in younger patients.

Treatment

For self-treatment of mild contact dermatitis, a 0.5 percent hydrocortisone topical preparation (ointment, cream or lotion) can be applied to the skin to relieve the itchiness, redness, scaling, and swelling. Because these formerly prescription-only medications had a good safety record, FDA approved them for over-the-counter (OTC) sale in 1979 on the recommendation of the Advisory Review Panel on OTC Topical Analgesic, Antirheumatic, Otic, Burn and Sunburn Prevention Treatment Drug Products. A petition to make 1.0 percent topical hydrocortisone drug products available for over-the-counter sale is currently being evaluated by the agency. [This petition has now been approved.]

The labeling of the OTC products states that if symptoms worsen or persist longer than seven days, a doctor should be consulted. (Occasionally, bacterial or fungal infections superimpose themselves on the dermatitis.) The labeling also cautions against internal use and use on children under 2 years old. Lubricating creams or lotions, preferably preservative- and lanolin-free, can be used to prevent cracking and dryness, especially of the hands, and the irritating factor or allergen should be avoided whenever possible.

Severe cases should be seen by a doctor. Stronger concentrations of topical corticosteroid preparations or oral corticosteroids, such as prednisone, may be prescribed. If there's a secondary infection, an oral antibiotic may be necessary.

When inflammation has gone on for a long time, an extended period of convalescence is often necessary. "I tell my patients it's like skin that's been burned after sitting on a hot stove," comments dermatologist Shelley. "You've got to allow time for the skin to heal itself."

Common Sensitizers

Among common sensitizers, poison ivy leads the pack. Estimates of Americans with poison ivy allergy range from 50 to 70 percent. Most of the rest of the population would develop poison ivy dermatitis on further exposures, though some people will never get it. Cross-sensitization to other members of the poison ivy family occurs, so that allergy can develop to poison oak, poison sumac, the oil in cashew nutshells, mango fruit peel and leaves, and the fruit of gingko trees. A severe airborne dermatitis can result from contact with the smoke from burning plants on exposed skin.

In mild cases, topical corticosteroids are used to relieve the itching, while severe cases are treated with oral or injected corticosteroids. In severe cases, hospitalization is sometimes necessary. Unfortunately, shots or medicines for desensitization to poison ivy have not been very effective and, in fact, can make poison ivy dermatitis worse.

Some common house and garden plants are not completely innocuous, either. Primroses and philodendrons cause allergic dermatitis in some people. Handling tulip bulbs may result in a sensitivity known as "tulip fingers." Asters, chrysanthemums, English ivy, castor beans, oleanders, geraniums, poinsettias, magnolias, lilacs, narcissus, and other bulb plants can be sensitizers, as can ragweed, some pollens, such as birch pollen (which can cross-sensitize to apples, carrots and celery), and the timber and sawdust of some trees.

Some vegetables may also cause a problem. Dermatitis can result from handling parsnips, garlic, onions, tomatoes, carrots, and ginger.

Nickel, the most common metallic sensitizer, produces more allergic dermatitis than all other metals combined. Other common sensitizers are permanent hair dyes containing the chemical paraphenylenediamine, rubber compounds, and the chemical ethylenediamine, found in dyes, insecticides, synthetic waxes, and used as a preservative in some medicines.

Preventing Skin Inflammation

Sensitive-skinned people, and even those with tougher hides, would do well to follow a number of measures to prevent contact dermatitis:

• Read the labels on cosmetics. FDA requires that all ingredients in cosmetics be listed on the label in descending order of predominance. If a cosmetic causes a problem, note the ingredients— fragrances and preservatives are the most likely suspects—and avoid similar cosmetic formulations in the future. (Specific fragrance components are not listed, so a switch to fragrance-free products should be tried if dermatitis persists.)

• Wash new clothing and bed linens several times before using. Contact dermatitis caused by clothing is usually due to formaldehyde released by chemicals in the finishing of fabrics, and sometimes to the dyes. Avoid polyester blends and cottons that are labeled "permanent press" and "wrinkle-resistant," and stick to natural fibers, such as cotton, linen and silk. (Though wool is a natural fiber, it can be irritating.)

• Use soaps or detergents specifically formulated for babies' wash if laundry products are under suspicion. Avoid fabric softeners and anti-static products, and double-rinse the wash.

• Wear heavy-duty vinyl gloves with cotton liners, if possible, when hands are in contact with harsh cleansers at home or chemical irritants at work. Avoid abrasive soaps for removing grease and oil. Remove rings when using soaps and detergents, because these materials can become trapped under rings and cause irritation. Keep the hands well-moisturized with a bland cream or lotion.

• Learn to recognize the leaves of poison ivy and poison oak, each three-leaved and poison sumac with its oval leaves and white berries. If exposed to them, wash hands and skin thoroughly after exposure, using any kind of soap. Before applying over-the-counter poison-ivy preparations, read the labels and use with caution medications containing zirconium, benzocaine, and diphenhydramine hydrochloride. Although most people have no problem with these, sometimes they may sensitize and produce a dermatitis on top of the poison ivy rash. Dermatitis can result from handling other plants, including vegetables such as parsnips, garlic, onions, tomatoes, carrots, and ginger.

- Don't self-treat too long. If the dermatitis is not better after a week or 10 days, see the doctor. The topical medications may be the problem, or the itching and rash may be the symptoms of something quite different. An intolerable itch may be a sign of Hodgkin's disease, or of scabies, transmitted by the itch mite, a parasite. Red, itchy rashes can also be caused by superficial fungal infections, such as candidiasis, or impetigo and other bacterial infections.

—by Evelyn Zamula

Evelyn Zamula is a free-lance writer in Potomac, Md.

Chapter 37

Atopic Eczema/
Atopic Dermatitis

The word eczema is used to describe all kinds of red, blistering, oozing, scaly, brownish, thickened, and itching skin conditions. Examples of eczema include **dermatitis** or **allergic contact eczema** such as allergies to poison ivy, sumac or oak, cosmetics, chemicals, dyes or detergents; **seborrheic eczema,** which is yellow-pinkish-brownish, thickened, greasy skin areas found most typically on the scalp and central face; and **nummular eczema,** which consists of round, oozing, crusting patches. This chapter will describe and discuss a different type of skin disease that is called atopic dermatitis or eczema.

Atopic Dermatitis or Atopic Eczema

The word "atopic" describes a group of allergic or associated diseases that often affect several members of a family. These families have allergies such as hay fever and asthma but also have skin eruptions called atopic dermatitis. About one patient in five with this condition does not have any other allergies or atopic diseases in himself or his family members.

Atopic dermatitis is very common in all parts of the world. It affects about ten percent of infants and three percent of the U.S. population overall.

The disease can occur at any age but is most common in infants to young adults. The skin lesions are very itchy and sometimes disfiguring.

©1987 American Academy of Dermatology, Revised 1991, 1993. Reprinted with permission.

407

The condition usually improves in early childhood or sometime before the age of 25. About 60 percent of patients keep some degree of dermatitis and some suffer throughout life. These cases can cause frustration to both the patient and the treating physician.

When the disease starts in infancy, it's sometimes called infantile eczema. This itching, oozing, crusting condition tends to occur mainly on the face and scalp, although spots can appear elsewhere. In attempts to relieve the itching, the child may rub his/her head and cheeks and other affected areas with a hand, a pillow, or anything within reach. Parents can be consoled with the fact that many babies improve before two years of age. Proper treatment can be helpful, sometimes controlling the disease until time solves the problem.

If the disease continues or recurs beyond infancy, the skin has less tendency to be red, blistering, oozing and crusting. Instead, the lesions become dry, red to brownish-gray, and the skin may be scaly and thickened. An intense, almost unbearable itching can continue, becoming severe during the night. Some patients scratch at their skin until the lesions become bloody and crusted.

In teens and young adults, the eruptions typically occur on the elbow bends and backs of the knees, ankles and wrists and on the face, neck and upper chest. Although these are among the most common sites, all body areas may be affected.

Recognizing Atopic Dermatitis

An itching rash as described above, along with a family history of allergies, may indicate atopic dermatitis. Proper, early and regular treatment by a dermatologist can bring relief and also may reduce the severity and duration of the disease.

There are instances when the disease does not follow the usual pattern. It also can appear on the palms or backs of the hands and fingers, or on the feet, where crusting, oozing, thickened areas may last for many years.

Questions and Answers About Atopic Dermatitis

Since this condition is associated with allergies, can certain foods be the cause?

Yes, but only rarely (perhaps 10 percent). Although some foods may provoke attacks, especially in infants and young children, eliminating them rarely will bring about lasting improvement or a cure. If all else fails, foods such as cow's milk, soy, eggs, fish, wheat, peanuts and other foods suggested by your dermatologist should be avoided at least for one to two weeks on a trial basis.

Are environmental causes important, and should they be eliminated?

Rarely does the elimination of contacted or airborne substances bring about lasting relief. Occasionally dust and dust-catching objects like feather pillows and down comforters, kapok pillows and mattresses, carpeting, drapes, some toys, and wool along with other rough fabrics, can cause the condition to worsen.

Are skin tests, like those given for hay fever or asthma, of any value in finding the causes?

Sometimes, but not as a rule. A positive test signals allergy only about 20 percent of the time. If negative, the test is good evidence against allergy. If these tests are desired, ask your dermatologist to recommend someone who has experience in administering them.

Are "shots" such as those given for hay fever and other allergies, useful?

Not as a rule. They may even make the skin condition worse in some patients.

What then should be done to treat this condition?

See your dermatologist for advice on relieving irritating factors in creams and lotions, rough, scratchy or tight clothing and woolens, rapid changes of temperature and any violent exercise that provokes sweating. Seek dermatological help for proper bathing and moisturizing advice and dealing with emotional upsets which make the condition worse.

Your dermatologist can prescribe external medications such as corticosteroids(cortisone) or tar creams, and internal medications such as antihistamines to control the itching. Sometimes oral antibiotics will be prescribed if there is also a secondary infection. For severe cases, your dermatologist may recommend ultraviolet light therapy.

409

Internally administered steroids should be avoided if at all possible. However, when all other measures have failed, your physician may prescribe systemic steroids.

Atopic dermatitis is a very common condition. With proper treatment, the disease can be controlled.

Chapter 38

Hand Eczema

What Causes a Hand Rash?

A hand rash—what your doctor might call "dermatitis"—can have many causes, but most of these usually fall into one of two types: an externally-triggered "contact" rash, or an internally-generated skin reaction.

Hand rashes are extremely common—many people start with dry, chapped hands that later become patchy red, scaly, and inflamed. The number of items which can irritate skin is almost limitless. A few of them are overexposure to water, or too much dry air, soaps and detergents, solvents, cleaning agents, chemicals, rubber gloves, or even ingredients in skin and personal care products. Once skin becomes red and dry, even so-called "harmless" things like water and baby products can irritate the rash, making it worse. It's very important to talk with your doctor and try to find out what substance in your everyday routine could be causing or contributing to the problem. Often your skin will get better by changing products or avoiding an ingredient completely.

A tendency to get skin reactions is often inherited. People with these tendencies may have a history of hay fever and/or asthma in combination with food allergies and a skin condition called atopic dermatitis or eczema. Their skin can turn red and itch after contact with many substances that might not bother other people's skin.

Can Stress Cause a Hand Rash?

While emotional "ups and downs" can play a role in many skin conditions, they are seldom the only cause of a hand rash. Stress may be involved when a person has a genuine psychological problem; these people may rub, wring, or scratch their hands constantly, or wash them 50 or 100 times a day. They may be more likely to consult a dermatologist for their "rash" than to consult a psychologist.

Finding the Culprit

The dermatologist will work with you to uncover and identify the possible causes of a hand rash. Like a detective, he or she will ask many questions about any previous rashes, whether you have hay fever or asthma, and any other medical problems. S/he will also want to know what creams or lotions you apply to your skin, whether and when you wear gloves, and what kinds of things your hands are exposed to all day long. The doctor will examine your feet and your skin as well as your hands in an effort to determine what's causing the rash. Your doctor may order special tests to see if you have a skin infection or other problems that might show up under a microscope.

If your doctor suspects the rash is due to an allergy to some external substance, a patch test may be done. This involves testing the skin on your arms or back to see what specific ingredients might be causing your skin to react. Your dermatologist will use these tests and probably will be able to suggest what substance or combination of factors might be responsible for your rash.

How Are Hand Rashes Treated?

Your dermatologist may offer a combination of methods to heal your skin. It's possible you may need an oral antibiotic if an infection is present. A soothing ointment or cream may be prescribed or recommended—be certain not to use this in combination with other hand creams. If this cream doesn't seem to be helping, tell your doctor right away. You can speed the healing yourself by keeping your hands out of harsh chemicals and away from other irritants. Your doctor will tell you what to avoid while your skin is healing.

Is Hand Protection Really Important?

Regardless of the cause of your rash, you'll want your hands to heal and to stay healthy. There are ways to pamper them, now and in the future, to lessen the chance of getting a rash again:

- Protect hands against soaps, cleansers and other chemicals by wearing vinyl gloves. Have four or five pair and keep them in the kitchen, bathroom, nursery and laundry areas. Have other pairs for non-wet housework and gardening. Avoid rubber gloves since many people are sensitive to them. Always replace any gloves that develop holes. Dry gloves out between cleaning jobs. Wear your gloves even when folding laundry, peeling vegetables, or handling citrus fruits or tomatoes.

- Use an automatic dishwasher as much as possible, and avoid hand-washing dishes or clothes as much as you can.

- When you wash your hands, use lukewarm water and very little soap. Remove rings whenever washing or working with your hands. They trap soap and moisture next to skin.

- When outdoors in cool weather, wear unlined leather gloves to protect against dry and chapped skin. Always use a dermatologist-recommended product to keep your hands soft and supple, and apply it as many times a day as you need it.

- If the type of work you do is affecting your hands, talk to your supervisor about ways that all employees can better protect their skin.

Hand rashes sometimes temporarily look worse while they're healing—and sometimes they just come back. Try to remember which substance or what activity triggered the recent "flare-up" and let your doctor know about it. Since many hand rashes can be stubborn, it's important to keep up with your medication, stay in contact with your doctor, and not get discouraged.

Chapter 39

Latex Allergies: When Rubber Rubs the Wrong Way

Every Thursday, Sue Lockwood's eyes would start to swell. Fridays were always the worst. Sometimes her eyes were so swollen she could hardly see. But, without fail, by the time Monday rolled around, the swelling was gone and her eyes were fine.

"I thought that I was allergic to the sand that I was playing volleyball in every Thursday," says Lockwood, who lives in Grafton, WI. "The sand would get in my eyes and [I thought] I was breaking out from the sand."

But, although Lockwood quit playing volleyball in August 1991, the problem with her eyes persisted into the fall.

Two ophthalmologists told her that her symptoms didn't indicate an eye infection. Finally, in October she went to see an allergist.

"After interviewing me and getting a medical history he told me he was sure I was latex sensitive. Sure enough, he drew blood and I tested positive."

What were the clues that led to the allergist's conclusion? First, Lockwood is a surgical technician. Like most health-care workers today, Lockwood practically lived in latex gloves at work.

Second, her work schedule was Tuesdays, Wednesdays, and every other Thursday. That explained the miserable Fridays and recovery by Monday.

And then there was the volleyball. "It turns out she didn't use a standard volleyball," says her allergist, B. Lauren Charous, M.D. "Her team used a red rubber volleyball."

FDA Consumer, September 1992.

Latex is the milky sap from the rubber tree *Hevea brasiliensis*. It doesn't cause problems for most people. But, like other things in nature—bee sting venom, poison ivy, peanuts—latex can cause problems for some people. Those problems can range from minor skin irritation to reactions so severe that emergency medical treatment is necessary to prevent death.

For those allergic to the rubber tree's sap the only sure solution is to stay away from it. But latex products are everywhere, especially in health-care settings. It is found in all kinds of medical devices, most notably the ubiquitous surgical and examination gloves that health-care workers wear. Most condoms and diaphragms are made of latex. And latex is found in many everyday items, including balloons, household gloves, underwear, and rubber bands.

Few know better than Lockwood the surprising places latex can show up. "I don't know what I'm going to run into next," she says. She's reacted to the new carpet in her mother's house (the carpet backing contained latex) and to her nieces' and nephews' rubber toys.

New Problem or Old?

The British first discovered latex in the mid-18th century, but it didn't come into wide use until about 50 years ago. It took several more decades before allergic reactions started to appear.

In 1979, a woman in Great Britain who reacted to her household rubber gloves was the subject of the first report of latex allergy in the medical literature. Between 1979 and 1988, about 50 cases were recorded in European medical journals. Then, things began to change.

In the fall of 1989, the Food and Drug Administration (FDA) started receiving reports of patients going into anaphylactic shock during radiologic examinations for lower gastrointestinal tract disorders. The patients had all received barium enemas, so at first the barium was suspected. But in some cases, the patients went into shock after the device, a latex-cuffed enema tip, was inserted but before the barium was administered. In all, 16 people died. The manufacturer of the barium enema tips voluntarily recalled all those on the market and started using tips with silicone cuffs instead. Because that manufacturer dominated the market, at that time FDA felt any further regulatory action was unnecessary.

Then, between March 1990 and January 1991, nine children at a children's hospital in Milwaukee had anaphylactic reactions within 30 minutes after general anesthesia was started but before any surgical incisions had been made. The latex connection was the anesthesia equipment and intravenous catheters. Fortunately, emergency procedures prevented any deaths. Eight of the children, however, required intensive care.

According to Michele Pearson, M.D., an epidemiologist with the national Centers for Disease Control, preliminary results of a nationwide survey of children's hospitals have identified at least 25 other institutions that have reported similar reactions since January 1990. All 75 children who had anaphylactic reactions had either spina bifida or other conditions involving the genitourinary tract.

What was happening? Were the allergic reactions a new phenomenon or just being recognized for the first time?

"I think it is something new," says Jay Slater, M.D., an attending physician in allergy and immunology at Children's National Medical Center in Washington, D.C. He explains that the symptoms and the connection to latex use are fairly easy for an allergist to identify, so it would have been noticed earlier if it had been occurring.

"I can't say that it never occurred before 1979, but I certainly don't think it was that much of a problem before '79."

Slater won't speculate about why allergy to latex has increased so dramatically in the last 13 years, but many others consider "universal precautions"—the use of latex gloves to protect against the AIDS virus—the culprit.

"There's lots of health-care technicians using gloves now who didn't use them before," says Jean Reeder, an Army nurse and immediate past president of the Association of Operating Room Nurses.

"Emergency workers are wearing gloves more often and for longer periods of time," says Jim Paturas, past president of the National Association of Emergency Medical Technicians.

Another possibility is that manufacturers aren't allotting enough time on the production line for washing the latex.

"We assume that more washing will make the latex safer," says Orhan H. Suleiman, Ph.D., chairman of FDA's latex sensitivity task group. Although FDA has no evidence that insufficient washing is an industry-wide problem, in May 1991, the agency outlined in a letter to all manufacturers of latex medical devices a two-step washing procedure—first during a step in the production process called leaching and again after the product is completed—that removes many of latex's allergenic proteins.

Testing for Latex Allergy

There are two ways to test for latex allergies. With one—the skin-prick test—tiny diluted amounts of latex or one of its proteins are injected under the skin or applied to a small scratch or puncture on the patient's arm or back. If the patient is allergic, a small, raised area surrounded by redness appears at the test site within about 15 minutes.

Laboratory analysis of a blood sample to detect antibodies is the other testing option. (The first time an allergic person is exposed to an allergen, the immune system produces a kind of antibody called immunoglobulin E—IgE for short.)

Slater says testing is both very important, and, unfortunately, imperfect. "It is clear that history alone is inadequate to screen some patients," he explains. (Some of the people who died from reactions to the latex barium enema tips had no history of latex allergy.) But, currently there is no FDA-approved extract for the skin-prick test or the blood test. Without an approved standard extract, the accuracy of the test results is not reliable.

The lack of an approved material that will identify latex-sensitive patients stems in part from latex's complexity. "We're comfortable that at least one of the proteins in latex is the problem," says FDA's Suleiman. But he adds that more than a dozen proteins have been identified in latex. "Which one of these actually initiates the [allergic] reaction? At this time, your guess is as good as mine."

He adds, however, that a tremendous amount of research has been stimulated by questions about latex's proteins.

In addition, latex from some sources, such as different brands of gloves, may cause more severe reactions than that from other sources, according to Harvard dermatology professor Ernesto Gonzalez in the February 1992 issue of the journal *Hospital Practice*.

Still, Slater says people in high-risk groups should be tested if they are concerned, as long as the tests are part of a through examination by an allergist who has the background to recognize possible allergens and exclude others based on an individual's history of allergic reactions. "It requires a fair amount of detective work," he says.

In addition, the allergist should be prepared with emergency equipment in case the skin-prick test itself causes a severe allergic reaction.

Slater warns that people shouldn't try to test themselves, by, for example, blowing up a latex balloon.

"That's a lousy idea," he says. "In fact, it's potentially very danger-ous." He explains that a truly allergic person could go into shock from such a "test."

Finally, Slater says people who are not in a high-risk group and who haven't had any history of reactions "need to sit tight."

Suleiman agrees. "Right now, unless someone is already sensitive [to latex] there's no reason to discontinue use. We especially don't want to scare people away from latex condoms."

While approximately 1 billion to 2 billion condoms are used per year in the United States, FDA has received only 44 reports of aller-gic reactions associated with condom use between October 1988 and the end of 1991.

Latex Free

Surgery is nothing new for 7-year-old Paul Reynolds, of Herndon, Va. He was born with spina bifida, and last September's hip opera-tion was his eighth. But, unlike the previous seven, this was his first surgery since he had developed an allergy to latex.

Paul's mother, Adriana Reynolds, says the doctors assured her the surgery would be latex free "as much as possible. I used to worry about the risks of anesthesia, but now I think this rubber allergy is my great-est concern."

Latex-containing devices fill the average surgical suite, and some-times even medical professionals aren't aware that a device has a la-tex component.

"What is needed in the anesthesia world is a list of devices that don't have latex," says Jane McCarthy, a nurse-anesthetist and mem-ber of FDA's latex task group. "The clinicians can only attempt at best to provide an environment that's latex free. There's been difficulty in doing that because the devices aren't labeled with or without latex."

In response to that need, several hospitals have developed their own lists of latex-free devices. In addition, two nurse-anesthetists, Charles R. Barton and Cynthia A. Roy, have developed a list of com-monly used medical devices that contain latex. (See Table 39.1).

To make sure a patient's latex allergy isn't overlooked, FDA sent a medical alert to approximately 1,000 leaders of health professional organizations in March 1991. The alert advised health professionals to:

- Include questions about latex sensitivity when taking a patient's health history. (Asking patients if they've ever experienced

itching, rash or wheezing after wearing latex gloves or inflating a toy balloon may be useful.)

- Flag the charts of patients who report signs of latex allergy.

- Counsel patients who have a suspected latex-related allergic reaction while under the professional's care, and recommend a latex allergy test to those individuals.

The agency also recommended that when health professionals are treating a latex-sensitive patient, they should wear a non-latex glove over a latex glove. If both the health professional and patient are sensitive, triple-gloving (wearing a glove liner or vinyl glove under a latex glove as well as a vinyl glove over the latex) is recommended.

To protect themselves, Slater recommends that people allergic to latex:

- Carry non-latex gloves (a medium size is their best bet) at all times for health professionals to use during both routine examinations and emergency procedures.

- Wear a Medic Alert bracelet.

- Carry an emergency epinephrine kit in case they are accidently exposed to latex and go into anaphylactic shock (epinephrine immediately counteracts the shock).

- Alert all health professionals they deal with about their latex sensitivity.

For Adriana Reynolds, worry over when and if her son could have another reaction is compounded by the lack of knowledge about latex allergies.

"It's all very new," she says. "You tell people that your son has a rubber allergy and they say 'rubber?' I've had to meet with the people at Paul's school several times to convince them that this is serious. I had to buy vinyl gloves for the school nurse [Paul has to be catheterized during the day] and remind them about things like rubber balls in physical education."

For Lockwood, the worst part of her allergy is the loss of her career as a surgical technician. Since she first started reacting to latex more than a year ago, her sensitivity has become so acute that even if she were to wear vinyl gloves during surgery, airborne latex from the rest of the surgical team's gloves would cause her problems.

"There's no way I can work in surgery anymore," she says. "I can't deal with that loss yet. I want my career back."

Who's At Risk

Common to all allergic reactions to natural substances is the body's need to recognize the substance. The more often the body comes in contact with the substance, the greater the opportunity to recognize and react.

For the general public, the risk of an allergic reaction to latex is less than 1 percent. But because of constant exposure to latex, two groups are at greater risk: health-care workers and children with spina bifida and other conditions involving multiple surgical procedures. Because latex-containing medical devices abound in surgical suites, dental offices, and other health-care settings, contact with latex is an occupational hazard for health-care workers. It is also part of daily health maintenance routines (for example, catheterization) and the many surgeries high-risk children undergo.

According to Jay E. Slater, M.D., attending physician in allergy and immunology at Children's National Medical Center in Washington, D.C., the risk is so high for children with spina bifida, "we should treat them as latex-allergic regardless, whether we know that they are or not."

He cites his own research as the basis for his statement. When he tested the blood of 64 spina bifida patients, he found 25 of the children had antibodies to latex.

"Among those who had the antibody, approximately half had a history of latex-associated reactions," he says. He adds that more and more of these kids will have reactions as time goes on.

Allergic reactions to latex can include:

- skin rash
- itching
- hives
- swollen red skin
- tears
- itching or burning eyes
- swollen lips and tongue with difficulty in breathing, wheezing
- shortness of breath

- dizziness
- fainting
- abdominal pain
- nausea
- diarrhea.

In rare cases, an allergic individual goes into shock; blood pressure plummets, the throat swells, and airways in the lungs constrict. Without immediate treatment, the person will die.

A shot of epinephrine—the same drug used to treat severe allergic reactions to bee stings—will counteract the shock if given immediately.

Commonly Used Latex Medical Products	Anesthesia Equipment Containing Latex
<ul><li>rubber gloves</li><li>elastic bandages</li><li>adhesive tape</li><li>urinary catheters</li><li>electrode pads</li><li>wound drains</li><li>stomach and intestinal tubes</li><li>condom urinary collection devices</li><li>protective sheets</li><li>enema tubing tips</li><li>dental cofferdams</li><li>rubber pads</li><li>fluid circulating warming blankets</li><li>hemodialysis equipment</li></ul> **(Source: *Journal of the American Association of Nurse Anesthetists,* (October 1991)**	<ul><li>rubber masks</li><li>electrode pads</li><li>head straps</li><li>rubber tourniquets</li><li>rubber nasal-pharyngeal airways</li><li>rubber oral-pharyngeal airways</li><li>teeth protectors</li><li>bite blocks</li><li>blood pressure cuffs</li><li>rubber breathing circuits</li><li>reservoir breathing bags</li><li>rubber ventilator hoses</li><li>rubber ventilator bellows</li><li>rubber endotracheal tubes</li><li>latex cuffs on plastic tracheal tubes</li><li>latex injection ports on intravenous tubing</li><li>certain epidural catheter injection adapters</li></ul>

Table 39.1. Medical devices often containing latex

Why Stick with Latex?

What is it about latex gloves? Why not just switch everyone to something else?

"We can't switch everybody out of latex," says B. Lauren Charous, M.D., chairman of the American College of Allergy and Immunology's task force on latex hypersensitivity. "There's no real reason to. We're still dealing with a very small percentage of health-care workers."

There are, however, real reasons to keep donning latex gloves. The main one is "latex is the barrier of choice [to protect against HIV]," says Orhan Suleiman, Ph.D., chairman of FDA's latex sensitivity task group.

"It's primarily a question of durability," says Thomas Arrowsmith-Lowe, D.D.S., deputy director for health affairs in FDA's Center for Devices and Radiological Health. "Within 15 minutes after putting on a vinyl glove, it starts to lose its barrier effectiveness. Latex maintains the barrier longer."

Of almost equal importance is latex's ability to stretch and conform to the shape of the hand. "You can stretch it to four or five times its original length and it will not tear," says Barry Page of the Health Industry Manufacturers Association. "There aren't many materials that will do that."

In addition, because latex gloves can be stretched so thin, they don't interfere with the sensitivity and fine manual dexterity required in many medical procedures.

"Latex gloves are better fitting and it's easier to feel veins and start IVs," says Vicki Freund, a paramedic/firefighter with the Montgomery County, Md., fire department. "So, I end up wearing those."

She also ends up with hives on the backs of her hands. "They itch like crazy." Sometimes her eyes swell up and itch and her nose starts running, too.

For now, because her reactions are relatively minor, Freund just lives with the problem.

But there are efforts to find an alternative for people like her. Several companies have developed latex-free gloves that the companies claim can stretch like latex and don't impair the wearer's sense of touch. As with all new products that make medical claims, these new gloves have to be reviewed by FDA before they can be sold.

Allergist Charous encourages people with mild reactions to try several different brands of gloves. He adds that "people who have only a history of mild latex glove eczema are not at risk [of a serious reaction] in any immediate sense. I want to emphasize that."

—by Dori Stehlin

Dori Stehlin is a staff writer for FDA Consumer.

Chapter 40

Cosmetic Allergies: When Beauty Aids Turn Ugly

Whether or not a permanent improves a person's appearance is a matter of opinion. But when Carolyn, a secretary in Rockville, MD, arrived at her wedding shower one May evening, it was easy to see that the permanent she got at a beauty salon the day before had not produced the desired results. While the chemical treatment did give her curly hair, it also gave her a red, swollen face.

"I tried to cover it up with makeup," she said, "but it didn't help much. I was so embarrassed at the shower. Thank goodness I didn't wait until right before the wedding."

Carolyn had a case of cosmetic contact dermatitis—an acute allergic inflammation of the skin caused by contact with various substances found in cosmetics. In addition to the redness and swelling, her skin was weeping and covered with papules (small, solid elevations of the skin)—all classic symptoms of contact dermatitis.

Cases of contact dermatitis from cosmetics are rarely painful or life-threatening, but they sometimes can be so uncomfortable the unhappy victim will seek a doctor's care. The frequency of adverse reactions to cosmetics that require a physician's care is approximately 210 per 1 million cosmetic products purchased, according to information from a Food-and-Drug-Administration (FDA) survey and a study of cosmetic reactions conducted by the North American Contact Dermatitis Group, a task force of the American Academy of Dermatology.

FDA Consumer, November 1986.

Skin-care products, such as facial cleansers and moisturizers, were associated with the largest number of cosmetic allergic reactions in the study, which ran from September 1977 to August 1983. Hair preparations in general, including hair dyes, formed the second largest group, and facial makeup, such as foundation and blusher, was third. Other problem products included nail preparations and fragrance products.

As for the types of ingredients that cause the allergic reactions, the study found that fragrances and fragrance ingredients were responsible for the greatest number. Preservatives were next, followed by phenylenediamine (found in hair dyes), lanolin, the hair-waving ingredient glyceryl monothioglycolate, and propylene glycol (a skin softener).

What caused Carolyn's reaction? It may have been a chemical in the permanent itself or one of the many ingredients in the other products she used before and after the permanent—the shampoo, conditioner, neutralizer. She never did find out, and she's still worried that the ingredient will be in some other products she may use.

"It is important to find out which ingredient causes an allergic reaction, so a consumer can look for that ingredient in other products," said Heinz Eiermann, director of FDA's Division of Colors and Cosmetics. Yet half of the patients and their dermatologists in the contact dermatitis group study did not at first realize that a cosmetic was responsible for the dermatitis. Dr. Robert M. Adams, clinical professor of dermatology at Stanford University and a member of the contact dermatitis group, called that an important—and surprising—finding.

Why don't the patients or doctors suspect a cosmetic? One possible reason is that a product can be used without a reaction for years before "suddenly" causing an allergic problem. Repeated exposure to the offending ingredient can build up sensitivity.

"A lot of people can walk through poison ivy without any kind of reaction, but after a while their cells start to recognize this antigen and they start to react to it," said John Sanders, a dermatologist with FDA's Center for Drugs and Biologics. "The same thing can happen with cosmetics. Patients will tell me 'I've been using this product for several years; it can't be.' But there's always a first time."

What should be done if a reaction occurs? First, stop using all cosmetics. To help relieve the itching, 0.5 percent hydrocortisone cream can be applied, several times a day if needed. Other treatments include wet compresses and *Aveeno* (an oatmeal preparation). (See "The Itch of the Great Outdoors" in the June 1986 *FDA Consumer*, reprinted in this volume as Chapter 47.)

Table 40.1.
Types of Cosmetics that Cause Allergic Reactions

This table shows the types of cosmetics that were found to have caused allergic reactions in a study of 713 patients between 1977 and 1983. The study was funded by FDA and performed by 12 dermatologists who were members of the North American Contact Dermatitis Group, a task force of the American Academy of Dermatology.

Product Category	Percent of Cases
Skin-care products (lotions, creams, etc.)	28
Hair preparations (including colors)	24
Facial makeup	11
Nail preparations (polish, remover, etc.)	8
Fragrance products (perfumes, colognes)	7
Personal cleanliness products	6
Shaving preparations	4
Eye makeup	4
Suntan and sunscreen products	3
Oral hygiene products	Less than 1 percent
Bath preparations	Less than 1 percent
Baby products	Less than 1 percent
Products not specified	4

A mild reaction should clear up in seven to ten days. For severe reactions or ones that last longer than ten days, a doctor may prescribe a stronger topical steroid preparation or oral medication.

Once the reaction is completely over, cosmetics can be tested, one by one, to find the guilty party. "Before putting a product all over the face and breaking out, place a little on the forearm and watch it for at least 24 hours," FDA's Eiermann advises.

Since consumers use an average of 12 cosmetic products, more or less, at the same time, it may take a while before the offending product is found. But there are a few things to watch for to make the detective work easier. Was a new product used only a few times before the reaction occurred? It should be tested first. Although sensitivity to an ingredient has to build up before a reaction occurs, just two

Table 40.2
Cosmetic Ingredients that Cause Allergic Reactions

This table shows the cosmetic ingredients that most often caused allergic reactions in the North American Contact Dermatitis Group study.

Ingredient	Percent of Cases
Fragrance ingredients	30
Preservatives (antibacterial)	28
p-Phenylenediamine	8
Lanolin and derivatives	5
Glyceryl monothioglycolate	5
Propylene glycol	5
Toluenesulfonamide/formaldehyde resin	4
Sunscreens and other ultraviolet absorbers	3
Acrylate or methacrylate	2
Others	10

applications of that ingredient may be enough. Even a new bottle or jar of a product used before can be the cause of the problem. Manufacturers are constantly reformulating cosmetics—a new ingredient may have just been added.

Cross-sensitization can also cause problems, particularly with new cosmetics. Cross-sensitization involves closely related chemicals, where a person sensitive to ingredient A may have an allergic reaction when chemically related ingredient B is applied.

After finding out which product was involved in the allergic reaction, the next step is finding out which ingredient actually caused it. FDA requires cosmetic ingredients to be listed in descending order of predominance; that is, the ingredient that makes up the largest part of the product is listed first. Color additives and ingredients that make up no more than 1 percent of the product are exceptions. They can be

---

Table 40.3
Parts of the Body Affected by Cosmetic Allergies

This table shows the parts of the body that were affected by allergic reactions to cosmetics in the North American Contact Dermatitis Group study.

Body Site	Percent of Cases
Face	37
Eyes	12
Forearms	12
Armpits	6
Ears	4
Entire body	4
Neck	3
Scalp	2
Mouth	2
Upper arms	2
Fingers	2
Fingernails or toenails	1
Other	6
Unknown	7

grouped together in any order. If the problem product lists an ingredient on the label that isn't in any other cosmetics you've used without incident, then that is probably the culprit and should be avoided, no matter what product it is in.

But what if a unique ingredient can't be found on the label of the reaction-causing product? It may be hidden behind the word "fragrance." Only the word fragrance—not the name of the actual scent-giving ingredient—is required on cosmetic labels. Avoiding fragrances, the leading cause of allergic reactions to cosmetics, requires careful label reading. In any case, this is when a dermatologist can do a series of ingredient patch tests.

In a patch test, a small amount of the suspect ingredient is applied to the skin and covered with a bandage. Tests are usually done on the back since there is enough room there to do a lot of tests at once. The patches are left in place for 24 to 48 hours to see if redness, rash or any other sign of allergic reaction occurs.

Because fragrance ingredients are the most likely cause of an allergic reaction, testing with those ingredients would be the most likely place for the dermatologist to start. But the process of fragrance testing is complicated. A perfume may consist of 10 to 300 separate components, and the formulas are secrets manufacturers don't want to (or have to) divulge. But manufacturers may, upon request, send a dermatologist different fragrance mixtures identified only by a letter. The dermatologist can then patch test each mixture, and get the separate components of any mixture that gives a positive result from the manufacturer and patch test with those. If a component gives a positive result, the physician can find out if that specific fragrance ingredient is in a specific product. But the manufacturers won't divulge every product that contains that fragrance.

Because of the secrecy, to play it safe those allergic to fragrances should only use products that are labeled "fragrance-free" or "unscented." But even these products sometimes contain small amounts of fragrances to mask the fatty odor of soap or other unpleasant odors in "unscented" antiperspirants and vaginal lubricants. They are also used in cosmetics labeled "lightly scented" and those with "nonlingering" fragrance. Many products are like the hair spray whose label says "unscented" on the front of the can, but lists "fragrance" as an ingredient . . . on the back. Although these fragrances make up less than 1 percent of the cosmetics they're in, they could cause problems.

If "fragrance-free" doesn't always mean that there isn't any fragrance in the product, what about the other claims aimed at people concerned about allergic reactions? Do "hypoallergenic" and "allergy tested" and other such label claims mean there's no chance of a reaction? Unfortunately, no. There's always a possibility that someone somewhere will have an allergic reaction.

The prefix "hypo" in this case means "less than." "Hypoallergenic" on the label means the product is less likely to cause an allergic reaction. But there are no standards on how a manufacturer decides when a product is hypoallergenic. Although some manufacturers do clinical testing, others may simply omit perfumes or other common problem-causing ingredients.

"Dermatologist-tested" is another common label claim on cosmetics. It only means that a skin doctor has tested the product to see if it will generally cause allergenic problems. Other label claims that, unfortunately, carry no guarantee that they won't cause reactions include "sensitivity tested," "allergy tested," and "nonirritating."

Replacing known allergens with chemicals that not only have a lower sensitizing potential but also are safe in other ways and don't alter the properties of the product is extremely difficult. The fragrance industry is trying to eliminate ingredients that cause adverse reactions. The International Fragrance Association has a list of chemicals they recommend not be used at all or at only limited concentrations. And the Cosmetic Ingredient Review Panel, a group of experts convened by the cosmetics industry, is reviewing the toxicology of the more than 4,000 ingredients used in cosmetics.

Yet, except for eliminating fragrances and known allergens such as lanolin, the basic ingredients in products both with and without hypoallergenic claims are the same. Although the differences between products with hypoallergenic claims and those without are small, sales of hypoallergenic cosmetics are no longer limited to people with serious skin problems, according to Advertising Age magazine. John Bard, President of Physicians Formula cosmetics (a line of hypoallergenic products), said that more than 50 percent of Americans think they have "sensitive" skin.

But how many people actually have allergic reactions to cosmetics? In the American Academy of Dermatology study, cosmetic ingredients were the cause of the contact dermatitis in only 713 out of 13,216 patients—just over 5 percent. But the actual incidence of reactions is hard to assess. Instead of going to a dermatologist and trying to pinpoint the ingredient that caused the reaction, many consumers just stop using the product they suspect is at fault. On the other hand, not every rash is an allergic reaction.

Everyone's skin is sensitive, in some degree, to the harsh materials in products such as depilatories (hair removers) and hair straighteners. The rashes these materials cause are usually not true allergic reactions—the skin is simply irritated.

For some people, the harsh ingredients that cause irritation must be completely avoided. However, others may still be able to use those products if they use less and don't leave it on as long.

Consumers and their dermatologists should report cosmetic adverse reactions to:

FDA's Division of Colors and Cosmetics,
200 C St., S.W.,
Washington, D.C. 20204.

"Although we may not be able to help the individual consumer," FDA's Eiermann said, "this information will tell us that there may be a problem with that product. If we do see a cluster of adverse reactions associated with a specific product, we can then investigate further and remove the product from the market, if warranted, to protect everyone."

The cosmetic manufacturers also want to hear about any allergic reactions to their products, according to Page Blankingship, manager of communications for the Cosmetic, Toiletry and Fragrance Association. "Most of the people in the cosmetic industry are pretty wise," FDA's Sanders said. "They've been around and they're not going to put a product out there that is going to cause reactions if they can help it."

Even with the cosmetic industry's efforts to eliminate problem ingredients, consumers who feel they may be prone to allergic reactions should still use some caution to avoid them. Here are some tips:

- A do-it-yourself patch test may be done with any new product. Put a small amount of the product on the inside of the elbow and cover it with a bandage. Do this on the same spot twice a day for four days. If a rash appears, don't use that product. Even if the patch test is negative, continue to watch for a reaction for a few days after starting normal use of the cosmetic.

- Don't try more than one new product at a time. Wash your hands, and use clean applicators when applying cosmetics to prevent contamination with bacteria. And never apply cosmetics to skin that is already irritated or inflamed.

- A patch test should be done a few days before any professional hair treatment, such as a permanent or hair coloring. It's worth the extra effort of making two trips to avoid an experience like Carolyn's. Although the ingredient labeling required on retail cosmetics isn't required on products sold to beauty parlors, that information may be available from the manufacturers. Tell your beautician of any ingredient you know you're allergic to.

- Read the label of any new cosmetic before you try it, and avoid any that contain an ingredient that caused a reaction in the past.

While even diligent label reading and patch testing can't guarantee reactions won't occur, don't give up hope. Carolyn didn't. A few months after her disastrous permanent, she decided to gamble on another. She went to a different beauty salon and made sure the beautician used a different brand of permanent. And she got a patch test. The test was negative, so she went ahead with the permanent. And this time she only got what she paid for—curly hair.

—by Dori Stehlin

Dori Stehlin is a member of FDA's public affairs staff.

Part Six

Asthma

Chapter 41

Asthma Myths and Statistics: Two Views of Respiratory Distress

The Myths of Asthma

The anguish experienced by asthma sufferers is only increased by common misconceptions about the disease. Few afflictions are enveloped by so many myths as asthma. While it is impossible to discuss all of them, a few of the more common fallacies should be dispelled:

Asthma isn't serious. After all, no one ever dies from it.

The 2,000 to 4,000 asthma deaths in the United States each year (more than 5,000 in 1989) refute this, as do the physical suffering, financial strain, and psychological and social problems discussed earlier.

Asthma is all in the mind.

As with any illness, there is a relationship between physical and psychological symptoms. Asthma is a respiratory disorder, however, and there is no convincing evidence that emotional factors actually cause the disease. The exact role of psychological events as triggers for asthma attacks remains unclear.

Excerpted from NIH Publication No. 80-388 and U.S. Department of Health and Human Services and National Heart, Lung and Blood Institute Data Fact Sheet: *Asthma Statistics, May 1992.*

Someone with asthma can bring it on any time s/he wants.

It is possible that a person may knowingly and willingly expose his or herself to something that can induce attacks, or may respond in certain situations with hyperventilation or overexertion. Whether a patient can precipitate an attack purely through thought processes is unproven. However, thoughts can initiate behaviors that may produce an asthmatic attack.

Asthma results from a faulty mother-child relationship.

This myth is found throughout psychological literature. In some cases, the mother-child relationship is psychologically unhealthy and contributes to the asthma but is not the cause. However, in many cases the mother-child relationship is psychologically healthy, and may assist in controlling the asthma.

Asthma does not require medical attention.

Unfortunately, many people still do not view asthma, especially in children, as an ailment that needs a doctor's care. They believe it can be treated with a variety of home remedies. Some of these folk "cures" presently in use in the United States include: rubbing tomato paste on the chest; petting a Chihuahua in a certain direction; a diet of chicken livers; drinking one's own urine; standing on one's head; and boiling herbs so the odor permeates the room. It is particularly sad when such useless rituals are the only treatments given to asthmatic children.

A child with asthma can have any short-haired pet.

True allergic reactions to animals are caused by dander—the small scales from an animal's skin—not its fur. Thus, if a person with asthma has an animal dander allergy, s/he should avoid animals of that species, even those with short hair.

Moving to another part of the country will cure your asthma.

Many asthmatic patients, or their parents, follow this advice and uproot themselves to settle in a different section of the country. A few may find relief if their asthma is due to local environmental factors; most do not.

Asthma Statistics

Asthma is a serious chronic condition, affecting almost 12 million Americans. People with asthma experience well over 100 million days of restricted activity annually, and costs for asthma care exceed $4.6 billion a year.

> The National Heart, Lung, and Blood Institute has initiated the National Asthma Education Program (NAEP) to educate asthma patients, health professionals, and the public about asthma and its treatment. To assist in planning and evaluation of the NAEP, and to encourage program planners, health administrators, and others to become more involved in asthma education, the NAEP has developed this information on Asthma Statistics to indicate the magnitude of the problem.

Prevalence

Asthma is much more prevalent among children than adults. Of the 12 million Americans that have asthma, about 4 million of them are under the age of 18. In 1989, the prevalence of asthma among persons under 18 was 6.1 percent compared with 4.8 percent among all other age groups (Figure 41.1). Overall, there is little difference in asthma prevalence by sex (almost 5 percent for both men and women). The percent of Blacks with asthma is higher than the percent of Whites with the condition (5.3 vs. 4.7 percent, respectively).

The reported prevalence of asthma is increasing. Between 1979 and 1989, the percent of the population with asthma increased by 60 percent (Figure 41.2). This represents an increase in prevalence from 3 percent of the population in 1979 to 4.8 percent in 1989. Increases in the prevalence of asthma have been reported in all age, race, and sex groups.

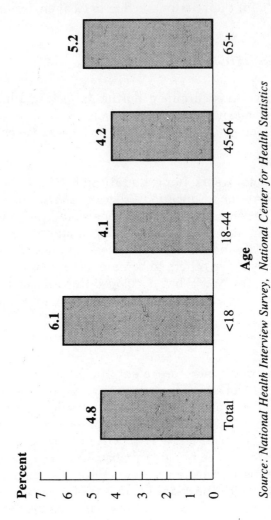

Figure 41.1. Prevalence of Asthma by Age, 1989

Source: National Health Interview Survey, National Center for Health Statistics

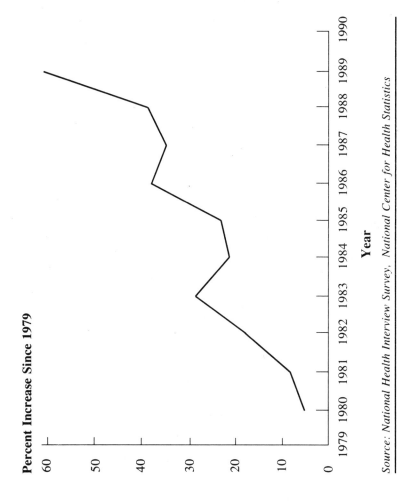

Figure 41.2. Trends in Asthma Prevalence: Percent Increase Since 1979

Percent Increase Since 1979

Source: National Health Interview Survey, National Center for Health Statistics

Physician Visits

In 1988 there were almost 15 million visits to physicians for asthma. About 35 percent of these visits were made by patients under 20 years of age. Figure 41.3 shows the distribution of physician visits for asthma according to the patients' age.

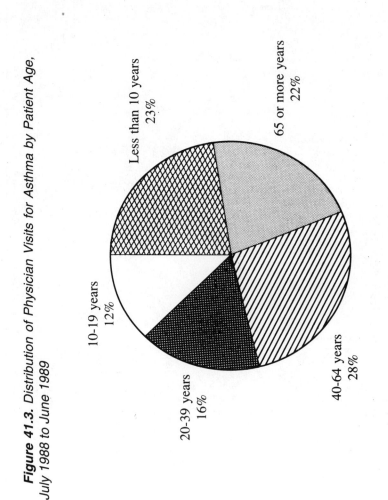

Figure 41.3. *Distribution of Physician Visits for Asthma by Patient Age, July 1988 to June 1989*

Less than 10 years 23%

65 or more years 22%

10-19 years 12%

20-39 years 16%

40-64 years 28%

Source: National Disease and Therapeutic Index, IMS America, Ltd.

Hospitalizations

In 1989, there were over 479,000 hospitalizations in which asthma was the first-listed diagnosis. Hospitalizations for asthma have been increasing among children. For example, from 1979 to 1989, the hospital discharge rate with asthma as the first-listed diagnosis rose 56 percent among children less than 15 years of age, from 19.8 to 30.9 discharges per 10,000 population (Figure 41.4).

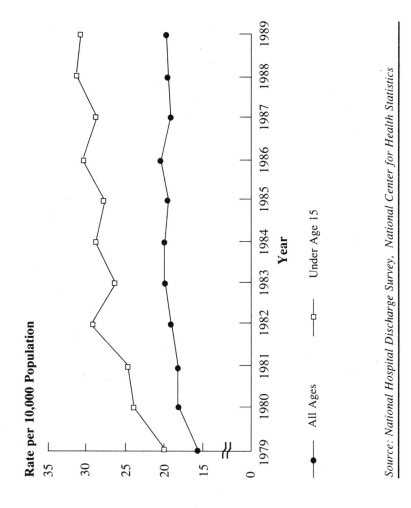

Figure 41.4. *Trends in Hospitalizations for Asthma*

Source: National Hospital Discharge Survey, National Center for Health Statistics

Mortality

In 1989, 5,150 people died from asthma in the United States. Asthma mortality has increased slightly over the past decade. The greatest increase in the asthma death rate has occurred in those older than 65 years of age.

In 1979, Blacks of both sexes were about twice as likely to die from asthma as Whites. Over the past decade this ratio has increased, and by 1988 the asthma death rate was almost three times greater among Blacks than Whites (Figure 41.5).

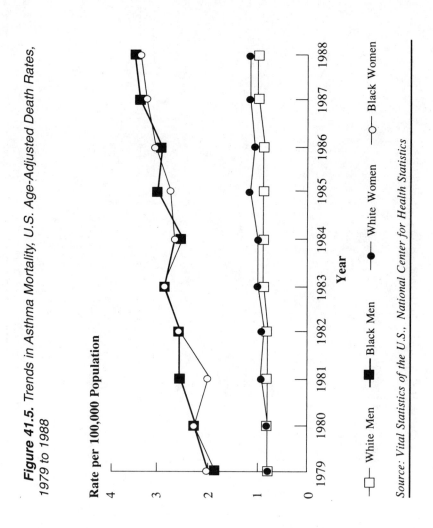

Figure 41.5. *Trends in Asthma Mortality, U.S. Age-Adjusted Death Rates, 1979 to 1988*

Source: Vital Statistics of the U.S., National Center for Health Statistics

Chapter 42

Asthma Mechanisms in Allergy

Not Just an Allergy

Millions of Americans suffer from asthma. For many of these individuals, the disease imposes the need for frequent visits to physicians and emergency rooms, constant medication, and restricted activity. In 1987, asthma was responsible for more than 4,000 deaths. In addition, asthma mortality rates are rising among non-Whites, especially inner-city residents.

Asthma is a disease in which an event such as contact with an allergen, viral infection, stress, or exercise triggers an acute asthmatic episode involving inflammation of the airways. Bronchoconstriction and excessive mucus secretion induce wheezing, choking, and varying degrees of suffocation.

Although asthma once was attributed to a dysfunction of nerves or muscles, it now is recognized as an immunologic-based disease. This recognition coincides with a heightened understanding of the immunologic processes of inflammation, including the interactions of cell types, the factors produced by these cells, and the events that trigger their production. Using this knowledge, scientists are developing more precise criteria for defining asthma as well as ways for diagnosing and treating the disease.

Excerpted from NIH Publication No. 91-2414.

Overview

No national data are available for estimating the true incidence of asthma in the United States. Moreover, the estimated number of persons who are affected with asthma varies according to epidemiologic definition of the disease. Data derived from the second National Health and Nutrition Examination Survey (NHANES II) indicate that in 1987 there were 25 million persons in the United States who currently had, or once had, asthma. The prevalence of persons with active asthma is estimated at 7.7 percent of the U.S. population—17.5 million people.

Asthma is associated with significant morbidity among Americans. It is responsible for more than 18 million restricted activity days annually. In 1985, asthma was the reason for 6.5 million visits to the offices of private physicians. Hospitalization rates for the disease appear to be increasing. In 1987, 4,360 reported deaths in the United States were attributed to asthma. Although deaths from asthma among non-Whites are infrequent, they appear to be increasing.

Extensive research findings have significantly altered our views about asthma. In the past, allergic, or "extrinsic," asthma was viewed simply as allergen-induced mast cell degranulation, which resulted in the release of mediators such as histamine and leukotrienes. These mediators, in turn, caused contraction of airway smooth muscle. "Intrinsic" asthma was considered to be a separate entity of unknown etiology. However, research findings now indicate that asthma, in both atopic and non-atopic subjects, is a chronic inflammatory disease that involves many interacting cells, which release a variety of inflammatory mediators. These mediators, in turn, affect several target cells in the airway, resulting in bronchoconstriction, microvascular leakage and edema, hypersecretion of mucus, and stimulation of neural reflexes. Although this response may be initiated in several ways, the inflammatory changes associated with asthma are observed even in patients who are only mildly asthmatic. These changes are characterized by infiltration with eosinophils, lymphocytes, and macrophages as well as shedding of airway epithelial cells. Furthermore, strong evidence indicates that inflammation also underlies bronchial hyper-responsiveness, which is a hallmark of asthma.

However, the precise relationship between airway inflammation, bronchial hyper-responsiveness, and asthmatic symptoms remains unclear. In addition, the standard tests of bronchial responsiveness, such as histamine or methacholine challenge, may not relate as closely to clinical symptoms as previously believed. Therefore, research that addresses these gaps in our basic understanding of asthma remains a high priority.

For the past two decades, immunologic research has been reductionist; that is, it has evaluated cell function, antibodies, interleukins, mediators, and other aspects of the immune system in the test tube and, to some extent, in animal models. However, there are only a few *in vitro* models and a limited number of animal models for studying asthma. To enhance our understanding of how these various systems function *in vivo*, scientists now need to study the ideal model, the human. Pursuit of the research opportunities delineated below should lead to major therapeutic advances in treating and preventing asthma, thus providing the clinical payoff from a previous investment in basic research.

Definition of Asthma

Attempts to define asthma by clinical or physiological criteria generally have failed. Preliminary evidence based primarily on bronchial lavage studies indicates that certain chemical moieties, such as mediators, inflammatory cells, and cytokines, or a combination of these elements, can be useful in defining the presence of asthma. Although a single underlying definition for all persons with asthma probably will remain elusive, it appears likely that different inciting agents encountering different hosts may produce similar pathological changes. Therefore, progress in evaluating new therapeutic advances can occur without objective criteria of definition. In the last two decades, scientists have described the structure and nature of the elements that are involved in asthma and have learned to measure them in clinically relevant situations. It now appears that this information can provide the basis for an objective assessment of persons with this disease.

Research Opportunity

- Develop biochemical criteria that will establish a diagnosis of asthma.

The Prevalence and Pathogenesis of Asthma

Evidence in the United States and the rest of the world indicates that the morbidity and mortality attributable to asthma are increasing, despite advances in medical care. To counter the rising incidence of disease, scientists first must define the prevalence of asthma in different populations. Recent research suggests that allergy, or IgE-related pathogenic events, may play an important role in asthma. In addition, viral infections appear to play a significant role in the pathogenesis of childhood asthma. Further study is needed to elucidate the emerging roles of allergy and infection in the disease.

Research Opportunities

- Define the prevalence of asthma in different populations by applying objective measures to appropriate patient populations.

- Elucidate the role of atopy and infection in the pathogenesis of asthma.

In vivo *Analysis of Inflammation In Asthmatic Patients*

Strong evidence indicates an inflammatory basis to asthma, rather than a pathogenesis based on dysfunction of nerves or muscle. Moreover, invasive techniques have permitted *in vivo* measurements in humans of each of the elements that are involved in asthma. Researchers now need to determine the combinations of inflammatory processes that lead to both the pathological and physiological changes that are noted in the disease. Specifically, scientists need to measure changes in cell surface markers that indicate activation of inflammatory cells and to define cell surface characteristics of infiltrating lymphocytes.

Research Opportunity

- Define the inflammatory cells, mediators, cytokines, and neuropeptides that are responsible for asthma symptomatology and bronchial reactivity, using primarily invasive techniques such as bronchial lavage and biopsy.

Therapeutic Modalities

Despite the evidence that there is an inflammatory basis for asthma, scientists have not yet begun to understand the immediate and long-term effects of appropriate drugs on each of the pathological changes that characterize asthma. After defining the mediators that are present during clinical disease, researchers have been able to develop receptor antagonists, which will allow further elucidation of the role of each mediator. Drugs such as steroids alter, or affect the function of, the infiltrating cells. By studying the effects of these drugs, scientists should be able to determine the role of each cell in the pathogenesis of asthma.

Research Opportunity

- Define the effects of anti-inflammatory drugs (e.g., steroids, cromolyn sodium cytotoxic agents, and enzyme inhibitors) as well as new receptor-blocking antagonists on the inflammatory cells, mediators, cytokines, and other elements involved in asthma; determine how these elements influence the progression of the disease.

Bibliography

Adelroth, E.; Hargreave, F.E.; Ramsdale, E.H. Do physicians need objective measurements to diagnose asthma? *American Review of Respiratory Disease* 134: 704-707, 1986.

Beasley, R.; Roche, W.R.; Roberts, J.A.; Holgate, S.T. Cellular events in the bronchi in mild asthma and after provocation. *American Review of Respiratory Disease* 139: 806-817, 1989.

Businco, I.; Cantani, A.; Farinella, F.; Businco, E. Month of birth and grass pollen or mite sensitization in children with respiratory allergy: a significant relationship. *Clinical Allergy* 18: 269-274, 1988.

Evans, R. III; Mullally, D.I.; Wilson, R.W.; Gergen, P.J.; Rosenberg, H.M.; Grauman, J.S.; Chevarley, F.M.; Feinleib, M. National trends in the morbidity and mortality of asthma in the United

States. Prevalence, hospitalization and death from asthma over two decades: 1965-1984. *Chest* 91: 65-74, 1987.

Frigas, E.; Gleich, G.J. The eosinophil and the pathophysiology of asthma. *Journal of Allergy and Clinical Immunology* 77: 527-537, 1986.

Gergen, P.J.; Mullally, D.I.; Evans, R. III. National survey of prevalence of asthma among children in the United States. 1976 to 1980. *Pediatrics* 81: 1-7, 1980.

Holgate, S.T.; Finnerty, J.P. Recent (1988) advances in understanding the pathogenesis of asthma and its clinical implications. *Quarterly Journal of Medicine* 66: 5-19, 1988.

Kay, A.B.; Hensen, P.M.; Hunninglake, G.W.; Irvin, C.; Lichtenstein, L.M.; Nadel, J.A. The role of inflammatory processes in airway hyper-responsiveness. In: *Cellular Mechanisms*, edited by S.T. Holgate. Oxford: Blackwell Scientific, p. 151, 1989.

Pearlman, D.S. Bronchial asthma. A perspective from childhood to adulthood. *American Journal of Childhood Diseases* 138: 459-466, 1984.

Sly, R.M. Mortality from asthma. *Journal of Allergy and Clinical Immunology* 82: 705-717, 1988.

Chapter 43

Asthma by Age Group

Childhood Asthma

Raising an asthmatic child can be both trying and heart-rending. As with any child suffering from a chronic disease, the youngster may be irritable, whiny, and easily exhausted. As the child grows older and enters school, new problems may arise. Absenteeism among asthmatic children is very high. Children with acute respiratory conditions, including asthma, lose 128,694,000 school days each year. This accounts for 61.3 percent of the total school days lost (209,781,000) because of illness or injury.

The pattern of absenteeism for children with asthma is also significant. Frequent, brief absences are more harmful academically than occasional long ones. And frequent absences are typical for many youngsters with asthma. As a result, they often fall behind healthier classmates and must constantly strive to "catch up." Frequent absences also hinder a child in learning the basic skills and work habits essential to success in school.

In addition, there may be limited participation in class outings, physical education, botany, and other classes that involve environmental stimuli that may trigger asthma attacks or other allergic reactions. In some instances, the child handicapped by asthma is further isolated by being assigned to special education classes or home-bound programs.

Excerpted from NIH Pub No. 80-388, and "Asthma Among the Elderly." ©Asthma and Allergy Foundation of America. Reprinted with permission.

451

Parents, and especially the mother, may find themselves fatigued and disheartened from the constant care and vigilance required by an asthmatic child. Hours may be spent housecleaning and preparing special diets to eliminate potential **allergens.** Finally, the parents must face their own frustrations about the little time they have for their own interests, activities, and friends, and the career implications of raising an asthmatic child. A promotion or overseas assignment may have to be declined because of inadequate medical care or an unfavorable geographic location. Many parents but especially women are forced to abandon or delay their own career or educational plans to care for a child with asthma or hay fever.

The brothers and sisters of an asthmatic child are affected also. They may feel jealous about the extra attention given to the sick child, or they may be overly anxious and tense about their sibling's health. Many youngsters develop guilt feelings because they assume they are responsible when an asthma attack occurs while they are playing with their asthmatic sibling. Some accept an excessively protective role and sacrifice normal childhood pleasures for the afflicted youngster.

Asthma in Adults

The problems of asthma are not limited to childhood. Adults with asthma and other allergic diseases find their lives affected. For example, asthma and hay fever are the third leading cause of restricted activity in persons under 45, and the fifth, for persons of all ages in this country. Asthma alone accounts for more than 90.5 million days of restricted activity each year. Social Security benefits of $400 million were allowed in just one year to workers disabled by asthma and other chronic respiratory diseases.

Asthma and hay fever have other work-related ramifications. For example, a worker usually must avoid jobs that entail exposure to tasks or substances that are likely to trigger an asthma attack or allergic reaction. Asthma also may limit promotion possibilities because the employer knows the worker may have to leave his job suddenly because of an attack.

Asthma Among the Elderly

Past "common knowledge" has had it that asthma is rare in the elderly. Today, we know this is not so.

A survey of the prevalence of asthma in Great Britain and Wales, for example, reported a broad increase in the illness among all age groups, more than doubling between 1955 and 1981 to 17.8 cases per 1,000. For people age 55 and above, the incidence of asthma grew faster than in other age groups.

Uncovering the Prevalence of Asthma in the Elderly

With the older segment increasing as a percentage of the American population over the foreseeable future, recognizing and dealing with asthma as a significant illness in the elderly will become an important challenge. About one-third of all asthma cases occur before the age of 16. The next peak in prevalence is usually seen in the third decade of life. Approximately 10 percent of asthma cases appear after age 65. About 20 percent of adults whose childhood asthma symptoms "disappeared" once they reached adulthood experience recurrence of the symptoms once past their mid-40s.

One interesting study of a group of elderly men and women suggests the actual magnitude of unrecognized and/or untreated asthma in this age group. Among 199 men and women living in a residential center, 128 (64 percent) had peak flow rates under 70 percent of the rate predicted for their age. Eighty-two percent improved their rates by at least 15 percent after being treated with an aerosol bronchodilator. However, only six percent of the entire group were receiving any medications for their respiratory disorders. It is becoming obvious that the estimate of 10 percent of people with asthma in the over 65 age group is too low.

Diagnostic Difficulties

Asthma in the elderly can range from mild and occasional episodes of attacks to chronic and life threatening illness. The disease can be difficult to pin-point in the elderly because there is usually a lack of the associated allergic conditions that makes diagnosis more easily

---

"Asthma Among the Elderly." ©Asthma and Allergy Foundation of America. Reprinted with permission.

recognizable in young people. For instance, chronic bronchitis, common in older patients, shares many symptoms with asthma and further complicates the diagnosis. There are several other reasons that explain why asthma is difficult to recognize in the elderly. One has to do with their relatively inactive lifestyles, causing asthma to be clinically associated with chronic cough and sputum production rather than with episodes of wheezing and breathing difficulty. As a result, some physicians may incorrectly make a diagnosis of chronic bronchitis, congestive heart failure, or other conditions which often coexist in the elderly. But changes in the lungs of elderly asthmatics are quite different from those associated with chronic bronchitis. For example, sputum from elderly individuals with asthma typically contains large amounts of eosinophils, a type of cell involved in the inflammation of lung tissue during asthma episodes. Also, when pulmonary function tests are performed on elderly patients, those with asthma have findings that are typical of airway obstruction. These patients then respond well to bronchodilator therapy.

Even if asthma is suspected in the elderly, poor compliance may prevent confirming the condition by home measurement of peak flow and bronchodilator therapy testing. Monitoring peak flow is important for the elderly person with asthma because it is easily performed and less likely to cause fatigue, a cause of unreliable pulmonary function results.

The elderly asthmatic patient presents several problems for the treatment of his or her disease. The cause of asthma may more often be related to recurring respiratory tract infections than to allergies. While asthma classically occurs as sudden attacks, in the elderly patient a chronic cough and breathlessness may be the major complaint. Night-time asthma problems present a special concern for the elderly. Yet, sleep disturbances may seem typical and too easily dismissed as a condition related to genital-urinary tract problems. Likewise, a constricted feeling in the chest and shortness of breath can easily be attributed to cardiologic problems.

Because of the complex health issues many elderly people experience, a careful diagnosis of asthma should include examination for respiratory tract infection, bronchitis, sinusitis, congestive heart failure, pulmonary embolism, chronic bronchitis and emphysema. Certainly, someone with chronic asthma will experience worsened symptoms if there is also a respiratory infection or a developing cardiac disease.

Treating the Elderly Asthma Patient

Treating the elderly asthma patient with drugs may be difficult for a variety of reasons:

- Other existing diseases may reduce tolerance to the stress imposed by an asthma attack.

- Medications being taken for other diseases may complicate treatment for asthma. For example, treatment of glaucoma with beta blockers may increase asthma symptoms.

- The elderly patient may become confused by the multiple drug therapy that is required, then fail to comply completely with directions.

- Mental confusion or an organic mental syndrome can also interfere with compliance with medication directions.

The ideal approach to drug therapy for most elderly people with asthma is for the physician to create an individualized treatment plan that accounts for the realities of the patient's needs. Treatment requirements should be designed with goals of controlling swelling of the membrane that lines the airways, bronchospasm, excessive secretion of mucus, and airway inflammation. To increase convenience, long-acting drug therapy is a worthwhile ideal. For example, a long-lasting oral theophylline medication may be the ideal initial drug to use to treat the elderly asthma patient. If this fails to bring relief, an inhaled bronchodilator medicine can be added with a maximum dose of two puffs four times a day.

Theophylline may be more acceptable to older patients with heart disease and musculoskeletal problems than other bronchodilating medications, since they are less likely to cause rapid heartbeat, tremor, or anxiety. Simple and reliable techniques to measure theophylline concentration in the patient's blood allow the physician to make appropriate adjustments to the dosage schedule. Nevertheless, the physician must be aware of the various factors that can influence theophylline metabolism, since the line between safe and effective use and sometimes dangerous toxicity is relatively slim. For example, when certain other medications are being used to combat viral and bacteriological infections, liver disease, obesity, and congestive heart

455

failure, the rate at which theophylline is cleared from the body can be slowed. Conversely, theophylline clearance can become too rapid as a result of tobacco smoking and high protein diets.

To control acute asthma flares, short periods of oral steroid therapy will normally be effective. Long-term oral steroid therapy should be avoided in the elderly asthma patient because of possible severe side effects, including bone deterioration (osteoporosis), ulcers, hyperglycemia (too much glucose in the blood), and high blood pressure (hypertension). It is absolutely essential for the elderly asthma patient to demonstrate for the physician that he or she is able to take the medications being prescribed. Often, the use of a spacer device will be very important in assuring effective use of an aerosol, since elderly patients may have difficulty in getting the timing right between breathing movements and activating the medication canister. When the patient has an associated arthritis condition, he or she may find it more difficult to use the aerosol canister, thus adding to the value of using a spacer device.

If asthma symptoms appear to be unresponsive to combined drug therapy, a brief course of systemic steroids followed by an added application of inhaled steroids may become necessary.

Should an acute episode of asthma be caused by respiratory infections, antibiotic therapy should begin before the results of any sputum cultures and sensitivity are made available. A broad spectrum antibiotic such as ampicillin is frequently adequate unless there is a history in the patient of penicillin allergy. When sinusitis is present, it too should be treated. If ignored, the sinusitis could transform a brief asthma flare into a chronic, smoldering attack.

Clinically-observed dehydration is also a common problem in any person with asthma, and more dangerous in the elderly patient. This condition should receive prompt treatment by fluid replacement and potassium supplements, if necessary. Should the elderly patient be unable to take adequate amounts of liquids by mouth, then hospitalization may be needed to guarantee proper treatment and speedy recovery.

A certain number of elderly asthma patients may have associated disorders such as hiatus hernia, causing what is commonly referred to as heartburn. Controlling these disorders may ease asthma symptoms as well.

Educating the Elderly Patient

Careful and thoughtful education of the elderly patient about how to use prescribed anti-asthma medications and what to expect from the drugs is very important. Patients' expectations for improved health should be discussed and examined in a realistic light. Patients should acquire a fair understanding of the drugs they are taking and how they work. Moreover, the patient must learn about which drug dosages can be modified without first consulting the physician, and which drugs must be taken according to a strict dosage schedule.

Side effects must also be a matter of frank discussion between the patient and the physician, and it is helpful for the elderly patient to be given simply written and clear information as well.

This information should not substitute for seeking responsible, professional medical care.

—by Howard J. Schwartz, M.D.

Dr. Schwartz, an allergist, is a clinical professor of medicine at Case Western Reserve University in Cleveland, Ohio.

Chapter 44

The Role of Eosinophils in Allergic Lung Reactions

A protein component of white blood cells known as eosinophils may play a direct role in constricting lung airways and in provoking increased airway sensitivity to allergens. These are reactions typically seen in patients with asthma and other allergic lung reactions, according to scientists at the Mayo Medical School in Rochester, Minnesota, and Boehringer Ingelheim Pharmaceuticals in Ridgefield, Connecticut. Their studies suggest that eosinophils are not beneficial in allergic reactions, as had been hypothesized, but rather are part of the problem, says Dr. Robert H. Gundel, principal scientist at the pulmonary inflammation laboratory, Boehringer Ingelheim Pharmaceuticals.

The Research

Dr. Gundel and Dr. Gerald J. Gleich, professor of immunology and medicine at the Mayo Medical School, Mayo Clinic and Foundation, collaborated to examine the effects of injecting purified proteins produced by human eosinophils directly into the tracheas, or windpipes, of anesthetized monkeys. The proteins are known as granule proteins because they combine to form microscopic dark-staining granules in the cell. The granule protein known as major basic protein (MBP) produced an immediate temporary constriction of the monkeys' bronchi, the tubes leading to the lungs, as well as a dose-related airway

Research Resources Reporter, March/April 1993.

hyper-responsiveness to inhaled methacholine, a chemical to which the airways of asthmatics are extremely reactive.

"This *in vivo* study shows for the first time that one of the granule proteins from the eosinophil has this biological effect. This is important because, until recently, the role of the eosinophil in asthma was unclear," says Dr. Gundel. Eosinophils are known to congregate in the air passages of asthmatics and release enzymes that reverse some aspects of allergic reactions; however, only in the past few years have the cells also been implicated as contributors to the symptoms of asthma.

Recent studies have shown a correlation between bronchial hyper-activity and increased numbers of airway eosinophils and increased levels of MBP in the lung fluid of primate models for asthma; similar findings were noted in patients with the disease, Dr. Gleich says. All these studies suggested that "some component of the eosinophil must play a role in asthma," he says.

To test this hypothesis, Dr. Gundel and his colleagues studied the ways human eosinophil proteins affected the respiratory tracts of five anesthetized cynomolgus monkeys. The scientists first monitored the animals' baseline airway function and then observed the effects when the monkeys inhaled increasing concentrations of aerosolized methacholine. Each animal subsequently received an intratracheal injection of an inert salt solution or one of the following diluted eosinophil granule proteins: MBP, eosinophil cationic protein, eosinophil peroxidase, or eosinophil-derived neurotoxin. Respiratory responsiveness to inhaled methacholine was monitored at one, two, and four hours after protein injection. In separate experiments extending over several months each animal received intratracheal injections of each of the four purified granule proteins.

Both MBP and eosinophil peroxidase produced an immediate constriction of the airways that was resolved after 60 minutes, the scientists say, but only MBP induced hyper-responsiveness to inhaled methacholine. The increased airway sensitivity to methacholine developed two hours after MBP was injected and returned to baseline values by four hours. The other eosinophil granule proteins tested had no effect on airway sensitivity or function. The investigators suggest that MBP may induce the release of chemical mediators that alter the responsiveness of the muscles of the airway and contribute to asthma and other inflammatory airway diseases.

"It is also interesting to note that MBP can cause hyper-responsiveness at subcytotoxic doses," Dr. Gundel says. Until recently, he says, these biological effects were believed to be related to the destruction of the cells lining the airway. However, in the primate study, hyper-responsiveness began two hours after the animals were exposed to the irritant and returned to normal after four hours, which suggests that no such cell deaths occurred.

Preventing or Reversing the Toxic Effects of MBP

The scientists recently completed a follow-up study that demonstrates how the toxic effects of MBP might be prevented or at least reversed. The investigators successfully blocked MBP toxicity in monkeys by pretreating the animals with polyglutamic acid aerosol inhalations. Because MBP has a very basic pH, the scientists speculated that a specific inhibitor of MBP—one that is as acidic as MBP is basic—might play a role in counteracting the toxicity of MBP. According to Dr. Gundel, an acidic subsection of newly synthesized MBP may initially neutralize the protein's toxicity, but this subsection and the protection it affords may be lost when MBP is incorporated into the eosinophil granule. Although the acidic subsection has not yet been isolated, Dr. Gundel and his colleagues were able to use polyglutamic acid to mimic its neutralizing action.

The researchers are now pursuing another approach that may lead to a new drug therapy for asthma. Knowing that MBP initially has a neutral pH, Dr. Gleich and his coworkers are looking for the enzyme responsible for cleaving off the acidic section of MBP. Once this enzyme has been identified, the scientists hope to find an inhibitor to block the enzyme's action, and the inhibitor may be used to treat patients who have asthma.

"To cure asthma one must deal not only with the broncho-constricting effects associated with the disease but also with the inflammation that is produced," says Dr. Gundel, whose area of expertise is inflammation. Some of his current research addresses the questions of how and why eosinophils enter the bronchi, release their toxic proteins, and alter airway function.

Several investigators are now studying the role played by T cells, a type of white blood cell that produces several substances that affect the activation of eosinophils. Dr. Gundel likens the T cell to a general who gives eosinophils their marching orders. "There are two possible approaches to therapy: We could look for inhibitors that will block the harmful effects of eosinophils once they are already in the

461

bronchi, or we could try to modulate T-cell function to block the release of substances that call for the release of eosinophils. The latter may be a better approach to therapy," he says.

Dr. Gundel and his colleagues are now examining substances called cytokines that are released by T cells and act as chemical messengers between cells. According to Dr. Gundel, cytokines promote growth and differentiation of eosinophils in bone marrow and activate those cells already present in the circulation and tissues. In patients with asthma certain cytokines are found in elevated numbers.

"Asthma has not been an easy disease to understand," says Dr. Gleich. In more than two decades of studying asthma, it took ten years to realize that the eosinophil is not beneficial, he says, and another decade to show how the eosinophil causes harm. "This work is a landmark in a long odyssey of work dealing with eosinophilia," he says.

Dr. Gleich speculates that the results of this study may have implications for understanding other inflammatory diseases. He hypothesizes that the MBP manufactured by eosinophils may produce similar effects in other organs, including the eye, the nose, the gastrointestinal tract, and possibly the bladder. "The mechanisms we observed in the lungs may also occur in other parts of the body. This granule protein may prove to be quite important," he says.

Additional Reading

1. Barker, R. L., Gundel, R. H., Gleich, G. J., et al., Acid polyamino acids inhibit human eosinophil granule major protein toxicity. *Journal of Clinical Investigation* 88:798-805, 1991.

2. Gundel, R. H., Letts, L. G., and Gleich, G. J., Human eosinophil major basic protein induces airway constriction and airway hyper-responsiveness in primates. *Journal of Clinical Investigation* 87:1470-1473, 1991.

3. Gundel, R. H., Gerritsen, M. E., Gleich, G. J., and Wegner, C. D., Repeated antigen inhalation results in a prolonged airway eosinophilia and airway hyper-responsiveness in primates. *Journal of Applied Physiology* 68:779-786, 1990.

4. Gundel, R. H., Gerritsen, M. E., and Wegner, C. D., Antigen-coated sepharose beads induce airway eosinophilia and airway

hyper-responsiveness in cynomolgus monkeys. *American Review of Respiratory Disease* 140:629-633, 1989.

The research described in this chapter was supported by the General Clinical Research Centers Program of the National Center for Research Resources, the National Institute of Allergy and Infectious Diseases, and the Mayo Foundation.

—*by L. Anne Hirschel, D.D.S*

Chapter 45

Research for the Future: Asthma and Allergic Diseases

Introduction

Allergic diseases were once brushed off as "just allergies," but we are now realizing the significant role that they play in the health and quality of life of people in this country and around the world. Among the major causes of chronic illness and disability in the United States, allergic diseases, including asthma, may affect as many as 50 million Americans, or one in five people. The economic burden of these diseases is staggering. For example, asthma was estimated to cost more than 6.2 billion health care dollars in 1990.

The National Institute of Allergy and Infectious Diseases (NIAID), a component of the National Institutes of Health, stands at the forefront of scientific research on allergic and immunologic diseases. NIAID scientists and those supported by NIAID are working to prevent a broad spectrum of disorders of the immune system, including asthma and allergies.

Until prevention is possible, an intermediate goal of the Institute's research programs is to determine how allergic diseases develop and to improve diagnosis and treatment. Achieving this goal will help reduce the impact these diseases have on health and quality of life as well as reduce the economic burden imposed on individuals, families, and the health care system.

NIH Publication No. 93-493.

At NIAID laboratories in Bethesda, Maryland, scientists are conducting basic and clinical investigations on asthma and allergic diseases. NIAID's Division of Allergy, Immunology, and Transplantation provides research grant, contract, and cooperative agreement support to scientists at universities and other research institutions throughout the United States.

Asthma

Epidemiology

Asthma is a serious respiratory disorder that affects an estimated 10 to 15 million people and claims more than 4,000 lives in the United States each year. Despite our increased knowledge about asthma, the epidemiology of this disease in the United States presents a dismal picture. During the last decade, the prevalence of asthma cases, hospitalizations, and deaths has been increasing. For example, in 1987 twice as many children and adults, ages 5 to 34, died from asthma than in 1969.

The statistics are particularly grim in minority populations in the United States. Non-Whites are almost three times as likely as Whites to die from asthma. A higher percentage of African Americans have asthma than do Whites. Minorities living in the inner cities seem to be at particular risk for developing asthma. For example, the rates of asthma among Puerto Rican children living in the New York City area are among the highest in the United States.

Socioeconomics

Of the $6.2 billion spent by Americans in 1990 on asthma-related care, almost $1.6 billion was for hospital care. Another $1 billion was spent on medications to treat and control asthma symptoms. Americans also lose billions of dollars in wages because of asthma-related problems. A recent study found that school absenteeism costs an estimated $1 billion in lost pay for parents who stayed home to care for asthmatic children. Adult asthmatics who stayed home from work because of illness lost wages amounting to $850 million.

Social factors influence the rising incidence of asthma, although the magnitude of these influences has not yet been determined. Certain factors, including poverty, family problems, inadequate treatment, and lack of access to health care, probably increase an asthma patient's risk of having a severe asthma attack or, more tragically, of dying from asthma.

Although good, consistent medical attention can reduce asthma-related hospitalizations, there are 500,000 asthma-related hospital admissions each year in the United States, with a higher percentage of African Americans and Hispanics being hospitalized than Whites. In New York City, for example, asthma-related hospitalizations and deaths cluster in poor, predominantly minority neighborhoods where there is often a lack of adequate primary health care.

Environmental factors can also adversely affect people with asthma. An example is indoor tobacco smoke, a well-known respiratory irritant that can cause serious problems for asthma patients. Asthmatic children with parents who smoke are at particular risk of suffering from the effects of inhaling second-hand tobacco smoke. The percentage of Americans who smoke cigarettes has been steadily decreasing, but smoking continues to remain highest among individuals who often have the least access to good health care.

Allergic Diseases

In the United States, an estimated 40 to 50 million people suffer from allergies. An estimated 33 million people have chronic sinusitis, the most prevalent allergy-related disease. Pollen allergy, commonly called hay fever, affects an estimated 19 million Americans and prompts 8 million office visits to physicians. Food allergies are believed to occur in 8 percent of children younger than 3 years old. In addition, each year billions of dollars are spent on treating allergic diseases in the United States.

When an allergic person comes in contact with an allergen (allergy-provoking substance), cells of the immune system produce an unusual class of antibody (disease-fighting protein). This class of antibody is called immunoglobulin E, or IgE, and it starts the classic allergic response. Among allergic individuals, how and to what extent their immune systems respond to a particular allergen is influenced by genetic as well as environmental factors.

While allergic reactions to airborne allergens such as pollen, mold, or dust usually cause relatively minor discomfort, sensitivity to substances such as penicillin, insect venom, or peanuts can cause anaphylaxis, a serious and potentially fatal allergic reaction. Anaphylactic reactions to penicillin are responsible for an estimated one to eight deaths per million population. An estimated one to two million people experience severe allergic reactions to insect stings each year. Moreover, severe, life-threatening allergic reactions to food may occur as frequently as those to insect stings.

Research

Although a variety of therapies have been developed to treat asthma and allergies, we still do not fully understand certain critical aspects of these diseases. To develop more effective therapies and devise methods for preventing these illnesses, researchers are attempting to discern how the immune system recognizes an allergen, why people respond differently to allergens, as well as what environmental, genetic, and other factors might be responsible for allergic diseases.

Allergy to latex has become an increasingly important health problem, especially among medical personnel who wear latex gloves to reduce exposure to human immunodeficiency virus (HIV), which causes AIDS, and hepatitis B virus. Although we know proteins derived from latex cause allergic reactions, better understanding of the structure and immunologic function of these proteins would help scientists devise ways to eliminate the cause of these potentially dangerous reactions.

NIAID-funded scientists have been at the forefront of discoveries and advances in the field of allergy. They were the first to identify the IgE antibody that is the key to the allergic response. NIAID intramural investigators and NIAID-supported investigators have now identified the complete structure of the IgE receptor, the molecule on the surface of mast cells and basophils to which IgE antibodies attach. (Mast cells in the tissues and basophils in the blood are cells that together cause allergy symptoms.) Blocking the function of the IgE receptor may eventually lead to a new therapy for allergies. Investigators have studied the events that occur after allergic reactions are initiated by allergen binding to IgE antibody on mast cells and basophils. Perhaps the most important breakthrough in studying allergic reactions is the identification by NIAID investigators of the biologic events responsible for the late phase reaction (LPR). LPR usually occurs four to six hours after an allergen has entered the body. The discovery that these late reactions involve inflammatory cells and that they resemble allergic reactions has led to the recent recognition that inflammation is a central feature of allergic diseases and asthma. This knowledge has provided a significant focus to asthma research—how the inflammation is produced, how it is regulated, and how it can be prevented. In addition, NIAID investigators discovered that inhaled corticosteroids inhibit LPR. That discovery contributed to the growing use of these drugs to successfully treat both allergy and asthma. The inflammatory process is highly complex, but the insights that have emerged highlight and expand this exciting area of research. One major key to this process is a group of powerful chemicals called cytokines, which are produced by certain cells of the immune system and which help regulate cell growth and function, including IgE antibody production and allergic and asthmatic inflammation. Substantial progress has been made recently in understanding how these chemicals are involved in most aspects of the development and function of inflammation.

Research studies have opened the door for developing promising alternative and innovative therapies such as new anti-inflammatory drugs and agents that block the actions of cytokines.

Research and the Community

National Cooperative Inner-City Asthma Study

The NIAID-supported National Cooperative Inner-City Asthma Study (NCICAS) is composed of eight units in seven cities that are studying the unusually high morbidity rates of asthma in inner-city children.

The objective of NCICAS phase I is to identify modifiable factors determining asthma severity and morbidity among inner-city children. A number of interesting findings have emerged from pilot studies. For example, allergen surveys of more than 80 inner-city homes revealed that cockroaches may be a more important trigger of asthma in this population than are house dust mites.

NCICAS is also evaluating the use of peak flow meters, plastic devices that can be used by patients at home to monitor their breathing. (Because of airflow obstruction in the lungs, asthmatics have trouble breathing air out.) From the patient's monitoring records, the doctor can tell when a person is doing well and when to take action, such as increasing medication to forestall trouble. The peak flow meter pilot studies showed that a two-week monitoring of the variability of peak air flow can be successfully and accurately carried out.

In addition, an innovative technique has been developed to measure the quality of asthma care delivered in inner-city emergency rooms.

Demonstration and Education Projects

To reduce asthma morbidity, Demonstration and Education (D & E) projects develop innovative ways to apply existing knowledge and programs. The main objectives of the projects are to teach better self-management skills to those with asthma and to increase asthma knowledge among health care providers.

Two school-based D & E projects involve new self-management skills. One project, carried out by investigators at Scripps Clinic in San Diego, California, is concerned with developing asthma intervention protocols in fourth through sixth graders in a predominantly Hispanic school district. The other, based at Johns Hopkins University in Baltimore, Maryland, is studying new evaluation tools for asthma in 13- to 18-year-olds in a predominantly African-American school district. In addition, a clinic-based project, a computer-driven asthma education aid for children, is in the final stages of development at Children's Hospital in Boston, Massachusetts. This program will teach asthma management skills to African-American asthma patients under age 15.

Asthma, Allergy, and Immunologic Diseases Cooperative Research Centers (AAIDCRCs)

NIAID established the Asthma, Allergy, and Immunologic Diseases Cooperative Research Centers (AAIDCRCs) to promote interaction among basic and clinical researchers and to enhance outreach and demonstration activities. These centers encourage close coordination between scientists studying fundamental concepts of immunology, genetics, biochemistry, and pharmacology and clinical investigators who treat allergic individuals. This approach will lead to both a better understanding of the complex mechanisms underlying asthma and allergies and the clinical application of this knowledge. Various allergic problems are under investigation at the AAIDCRCs: asthma; skin diseases, such as atopic dermatitis; urticaria; angioedema; and allergic reactions caused by insect stings, foods, drugs, and airborne allergens.

Studies also focus on the basic mechanisms involved in immune system function and reactions, including research on antibodies, particularly IgE, and on the inflammation-inducing chemicals released during an allergic attack.

Future

The remarkable advances during the last ten years in our understanding of the structure and functions of the immune system are paving the way to an exciting and hopeful future for diagnosing, treating, and preventing asthma and allergic diseases.

Recent discoveries using modern molecular technology are providing a stimulus for allergic disease research. For example, scientists have developed a genetically altered mouse that produces large amounts of the cytokine interleukin-4 (IL4). Such mice express an inflammatory response in several tissues that resembles human allergic inflammation, and they also can produce large amounts of IgE antibody. This type of approach will lead to a clearer understanding of which genes are responsible for allergic responses.

We are now beginning to understand how cytokines regulate the production of adhesion molecules that bind inflammatory cells to the sites of allergic disease, such as the nose, skin, and lungs. These and other findings suggest that molecules directed against critical targets in the allergic process—such as cytokines and adhesion molecules—may lead to a new means of therapy to better treat asthma and allergic diseases.

One of the most exciting areas of research involves unraveling the genetic mysteries of asthma and allergic diseases in conjunction with studying how allergens and other environmental factors induce these diseases. By identifying the genes responsible for them, prenatal diagnostic tests could be developed to identify persons at risk for allergic disease. This early diagnostic knowledge could be used to manipulate the environment or to start early intervention therapy, thereby eliminating or altering the severity of the disease process in these individuals. Thus, the overall quality of life would be greatly improved for these patients.

Recent studies in understanding how and why the immune systems of allergic individuals produce IgE antibodies to allergens may lead to innovative vaccine therapy. In preliminary clinical trials, scientists are evaluating an approach that could stop the immune system from responding to allergens. Called **peptide-induced anergy,** this process could be the "allergy shot" of the future. Finally, researchers are working to better understand the actions of the cells and molecules associated with the inflammatory process in asthma and allergic diseases. Knowing more precisely how these cells travel to the site of inflammation in the lungs, nose, gastrointestinal tract, or skin should pave the way for new drugs that block this cascade of events.

471

With the quickening pace of research on asthma and allergic diseases and on the immune system, we may be able to cure—or even prevent—these chronic, often severe, and sometimes life-threatening diseases by the end of the decade.

Information Resources

Allergy and Asthma Network/Mothers of Asthmatics, Inc.
3554 Chain Bridge Road, Suite 200
Fairfax, VA 22030
1-800-878-4403

American Academy of Allergy and Immunology
611 East Wells Street
Milwaukee, WI 53202
1-800-822-ASMA

American College of Allergy and Immunology
800 E. Northwest Highway
Suite 1080
Palatine, IL 60067
708-359-2800

American College of Chest Physicians
3300 Dundee Road
Northbrook, IL 60062-2340
708-498-1400

American Lung Association
American Thoracic Society
1740 Broadway
New York, NY 10019-4374
212-315-8700

Asthma and Allergy Foundation of America
1125 15th Street, N.W., Suite 502
Washington, DC 20005
1-800-7-ASTHMA

National Asthma Education Program Information Center
P.O. Box 30105
Bethesda, MD 20824-0105
301-251-1222

Part Seven

First Aid for
Allergy Symptoms

Chapter 46

Easing the Itch of the Great Outdoors

On these hot summer days, when the realization dawns that the tiny blisters on legs or arms or wherever can only have come from a brush with poison ivy, there may be some small comfort in knowing that you are not alone. Most Americans are sensitive in some degree to this ubiquitous three-leafed plant. Only about 15 percent of the population is not affected.

Poison ivy and its cousins, poison oak and poison sumac, are responsible for more of those itchy, oozing blisters (a condition known medically as allergic contact dermatitis) than any other cause, including industrial chemicals, household products, and cosmetics. While it may be only a summer annoyance for some, for others poison ivy dermatitis can be disabling and is responsible for a considerable amount of time lost from work. Firefighters are particularly vulnerable. They not only come in contact with the plants themselves, but are exposed to smoke carrying plant particles, which when inhaled can have severe internal as well as external effects.

Despite the toll it takes in discomfort and disability, no one has come up with a way—other than avoidance—to prevent or cure this condition known simply as "poison ivy."

However, there are some things you can do.

Start Treatment Immediately

If you suspect you've gotten into poison ivy, the first thing to do is to thoroughly wash the exposed areas. Washing may not stop the initial

FDA Consumer, June 1986.

outbreak of the rash if too much time has elapsed, but it can help prevent further spread.

Harold Baer, an FDA expert on poison ivy, advises washing with soap. The sap of the ivy and oak plants is very sticky and not very water soluble. Soap helps to break it down so that it can be removed, Baer says. Myth has it that a strong yellow soap is required. Not so, according to Baer. Any soap will do.

Clothing that has picked up the sticky sap should also be washed as soon as possible. Be sure to handle it carefully, with gloves, if necessary, to prevent any more exposure to the sap.

Considering that poison ivy has been recorded since the days of Captain John Smith, it is not surprising that a wealth of home remedies has evolved to treat this dermatitis. Not the least creative— though hardly to be recommended—are bathing in horse urine, cleaning the skin with gasoline or strychnine, and rubbing on a variety of products such as ammonia, hair spray, clear nail polish, meat tenderizer, or mouse-ear herb boiled in milk. The juice of crushed leaves of plantain, a common weed found in many yards, is favored by many hikers today. There is no scientific proof that it works.

When all is said and done, the simplest treatment is still the best. Mild cases of poison ivy may require no more than wet compresses or soaking in cool water to relieve the itching. Dilute aluminum acetate (Burrow's solution), saline (salt), or sodium bicarbonate (baking soda) solutions are often recommended to dry up the oozing blisters.

Oatmeal is a drying agent as well as a cereal. You can buy an oatmeal preparation (*Aveeno*) for use in a bath or make your own by tying up about half a cupful of uncooked oatmeal in a clean cloth, such as a large handkerchief, and soaking it in water. Squeezing releases an oatmeally solution that will help dry up oozing blisters. Be warned, however, that it is messy and can make the tub extra slippery.

A variety of nonprescription drug products is also available to dry up the oozing and weeping blisters. Among the skin protectant ingredients FDA's expert advisors say are safe and effective are aluminum hydroxide gel, calamine, kaolin, zinc acetate, zinc carbonate, and zinc oxide. These ingredients were given the green light by the Advisory Review Panel on OTC Topical Analgesic, Antirheumatic, Otic, Burn, and Sunburn Prevention and Treatment Drug Products, one of 17 panels of outside experts assisting FDA in its massive review of all OTC (over-the-counter) drug products.

The same panel recommended, and FDA has concurred, that hydrocortisone preparations—hydrocortisone 0.25 and 0.5 percent and hydrocortisone acetate 0.25 and 0.5 percent—be used for the temporary relief of itching associated with poison ivy, poison oak, or poison sumac.

Other external analgesics considered by the panel and FDA as safe and effective to relieve itching associated with minor skin irritations include "caine"-type local anesthetics, such as benzocaine, lidocaine or tetracaine; alcohols, including benzyl alcohol, menthol and resorcinol; and the antihistamines diphenhydramine hydrochloride and tripelennamine hydrochloride. (Final standards for skin protectant and external analgesic drug products are under consideration by FDA.)

All these OTC drug products are intended only for the treatment of minor symptoms of poison ivy and should not be used for more than seven days. Some ingredients should not be used over large areas of the body or on raw surfaces or blistered areas and therefore would not be good for poison ivy blisters. A few ingredients are not recommended for use on young children without consulting a doctor. Always check the label of OTC drug products for specific instructions for use.

Severe poison ivy dermatitis should be treated by a doctor, who may prescribe a stronger topical steroid preparation or oral medication to be used for several days. Because side effects can be serious, such treatment is not given lightly.

Preventing poison ivy miseries should be easy—just stay away from plants. However, this is not always possible for those whose work takes them into the woods and fields where the oak and ivy grow. Unfortunately, there are no OTC products that can prevent poison ivy, oak or sumac dermatitis, according to the Advisory Review Panel on OTC Miscellaneous External Drug Products.

Another approach to preventing, or at least lessening, the consequences of poison ivy is desensitization with extracts of the plant itself. American Indians are said to have eaten poison ivy leaves for protection against the sap. This is not a practice to be recommended, however, for a nasty side effect is dermatitis at both ends of the gastrointestinal tract—the mouth and the anus. (The middle portion seems to be immune to these effects.)

Researchers at the University of California, San Francisco, are working on a potential vaccine. They claim to have found a way to neutralize the urushiol molecules, thus eliminating the itching. More testing is needed to see if the vaccine is truly safe and effective.

Because of severe reactions, injections with plant extracts (called **oleoresins**) to prevent poison ivy are not recommended FDA noted in a proposal to establish standards for allergenic products. The proposal was based on the recommendations of the Advisory Panel on Review of Allergenic Extracts. The agency also said no injectable or oral oleoresins should be given once dermatitis has developed, because severe local or systemic reactions may occur.

There is good evidence that oral oleoresins can reduce the severity of the dermatitis—but not prevent it entirely—if the dose is strong enough and it is given for long enough before contact with the plant, said FDA. It is important that the doctor adjust the dose in response to the patient's reactions to the plant material. Sensitivity to the poison plants returns when the treatment is stopped. Currently available products in both liquid and tablet form are safe enough to remain on the market, but FDA recommended further tests to establish effectiveness.

A number of skin tests to confirm a diagnosis of poison ivy dermatitis are available. However, FDA has recommended that additional studies are needed to standardize these products.

A two-stage patch test to determine who is sensitive to poison ivy is being developed by the Forest Service of the U.S. Department of the Interior, to aid in assigning firefighters. The more sensitive people can be assigned to areas where there is less chance of exposure to the plants.

Until effective vaccines are available, the bottom line still remains—if you want to prevent poison ivy dermatitis, avoid the offending plants. Learn to recognize them in all seasons. If you're going to be in areas where they are likely to lurk, protect yourself by wearing long pants and long sleeves.

As soon as you realize that you have been in contact with poison ivy, oak or sumac, thoroughly wash all exposed areas of skin. Launder your clothes and wipe off footwear, tools and other items that may have been in contact with the sap as soon as possible.

Summertime doesn't have to be spoiled by poison ivy itches if you stay alert.

—by Annabel Hecht

Annabel Hecht is a member of FDA's public affairs staff.

Chapter 47

It's Spring Again and Allergies Are in the Bloom

Chances are that you would just as soon not think about your nose. As long as it lets air in and out fairly easily, sniffs a nice aroma now and then, and keeps eyeglasses in place, a nose is, well, forgettable.

But for 25 million to 30 million Americans who suffer from *seasonal allergic rhinitis*—better (if inaccurately) known as *hay fever*—it is sometimes hard to think of anything but their noses. When a hay fever victim's particular nemesis is in the air, he or she is apt to be preoccupied by a constant struggle against the ailment's classic symptoms: watery nasal discharge, runny eyes, violent fits of sneezing, and itching that can affect not just the nose, but the roof of the mouth and even the Eustachian tubes connecting the inner ear to the back of the throat.

If tree pollen is the culprit, this all-out barrage against the nose and its neighbors usually strikes in early spring. Grass pollen tends to be troublesome in late spring and summer, and the deservedly notorious ragweed pollen is most abundant in the fall. Depending on where they live, hay fever victims who react to all three types of pollen may get a respite only in mid-summer and the dead of winter.

On the other hand, a hay fever sufferer who is allergic to molds, house dust, or animals may have to contend with symptoms the year 'round. So do people whose attacks are triggered by industrial pollutants, cigarette smoke, and other airborne irritants and allergens where they live or work. These unfortunate souls have "perennial allergic rhinitis." Their hay fever never lets up.

DHHS Publication No. (FDA)90-1161. Reprint of *FDA Consumer*, May 1989.

If that is the bad news, the good news is that a lot can be done to help hay fever sufferers cope with the disease. Better understanding of the complex events involved in an allergic reaction has made possible substantial improvement in the care of allergy patients, whether they have hay fever, asthma, food allergies, or any of a wide range of distressing and sometimes life-threatening allergic diseases. Medical science cannot cure allergies the way it can pneumonia. But advances in treatment and prevention allow millions of people to avoid the torment that can plague anyone unfortunate enough to "have allergies."

Allergies or a Cold?

Allergists (physicians who specialize in treating allergies) think that a good deal of allergic disease is unrecognized and therefore untreated. One reason is that seasonal allergies can easily be mistaken for a cold. Careful observation and common sense are useful guides to whether a stuffy, runny nose and sneezing signal a cold or an allergy. If the symptoms last more than a week or so, if they go on virtually all of the time, if they start and stop at the same time every year, flare up around cats or horses (principal causes of animal allergy), or otherwise follow a consistent pattern, allergy ought to be suspected. To be more certain, however, appropriate tests should be done by a physician, preferably an allergist.

The diagnosis of allergic rhinitis—the medical term for the inflamed, runny nose that's the main symptom of "allergies"—is based on a detailed patient history and examination of the nose. But the most critical step is skin testing. Tiny, diluted amounts of suspected allergens are injected under the skin or applied to a small scratch or puncture on the patient's arm or back. Within about 15 minutes, if the patient has IgE antibodies to an allergen being tested, a small raised area surrounded by redness—the "wheal and flare" reaction—will appear at the test site. The size of the skin reaction indicates how sensitive the patient is to the allergen that caused it.

Paul C. Turkeltaub, M.D., of FDA's Center for Biologics Evaluation and Research, and researchers at the National Center for Health Statistics examined information on allergen skin testing collected between 1976 and 1980 in the Second National Health and Nutrition Examination Survey. Among more than 16,000 people aged 6 to 74, about one in five had skin reactions to at least one allergen. Ryegrass and ragweed pollen each produced reactions in over 10 percent of the people tested, 6.2 percent were sensitive to house dust, and 2.3 percent showed a reaction to cats. More than twice as many people reacted to allergens found outdoors than to those found indoors.

Not everyone who tests positive for specific IgE antibodies necessarily has allergy symptoms. Nevertheless, many allergists think that allergic disease of one kind or another—hay fever, asthma, drug allergy, or an allergic reaction to certain foods or insect stings—is likely to appear sooner or later in a person who has no symptoms but who has a positive skin test. About 80 percent of people who develop allergic rhinitis do so before the age of 30. But the disease has also first appeared in people in their seventies or eighties.

Shots and Other Relief

Before the 1940s brought the general availability of antihistamines, hay fever sufferers could get little help from the pharmacy. A hundred and fifty years ago, the English clergyman, wit, and hay fever victim Sydney Smith—he said his sneezes could be heard for six miles—put opium in his nostrils to relieve "this little upstart disease." Today allergic rhinitis can be controlled by more effective and much less dangerous drugs.

Antihistamines. Antihistamines, available both over the counter and by prescription, remain the most widely used agents to treat hay fever symptoms. They can be highly effective in controlling itching and sneezing, but do less well in clearing nasal congestion. Antihistamines are most effective when used regularly rather than sporadically. Their chief undesirable side effects are drowsiness and excessive drying of tissues. Newer antihistamines, such as the prescription medication Seldane (terfenadine), are less apt to cause these side effects.

Nonprescription decongestants. Nonprescription decongestants that shrink blood vessels in and around the nasal passages may help relieve nasal stuffiness. Decongestants are often sold in combination with antihistamines in the form of tablets, capsules, caplets and liquids. Others are sold as nose drops or sprays. While very effective for short-term use (a few days at most) over-use of nose drops and sprays can cause a "rebound" effect in which the congestion comes roaring back worse than ever. Patients can get caught in a vicious circle of use, relapse, and more use. The only solution is to stop using the drug altogether.

Intal or Nasalcrom inhalers (active ingredient cromolyn sodium), available by prescription, were first used against asthma and are proving useful in treating hay fever as well. For most people, inhaled cromolyn has few if any side effects, but must be taken frequently— every four hours—to be of maximum benefit. The corticosteroids, hormone-like drugs that suppress the immune response, may also be useful in relieving allergy symptoms. They are usually administered as sprays, but are sometimes taken by mouth. While long-term use of oral corticosteroids can depress the activity of the adrenal glands, resulting in diminished resistance to infection, and cause other serious side effects; the nasal preparations used to treat allergic rhinitis are not thought to have any effect on the body as a whole. Corticosteroids are available only by prescription.

Allergen immunotherapy. Allergen immunotherapy—"allergy shots"—offers another effective approach to controlling hay fever symptoms. First employed in the 1920s, immunotherapy consists of injecting gradually larger amounts of the allergens that cause the patient's allergic response. At the beginning of the treatment the dose is intentionally much too small to cause a reaction.

The dose is gradually increased to a level that protects the patient from whatever is causing the allergy. It usually takes 6 to 12 months to reach a protective dose. Once protection has been achieved, patients are given maintenance shots at four- to six-week intervals to keep symptoms under control. Whether or not the patients can successfully stop receiving allergy shots is uncertain. Studies suggest that protection fades if the shots are discontinued. For that reason, some allergy specialists recommend that they be continued indefinitely.

Aiming for Improvements

FDA is actively seeking to standardize the commercially available extracts used in skin testing and immunotherapy to improve their safety and effectiveness. The agency has two main objectives:

- expanding the availability of single-allergen extracts (individual kinds of pollen, for example, rather than extracts containing mixtures of several allergenic pollens); and

- standardizing extracts on the basis of how strong a skin reaction they produce.

Table 48.1.

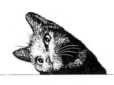

Ready Relief from Nasal Warfare: Nonprescription Allergy Medicines

FDA has proposed these ingredients as safe and effective for use in over-the-counter medications to relieve certain allergy symptoms:

Antihistamines (relieve runny nose and sneezing)

Brompheniramine maleate
Chlorcyclizine hydrochloride
Chlorpheniramine maleate
Dexbrompheniramine maleate
Dexchlorpheniramine maleate
Diphenhydramine hydrochloride
Doxylamine succinate
Phenindamine tartrate
Pheniramine maleate
Pyrilamine maleate
Thonzylamine hydrochloride
Triprolidine hydrochloride

Decongestants (relieve stuffy nose)

Oral:

Phenylephrine hydrochloride
Pseudoephedrine hydrochloride
Pseudoephedrine sulfate

Topical:

1-Desoxyephedrine
Ephedrine
Ephedrine hydrochloride
Ephedrine sulfate
Racephedrine sulfate
Racephedrine hydrochloride
Naphazoline hydrochloride
Oxymetazoline hydrochloride
Phenylephrine hydrochloride
Propylhexedrine
Xylometazoline hydrochloride

For more information, including labeling claims, dosages and warnings, see the proposed standards published by FDA in the Federal Register:
• Antihistamines: Jan. 15, 1985, and Aug. 24, 1987
• Decongestants: Jan. 15, 1985

Studies have shown, for example, that weed and grass pollen extracts are more than 10,000 times as potent in producing skin reactions as extracts made from white pine and mountain cedar pollen. The labeling of standardized extracts reflects such differences in terms of "allergy units." Using single-allergen, standardized extracts, physicians are better able to tell precisely what causes a patient's symptoms and to plan, if necessary, the most effective course of allergy shots.

Immunotherapy has proven effective in hay fever sufferers and can be little short of miraculous for some patients who cannot get adequate relief either from avoiding allergens or from medication. Allergy shots are, however, time-consuming and costly and entail a slight risk of causing the kind of reaction they are meant to prevent. Because such a reaction can be serious, doctors like to monitor patients for at least 20 minutes after giving the shot.

The best course of action in treating hay fever is to get a careful diagnosis and discuss treatment options with an allergist. Once a hay fever sufferer's problem has been diagnosed, a doctor often can show how symptoms can be controlled by avoidance of the allergen or allergens involved or by the careful use of over-the-counter antihistamines and decongestants. If prescription drugs or immunotherapy are called for, a physician can recommend the most appropriate course of treatment. The important thing is that virtually every hay fever sufferer can be helped by prevention and treatment.

Noses are remarkable. They filter the air we breathe, warm it when it's too cold, and moisten it when it's too dry. They alert us when food might be unsafe to eat, and some noses can even smell a rain storm coming. Yet, with the possible exception of Bob Hope, we would all be grateful if noses went about their impressive variety of tasks unnoticed. For hay fever victims, that would be a blessing. Thanks to medical science, it's a blessing millions of them can enjoy.

An Over-Achiever Immune System

Seasonal allergic rhinitis—hay fever—is the most common allergic disease. Its medical name means inflammation of the membrane lining the nose caused by exposure to an allergen at specific times of the year. (Hay is almost never its cause, and fever is not one of its symptoms, but the misnomer has stuck since it was coined more than 160 years ago.) Research, most of it in the 20th century, has demonstrated that allergy is actually an altered or exaggerated immune response. In an allergy-prone person the immune system reacts powerfully to foreign substances, such as pollen, that simply do not bother most of us.

The phenomenon of immunity has long been recognized. Ancient scribes reported that survivors of plague seemed to be protected if the disease struck again. Fifteenth century Chinese and Arab physicians tried injecting people with pus taken from smallpox victims. Sometimes the result was a mild case of smallpox that protected against the more serious form of the disease. Sometimes, too, the outcome was severe smallpox and death.

Two centuries ago, an English physician named Edward Jenner successfully immunized a young boy against smallpox by injecting him with a fluid from a cowpox sore—hence the term vaccination—from *vacca*, Latin for cow. But it was not until the late 19th and early 20th centuries that scientists began to explore the immune system and discover that it is responsible for a number of illnesses, including allergies.

The mechanisms by which the human body recognizes its own components and distinguishes them from foreign substances are among the most elegant products of evolution. Although they do not understand it fully, scientists believe the immune system consists of two main branches. One works through the action of white blood cells called T lymphocytes, or simply T cells. T cells attack foreign materials directly and also produce substances that summon other parts of the immune system to help destroy an invader. A deficit of T cell-mediated immunity is characteristic of acquired immune deficiency syndrome (AIDS).

The other branch of the immune system is the one we associate with antibodies (highly specialized proteins manufactured by B lymphocytes) and antigens (enzymes, toxins, or other foreign substances that provoke a response from the body). When B cells encounter antigens, such as those on the surface of bacteria, they multiply and produce antibodies that destroy the invading germ or make it vulnerable to attack by other parts of the immune system. Once B cells have learned to make an antibody against a specific antigen, they go on making it indefinitely. This is why vaccines can induce permanent immunity against some diseases.

Ironically, it is the immune system's ability to maintain constant readiness against a repeat onslaught by an antigen that makes millions of people susceptible to allergic disease. For reasons that are not entirely clear, some antigens cause B cells to make a kind of antibody called immunoglobulin E (IgE for short). (Antigens that provoke IgE formation are referred to as allergens because they can cause an allergic reaction.) The first time an allergy-prone person is exposed to an allergen—pollen or house dust for example—the B cells respond by making IgE antibodies tailored to counteract the allergen. These IgE antibodies attach themselves to mast cells that are abundant in the respiratory tract, digestive system, and skin and to basophils, cells circulating in the blood.

The next time an allergen and its IgE antibodies come together, mast cells and basophils release powerful substances called mediators, among them histamine, that cause the allergic reaction. These mediators are fairly rapidly neutralized by the body. But as long as the allergen is present, histamine and other mediators will continue to be released from mast cells and basophils, and the patient's allergy symptoms will persist.

No one knows for sure why some people have allergies while most do not. Genetics appears to play a part; people who suffer from allergies usually have a close relative with similar problems. Susceptibility seems to be related to a person's capacity to produce IgE antibodies. Yet only 30 percent to 40 percent of people with allergic rhinitis have high IgE levels, and individuals with low IgE levels can still suffer from hay fever and other allergies.

In view of all the grief they cause, you have to wonder if IgE antibodies are good for anything. The answer may well be yes. Studies suggest that several kinds of human parasites provoke the formation of IgE antibodies and are rapidly destroyed by them. (These amoebas and worms are no longer common in this country, but they still cause serious health problems in under-developed parts of the world.) Looking at this intriguing discovery, a Swedish immunologist has speculated that "pollen allergy might partly be an undesirable consequence" of modern society's success in ridding itself of parasites and the diseases they cause.

Absence Makes the Nose Grow Fonder

Once hay fever has been diagnosed and the responsible allergen or allergens identified, the first line of defense is prevention—avoiding the pollen, house dust, mold spores, scales shed by the skins of animals (dander), or other substances that provoke an allergic reaction.

Sometimes this can be fairly easy. A patient may hate to part with a pet cat or give up horseback riding, but that may be all it takes to be free of symptoms. People allergic to mold spores may solve their problem by keeping out of damp, musty areas. They may also be well advised to avoid foods such as peanuts that may contain mold spores and not to take penicillin and similar drugs that can cause an allergic reaction in mold-sensitive people.

If house dust is the problem, frequent and thorough cleaning of the floors, fabrics such as carpets and curtains, upholstered furniture, and bedding can be beneficial. So can the use of high-efficiency indoor air-filtering devices (not those built into ordinary heating and air conditioning systems) that trap dust particles. (Filtering devices that really help don't come cheap. Beware of inexpensive—and ineffective—substitutes.) Persuasive evidence points to microscopic mites as the prime offenders in house dust allergies. While these spider-like creatures thrive during warm summer months, they may actually be more troublesome in colder weather when fragments of dead mites are more readily dispersed in the air and inhaled.

It is more difficult to avoid pollen and other outdoor airborne allergens. Air conditioning helps in homes, automobiles and workplaces. Simply keeping doors and windows closed can lower the allergen content of indoor air. Hay fever symptoms can be brought on by pollen concentrations as low as 20 grains per cubic meter of air; so during certain seasons, no outdoor area can be assumed pollen-free. Yet it is wise to be especially wary of areas known to have high concentrations of allergens. Another prudent measure for allergic rhinitis sufferers is to avoid irritants such as tobacco smoke, fumes, polluted air, and hair sprays.

It is seldom helpful to move someplace else to escape hay fever-causing pollen. Every part of the country has varieties of trees, weeds and grasses that shed allergenic pollen. People who try moving to the West Coast to escape ragweed pollen (ragweed does not grow in California, Oregon or Washington) may discover that they are allergic to a pollen found in the new location. Furthermore, pollen grains have been found in air samples collected as far as 400 miles at sea. The adage "you can run but you can't hide" is all too true for most hay fever sufferers.

—by Ken Flieger

Ken Flieger is a free-lance writer in Washington, D.C.

Chapter 48

Topical Nasal Sprays: Treatment of Allergic Rhinitis

Abstract

Topical nasal sprays, especially steroids, have regained favor as treatment for allergic rhinitis. Nasal steroids are widely used and are as safe and effective as antihistamines in controlling symptoms of rhinitis. However, if improperly used, steroids can have side effects. It is essential that patients learn correct techniques for administering nasal steroids and understand complications that can result from nasal steroid use. New steroid drugs, such as budesonide, tripedane and fluticasone, are being evaluated and will be available in the near future. Other topical drugs, such as cromolyn and ipratropium, are also effective. Over-the-counter decongestants are helpful in reducing nasal congestion and allowing other topical medicines to penetrate effectively into the nasal cavity, but their use should be limited to no more than three days. Prolonged use of topical nasal decongestants has no place in the treatment of allergic rhinitis and can be associated with significant side effects.

Choices: Old and New

Combination oral antihistamine/decongestants have been the mainstay of therapy for allergic rhinitis since the post-World War II era.[1] Because of the sedating effect of conventional antihistamines,

---

non-sedating antihistamines such as loratadine (Claritin), terfenadine (Seldane) and astemizole (Hismanal) were developed and are used with increasing frequency. Recently, however, concern about cardiac arrhythmias and reports of a few deaths associated with these agents have raised reservations about their widespread use.[2,3]

Immunotherapy, a time-honored treatment for allergies, has been in use for more than 80 years, beginning in 1911 with the administration of boiled grass-pollen extracts to patients with hay fever.[4] Immune modulation can result in decreased allergic response and, in many patients, significant relief. Unfortunately, in its current state, immunotherapy is time-consuming, inconvenient, requires months before benefits are seen and can be associated with allergic reactions.

The desire to attain safe, effective, convenient and rapid relief of symptoms has rekindled interest in topical intranasal medications for allergic rhinitis and other nasal problems (Table 48.1). Advantages of this kind of medication include fewer side effects, delivery of medication directly to the target tissues and costs competitive with those of other treatment forms. Nonetheless, their use is still limited because of uneasiness about treatment with steroids, combined with limited long-term experience with these drugs and a concern about patients becoming "addicted" to nasal sprays.

TABLE 48.1.

Conditions for Which Topical Nasal Sprays Are Beneficial

- Allergic rhinitis, both seasonal and perennial
- Nonallergic rhinitis with eosinophils (using topical corticosteroids)
- Preventing recurrence of nasal polyps following surgical removal (using topical corticosteroids)
- Vasomotor rhinitis (ipratropium [Atrovent] may be more effective than topical corticosteroids)
- Conditions for which topical nasal sprays may contribute to overall disease control:
    — Preventing sinus infections
    — Preventing serous and suppurative otitis media
    — Bronchial asthma

Pathophysiology of Allergic Rhinitis

Allergic rhinitis is a chronic condition characterized by sneezing, nasal itching, thin, watery rhinorrhea and congestion. Typically, the conjunctivae and pharynx are also involved. Seasonal and perennial forms occur, and it is not uncommon for patients to have both forms.

In allergic (sensitized) persons, airborne allergens come into contact with mucosal-bound mast cells and basophils with IgE-specific antibodies on their membrane surfaces. This contact results in degranulation of mast cells and basophils, with release of preformed (e.g., histamine, tryptase) and synthesized (e.g., leukotrienes, prostaglandins) mediators.[5,6] These chemical mediators can cause immediate sneezing, itching, congestion and mucus secretion, with mucosal edema.

In many cases, "late-phase" mast-cell mediated reactions occur four to 12 hours later, with characteristic cellular infiltration with basophils and eosinophils.[7] Congestion is typical, along with "stuffiness" that is poorly responsive to antihistamine/decongestants. In some persons, a "priming" effect occurs: recent or ongoing exposure to allergens causes heightened sensitivity, so that, subsequently, smaller amounts of allergen provoke symptoms.[8]

Types of Nasal Sprays

A variety of nasal sprays are available to treat allergic rhinitis. Corticosteroid sprays are probably the most effective but may be underutilized; decongestant sprays are the most widely used but are not as effective.

Topical Steroids

Topical steroids have been in use for more than three decades; older preparations containing hydrocortisone, prednisolone, dexamethasone and betamethasone were found to sometimes cause adrenal suppression. The newer steroid preparations are safer,[9] have a longer duration of action and are less irritating to the nasal mucosa than the older agents.

Topical steroids are effective in treating both allergic and nonallergic rhinitis and, although they do not alleviate eye symptoms, may be more effective than systemic antihistamines for nasal

491

symptoms.[10,11] The effect of intranasal steroids appears to be achieved by causing decreased capillary permeability, decreased mucus secretion and inhibition of inflammation and inflammatory cell migration.[12]

In general, topical nasal steroids are comparable and selection may be a matter of patient and physician preference. An aqueous solution, such as Vancenase AQ, Beconase AQ, or Nasacort Aqueous (the latter is not currently available in the United States), may be more soothing to nasal tissues and cause less burning, irritation, dryness and epistaxis. However, some patients prefer a low-pressure powdered spray, such as Vancenase Pockethaler.

In general, all of the steroid sprays are well tolerated, even by children. Cost and patient preference (aqueous versus propelled dry powder) should be used as a guide for product selection (Table 48.2). Other topical steroids are currently being tested and will become available in the near future; these include fluticasone, tripedane and budesonide. Whether these agents will offer advantages over currently available drugs remains to be demonstrated.[13]

Although topical steroids are generally safe and effective,[9,14] side effects may occur[15,16] (Table 48.3). The most common side effects are nasal irritation, nosebleeds and sore throat. Rare but serious complications include nasal septal perforation,[17,18] candidiasis and cataracts.[19,20] Systemic absorption at recommended dosages is minimal; however, at higher doses, absorption may occur and generalized side effects are possible.[16] Side effects from long-term usage are unknown. Therefore, caution is advised, and periodic assessment for nasal irritation, perforation and cataracts is recommended.

If nosebleeds occur, the patient should be advised to discontinue using the steroid nasal spray for a week or so and substitute a nasal saline spray. Patients should also apply a thin layer of petroleum jelly with a cotton swab. It may also be helpful to give the patient additional instruction about proper use of the topical nasal steroid or substitute an aqueous preparation. The safety of steroid nasal sprays in young children is unknown, since most studies have involved short observation periods with subjects only as young as four to six years of age.[21,22] The safety of these preparations in persons over 65 years of age and in pregnant women is also unknown. It is possible that topical steroids may be safer than systemic antihistamines/decongestants in these groups, but it is not yet known. Therefore, some physicians may prefer to give persons in the latter groups a nontoxic agent such as cromolyn (Nasalcrom).

Table 48.2. Cost Comparison of Topical Nasal Sprays.

Steroid Product	Dose per Actuation	Actuations per Canister	Usual Dose per Nostril	Canister Supply	Average Wholesale Price per Canister*	Cost per Month*
Nasalide (flunisolide)	25 µg	200	>14 years: two sprays twice daily 6 to 14 years: one spray three times daily	25 days 33 days	$25.52	$30.62 $23.20
Nasacort (triamcinolone acetonide)	55 µg	100	≥12 years: two sprays once daily	25 days	$36.16	$43.39
Vancenase AQ (beclomethasone)	42 µg	200	≥12 years: two sprays twice daily 6 to 12 years: one spray twice daily	25 days 50 days	$31.01	$37.21 $18.61
Vancenase Pockethaler (beclomethasone)	42 µg	200	>6 years: one spray three times daily	33 days	$28.72	$26.11
Beconase AQ (beclomethasone)	42 µg	200	>12 years: two sprays twice daily 6 to 12 years: one spray twice daily	25 days 50 days	$31.01	$37.21 $18.61
Beconase aerosol (beclomethasone)	42 µg	200	>6 year: one spray three times daily	33 days	$28.72	$26.11
Nasalcrom (cromolyn)	5.2 mg	200	>6 years: one spray three to four times daily	33 days	$37.74	$34.31
Atrovent (ipratropium)	18 µg	200	One spray three times daily	33 days	$27.00	$24.55

*Costs based on average wholesale prices according to *Red Book*, 1994, April Update. Montvale, N.J.: *Medical Economics Data*, 1994.

Table 48.3.
Complications of Topical Nasal Sprays

Steroid Sprays

Local reactions
- Nasal burning and stinging
- Sneezing, nasosinus congestion, watery eyes, throat irritation, bad taste in the mouth
- Drying of the mucous membranes with epistaxis or bloody discharge
- *Candida albicans* infection of the mucous membranes (rare)
- Perforation of nasal septum (rare)

Systemic reactions

Common (>5% incidence)

- Headaches

Uncommon (<5% incidence)

- Nausea and vomiting
- Loss of sense of taste and smell
- Dizziness and light-headedness

Rare

- Increased intraocular pressure
- Anaphylaxis, urticaria, angioedema, bronchospasm

Anticholinergic Agents

- Nervousness, palpitations, blurred vision, dry mouth

Decongestant Nasal Sprays

Local reactions
- Stinging, burning and irritation of the nasal mucosa
- Rebound and rhinitis medicamentosa as a result of over-use

Systemic reactions
- Tremors, palpitations, insomnia
- Urinary retention from prostatic constriction
- Hypertension

Cromolyn

Local reactions (<10%)
- Burning, stinging, sneezing or irritation

Cromolyn and Other Mast-cell Stabilizing Agents

Because of its safety margin, cromolyn is widely used in children and adults.[23,24] Cromolyn appears to work by stabilizing mast cells, thus preventing mediator release.[25] This drug may be especially effective in attenuating the signs and symptoms of seasonal allergic rhinitis when it is used before exposure to allergens.

Cromolyn is effective in controlling both early- and late-phase allergic reactions; however, its delayed onset of action, short duration of activity (to be effective, cromolyn should be used four times or more a day), high cost and inferior efficacy compared with steroids[24,27] are relative shortcomings. Cromolyn is not effective in treating nonallergic rhinitis and has limited effectiveness in patients with nasal polyposis.

Anticholinergic Agents

Anticholinergic agents such as atropine have been used for decades to treat allergic rhinitis; however, the limited duration of action and multiple side effects of atropine have curbed its use. Recently, ipratropium (Atrovent), a quaternary derivative of atropine, has been used in patients with excessive rhinorrhea; however, this drug has not yet been manufactured in an intranasal form.[28]

Saline, Steam and Other Wetting Agents

Saline nose sprays such as SalineX, Ocean Nasal Mist and NaSal can be helpful in soothing irritated nasal tissues, dislodging thickened mucus and moisturizing dry mucous membranes. Saline nose sprays are generally very safe but tend to be under-utilized.

Steam appears to provide short-term relief for nasal congestion. A number of simple and safe steam-emitting devices are available.

Nasal Decongestants

Nasal decongestant sprays and drops are potent alpha-adrenergic agonists that cause vasoconstriction. Decongestants have long been available over the counter and include oxymetholone (Afrin, Dristan), phenylephrine hydrochloride (NeoSynephrine), xylometazoline (Otrivin) and naphazoline (Privine). Although these products are highly effective and act rapidly in relieving nasal stuffiness, over-use can result in side effects. Frequent administration results in tachyphylaxis, and decreased efficacy prompts the patient to use the medication at progressively shorter intervals. If nasal decongestants are used for a week or longer, rebound nasal congestion results when the drug is discontinued.

Prolonged use of nasal decongestant sprays can lead to rhinitis medicamentosa, characterized by inflammation and irritation of the nasal mucosa. Treatment is complicated by the fact that the patient experiences immediate relief of nasal obstruction with continued use; weaning over a period of one week, often combined with oral steroids (0.5 to 1.0 mg per kg per day) tapered over seven to ten days, is necessary. Rarely, exacerbation of hypertension, cardiac arrhythmias or urinary obstruction can occur.

In summary, use of topical decongestants is appropriate only on a short-term basis (three days or less) and then primarily to "open up" the nasal passages to allow other topical medications, such as cromolyn or steroids, access into the nasal cavity. Long-term use of topical decongestants has no place in the treatment of allergic rhinitis.

Treatment of Allergic Rhinitis

Allergen Avoidance

The mainstay of therapy for allergic rhinitis is identification and avoidance of offending allergens. When the allergen is animal dander, house dust or mold spores, avoidance is possible and should be strongly encouraged. Even in the case of airborne allergens such as pollen, some avoidance is possible. It may be effective, for example, to use simple measures such as air conditioning in the home or office, staying indoors on dry, windy days, using a clothes dryer rather than hanging clothes outside to dry when pollen and mold spore counts are high, and avoiding pets that come in from the outside covered with pollen. Even in the case of occupation-related allergies, avoidance is sometimes possible and should be encouraged.

Antihistamines and Decongestants

Antihistamines and decongestants are considered first-line pharmacotherapy for allergic rhinitis. Many over-the-counter agents are beneficial for patients with mild to moderate symptoms. Chlorpheniramine (Chlor-Trimeton) and Brompheniramine (Dimetapp, Dristan Allergy) have a wide safety margin with less sedation and fewer cholinergic side effects than other commonly used antihistamines.

Other over-the-counter medications, such as clemastine (Tavist), are also useful. Diphenhydramine (Benadryl) is modestly effective but is associated with considerable sedation; however, its margin of safety is well established.

Combination antihistamine/decongestant preparations can occasionally be used, especially if congestion is a complicating feature. Brompheniramine and Chlorpheniramine are commonly available, either over the counter or by prescription, in combination with a systemic decongestant such as pseudoephedrine or phenylephrine.

Second-generation antihistamines should be tried only if intolerance to different classes of first-generation antihistamines is encountered. However, second-generation antihistamines, including loratadine, astemizole and terfenadine, are expensive. Overdosage or drug interactions with terfenadine and astemizole have resulted in cardiac arrhythmias such as *torsade de pointes*, and death.[2,3] Patients with impaired liver function or known cardiac arrhythmias, those taking medications that increase QT intervals or those taking macrolide antibiotics such as erythromycin, clarithromycin (Biaxin) and azithromycin (Zithromax), or antifungal agents such as fluconazole (Diflucan) and ketoconazole (Nizoral), should avoid using second-generation antihistamines.

Topical Nasal Sprays

Topical nasal sprays are typically reserved for patients with chronic allergic rhinitis and moderate to severe symptoms (Table 48.4). Many of these medications are expensive (Table 48.2). In patients with more severe symptoms, combination treatment with antihistamines and topical nasal sprays may be useful. Topical nasal sprays are efficacious, but their long-term effects are not well defined. They are generally thought to be quite safe, but long-term data are lacking.

Immunotherapy/Immune Modulation

Immunotherapy remains a highly effective method of treating seasonal and perennial allergic rhinitis.[29-31] Eighty years of experience with this technique are available, and mechanisms and efficacy are under investigation. However, expense, inconvenience and the time required before results are seen (2 to 12 months) cause this form of

Table 48.4. Topical Nasal Sprays

Agents	Clinical use	Comments
Steroids	Seasonal allergic rhinitis, perennial allergic rhinitis, nasal polyps, non-allergic rhinitis	More effective than cromolyn. Generally safe. Most preparations not approved for use in children. Dosing frequency is typically twice daily, occasionally once daily. Not useful for eye symptoms but may decrease asthma symptoms. Information on long-term safety is sparse.
Cromolyn (Nasalcrom)	Seasonal allergic rhinitis, perennial allergic rhinitis, acute prophylaxis	Safe in children and others when side effects are a concern. Effective in immediate and late phase reactions. Must be used frequently (4 times daily). Non-labeled use for eye symptoms
Anticholinergic agents	Perennial allergic rhinitis, seasonal allergic rhinitis, excessive rhinorrhea	Atropine has been used; side effects are common and duration of action is short. Ipratropium (Atrovent) has been helpful for rhinorrhea.
Saline solution	Seasonal allergic rhinitis, perennial allergic rhinitis, nasal irritation and dryness, mucosal atrophy	Safe, may be used frequently. Helpful in soothing irritation and inflammation. May be used to irrigate and remove tenacious mucus. Occasionally used immediately before steroids to prevent irritation.
Decongestants	Significant congestion	Available in many over-the-counter preparations. Effective in rapid relief of nasal congestion. Abuse is common. Has no place in the treatment of chronic allergic rhinitis.

therapy to be reserved for patients with chronic moderate to severe symptoms, when medications have not been tolerated or have been ineffective.

References

1. Simmons FE, Simmons KJ. Antihistamines. In: Middleton E Jr, Reed CE, Ellis EF, eds. *Allergy, principles and practice.* 4th ed. St. Louis: Mosby, 1993: 856-92.
2. Monahan BP, Ferguson CL Killeavy ES, Lloyd BK, Troy J, Cantilena LR Jr. Torsades de pointes occurring in association with terfenadine use. *JAMA* 1990;264:2788-90.
3. Simons FE, Kesselman MS, Giddins NG, Pelech AN, Simons KJ. Astemizole-induced torsade de pointes [Letter]. *Lancet* 1988;2(8611):624-5.
4. Bierman CW, Pearlman DS, Berman BA. Injection therapy for allergic diseases. In: Bierman CW, Pearlman DS, eds. *Allergic diseases from infancy to adulthood.* 2d ed. Philadelphia: Saunders, 1988: 279-93.
5. Naclerio RM, Meier HL, Kagey-Sobotka A, Adkinson NF Jr, Meyers DA, Norman PS, et al. Mediator release after nasal airway challenge with allergen. *Am Rev Respir Dis* 1983;128:597-602.
6. Naclerio RM, Proud D, Togias AG, Adkinson NF Jr, Meyers, DA, Kagey-Sobotka A, et al. Inflammatory mediators in late antigen-induced rhinitis. *N Engl J Med* 1985;313:65-70.
7. Bascom R, Pipkorn U, Lichtenstein LM, Naclerio RM. The influx of inflammatory cells into nasal washings during the late response to antigen challenge. *Am Rev Respir Dis* 1988;138:406-12.
8. Connell JT. Quantitative intranasal pollen challenges. 3. The priming effect in allergic rhinitis. *J Allergy* 1969;43:33-44.
9. Naclerio RM. Allergic rhinitis. *N Engl J Med* 1991;325:860-9.
10. Beswick KB, Kenyon GS, Cherry JR. A comparative study of beclomethasone dipropionate aqueous nasal spray with terfenadine tablets in seasonal allergic rhinitis. *Curr Med Res Opin* 1985;9:560-7.
11. Robinson AC, Cherry JR, Daly S. Double-blind cross-over trial comparing beclomethasone dipropionate and terfenadine in perennial rhinitis. *Clin Exp Allergy* 1989;19;569-73.

12. Pauwels R. Mode of action of corticosteroids in asthma and rhinitis. *Clin Allergy* 1986;16:281-8.
13. Ratner PH, Paull BR, Findlay SR, Hampel F Jr, Martin B, Kral KM, et al. Fluticasone propionate given once daily is as effective for seasonal allergic rhinitis as beclomethasone dipropionate given twice daily. *J Allergy Clin Immunol* 1992;90(3 Pt 1):285-91.
14. Orgel HA, Meltzer EO, Bierman CW, Bronsky E, Connell JT, Lieberman PL, et al. Intranasal fluocortin butyl in patients with perennial rhinitis: a 12-month efficacy and safety study including nasal biopsy. *J Allergy Clin Immunol* 1991;88:257-64.
15. Norman PS, Winkenwerder WL, Agbayani BF, Migeon CJ. Adrenal function during the use of dexamethasone aerosols in the treatment of ragweed hay fever. *J Allergy* 1967;40:57-61.
16. Stead RJ, Cooke NJ. Adverse effects of inhaled corticosteroids. *BMJ* 1989;298:403-4.
17. Soderberg-Warner ML. Nasal septal perforation associated with topical corticosteroid therapy. *J Pediatr* 1984;105:840-1.
18. Schoelzel EP, Menzel ML. Nasal sprays and perforation of the nasal septum [Letter]. *JAMA* 1985; 253:2046.
19. Fraunfelder FT, Meyer SM. Posterior subcapsular cataracts associated with nasal or inhalation corticosteroids. *Am J Ophthalmol* 1990;109:489-90.
20. Karim AK; Thompson GM, Jacob TJ. Steroid aerosols and cataract formation [Letter]. *BMJ* 1989; 299:918.
21. Welch MJ, Bronsky EA, Grossman J, Shapiro GG, Tinkelman DG, Garcia JD, et al. Clinical evaluation of triamcinolone acetonide nasal aerosol in children with perennial allergic rhinitis. *Ann Allergy* 1991; 67:493-8.
22. Kobayashi RH, Tinkelman DG, Reese ME, Sykes RS, Pakes GE. Beclomethasone dipropionate aqueous nasal spray for seasonal allergic rhinitis in children. *Ann Allergy* 1989;62:205-8.
23. Schwartz HJ The effect of cromolyn on nasal disease. *Ear Nose Throat J* 1986;65:449-56.
24. Murphy S. Cromolyn: basic mechanisms and clinical usage. *Pediatr Asthma Allergy Immunol* 1988; 2:237-44.
25. Chandra RK, Heresi G, Woodford G. Double-blind controlled crossover trial of 4% intranasal sodium cromoglycate solution in patients with seasonal allergic rhinitis. *Ann Allergy* 1982;49:131-4.

26. Hillas J, Booth RJ, Somerfield S, Morton R, Avery J, Wilson JD. A comparative trial of intra-nasal beclomethasone dipropionate and sodium cromoglycate in patients with chronic perennial rhinitis. *Clin Allergy* 1980;10:253-8.
27. Welsh PW, Stricker WE, Chu CP, Naessens JM, Reese ME, Reed CE, et al. Efficacy of beclomethasone nasal solution, flunisolide, and cromolyn in relieving symptoms of ragweed allergy. *Mayo Clinic Proc* 1987;62:125-34.
28. Mygind N, Borum P. Anticholinergic treatment of watery rhinorrhea. *Am J Rhinol* 1990;4:1-5.
29. Creticos PS, Adkinson NF Jr, Kagey-Sobotka A, Proud D, Meier HL, Naclerio RM, et al. Nasal challenge with ragweed pollen in hay fever patients. Effect of immunotherapy. *J Clin Invest* 1985;76: 2247-53 [Published erratum appears in J Clin Invest 1986;78:1421].
30. Creticos PS, Marsh DG, Proud D, Kagey-Sobotka A, Adkinson NF Jr, Friedhoff L, et al. Responses to ragweed-pollen nasal challenge before and after immunotherapy. *J Allergy Clin Immunol* 1989;84: 197-205.
31. Ewan PW, Alexander MM, Snape C, Ind PW, Agrell B, Dreborg S. Effective hyposensitization in allergic rhinitis using a potent partially purified extract of house dust mite. *Clin Allergy* 1988;18:501-8.

Roger H. Kobayashi, M.D.,
University of California
Los Angeles,
School of Medicine,
Los Angeles, California

Frederic Kiechel III, M.D.,
Ai Lan D. Kobayashi, M.D.
Morris B. Mellion, M.D.,
University of Nebraska
Medical Center,
Omaha, Nebraska

The Authors

Roger H. Kobayashi, M.D. has a private practice in allergy, immunology and asthma in Omaha and is also an associate clinical professor of pediatrics at the University of California, Los Angeles, School of Medicine. After graduating from the University of Nebraska College of Medicine, Omaha, Dr. Kobayashi completed pediatric training at the University of Southern California School of Medicine, Los Angeles, and served a fellowship in immunology research at the UCLA School of Medicine.

Frederic Kiechel III, M.D. has a private practice in the treatment of allergy and asthma in Lincoln, NB, and is an assistant clinical professor of pediatrics at the University of Nebraska College of Medicine. Dr. Kiechel graduated from the University of Virginia School of Medicine, Charlottesville, and completed pediatric training at Babies Hospital, Columbia University College of Physicians and Surgeons, New York City, and a fellowship in allergy and asthma at the National Jewish Center for Immunology and Respiratory Medicine, Denver.

Ai Lan D. Kobayashi, M.D. has a private practice in pediatrics and adolescent medicine in Omaha and is an assistant clinical professor of pediatrics at the University of Nebraska College of Medicine, where she obtained her medical degree. Dr. Kobayashi completed pediatric training at the University of Southern California School of Medicine, Los Angeles.

Morris B. Mellion, M.D. has a private practice in Omaha and is clinical associate professor of family practice in orthopedic surgery (sports medicine) at the University of Nebraska Medical Center, Omaha. Dr. Mellion is also adjunct associate professor in the School of Health, Physical Education and Recreation, and team physician for men's and women's sports in the Athletic Department at the University of Nebraska at Omaha. He graduated from Yale University School of Medicine, New Haven, Conn., and completed a residency in family medicine at the University of Vermont College of Medicine, Burlington. Dr. Mellion is a past president of the American Academy of Family Physicians.

Chapter 49

"Over-the-Counter" Medications: Do They Work for Allergies?

So, it's getting to be that time of the year again for you. Days are longer, birds are chirping, trees are budding and the grass is beginning to turn green once again. Oh, oh! That spells the beginning of allergy season. If you suffer from allergies, you are probably not looking forward to the many uncomfortable days and nights you may have to endure over the next several months.

However, you can do something to make allergies more bearable. There are many "over-the-counter" (OTC) medications you can purchase without a prescription. This chapter will focus on which OTC drugs are available, where and when not use these products, and when it would make good sense to seek professional help from your doctor.

Hay fever is a chronic condition characterized by sneezing, nasal congestion, runny nose, and itching of the nose, palate, ears and eyes. If these are your only symptoms and they occur for a short period of time (two months or less) and you are healthy otherwise, using OTC medications might be all you need to do.

The two major classes of OTC medications are antihistamines and decongestants. Antihistamines are the mainstay of treatment. They help relieve the sneezing, itching and runny nose. They work best if you take them on a regular basis rather than waiting until you're severely suffering. Most people tolerate antihistamines well, although 20 percent will experience drowsiness.

Hay fever sufferers might try one from each of the three antihistamine classes to see which works best. The first class is alkylamines.

©Asthma and Allergy Foundation of America. Reprinted with permission.

The second class is ethanolamines. These are readily available by brand and generic names. The newest OTC antihistamine is clemastine and offers a third class to try. Long-acting (8- to 12-hour) types give more prolonged relief and can help you get through the night. The 4-hour type begins working faster (usually within 20 minutes) and lasts a shorter time.

Do not take any of these medicines if you have glaucoma, because they can raise your eye pressure. They should not be used if you have difficulty urinating due to prostate problems. Avoid them if you have emphysema or chronic bronchitis, as they may dry the mucus in your chest and cause breathing problems. Combining them with antidepressants, tranquilizers or sleeping pills is not recommended.

Speak with your doctor before using any medications. If you become drowsy with all three classes of antihistamines or fall into the group of people who have another reason not to take these drugs, talk to your doctor about the newer, non-sedating antihistamines. These drugs require a doctor's prescription.

Most antihistamine packages warn not to use antihistamines if you have asthma. Theoretically, they could dry the mucus in the lungs and worsen the asthma. If you wish to use these medications and you have asthma, check with your doctor first, but I believe antihistamines can be used safely to treat nasal and eye allergies in asthmatics.

Decongestants are the second type of OTC medication useful in treating nasal and eye allergies. They are available in topical forms, eye and nose drops and sprays, and oral (liquid and tablet) forms. Such nose drops and sprays should be used for no more than three days maximum! They lead to physical addiction with rebound swelling in the nose if you try to stop them after three days. Be careful! They can raise your blood pressure even if you have normal blood pressure.

Each year, several otherwise healthy adults develop very high blood pressure due to decongestant nose sprays. Their blood pressure returns to normal when they finally get off the nose sprays.

Eye drops are safer, but inasmuch as the OTC preparations do not contain antihistamines, they are not nearly as effective as combination antihistamine/decongestant eye drops available from your doctor with prescription.

The oral decongestants certainly help the nasal stuffiness and drainage, but do nothing for the itching and sneezing. They frequently cause jittering, tremors, insomnia, fast heartbeat and rapid pulse. They should not be used by people who have high blood pressure, heart problems, thyroid disease, diabetes or prostate problems.

Antihistamine/decongestant combinations, for those people who can take them, are uniformly the most effective OTC medications available for nasal and eye allergies. Beware of such combinations which also contain a pain reliever, such as acetaminophen or aspirin. Chronic use of these can lead to inflammation in the liver and bleeding from your stomach or intestine.

It is perfectly acceptable to treat nasal and eye allergies with OTC medications unless complications develop. These include recurrent sinus infections, ear infections, headaches, cough, any wheezing or difficulty with exercise. Prompt consultation with a physician is then indicated to determine the significance of the complication and to make recommendations for management. The physician can prescribe drugs that may provide relief not afforded by the OTC medications. Other recommendations may include referral to an allergy specialist who can frequently stop the worsening of the allergic condition and often times reverse the problems.

OTC medications are also available to treat asthma. These include epinephrine inhalers and oral theophylline-ephedrine combinations. However, asthmatics should not direct their own treatment. If OTC drugs are used inappropriately, they could lead to increased blood pressure, stroke, heart attack or convulsion. In the face of huge advancements in treating asthma, it is possible to reduce hospitalizations and death rates. This is one disease where the directions by a physician and a proven treatment program could literally save your life.

This information should not substitute for seeking responsible, professional medical care.

—by Joel M. Karlin, M.D.

Joel M. Karlin, M.D., FAAI, FACAI, is Assistant Professor of Medicine and Pediatrics at the University of Colorado School of Medicine. He is also Senior Physician, Denver Allergy and Asthma Associates, PC.

Chapter 50

Immunotherapy: Avoiding Allergies Is Worth a Shot

Isn't it a beautiful spring day?

Those words used to drive me insane. Beautiful spring days in Maryland mean warm sunshine and gentle breezes. But drifting in those spring breezes is pollen. So much pollen, mostly from trees, that the air becomes hazy, making life miserable for people with pollen allergies like my son Paul.

Two years ago, sunny spring days didn't mean riding bikes and playing ball for 5-year-old Paul. They meant recess in the school library, a box of tissues at his desk, and eyes nearly swollen shut by the end of the school day. Once home, he took off his pollen-covered clothes, put on clean clothes, and spent his afternoons inside a closed house with air conditioning running even if it was a balmy 70 degrees Fahrenheit (21 degrees Celsius) outside.

Only rainy days were beautiful spring days to Paul.

But last spring wasn't as bad for him, and this spring—after nearly two years of allergy shots—he may finally be able to enjoy sunny spring days outdoors.

One treatment for people with allergies is injections of small amounts of the substances they're allergic to. This is called immunotherapy. Over time as the dose is increased, the patient becomes hyposensitized (less allergic) to the allergens because the body, for reasons not yet fully understood, becomes more tolerant to the offending substances. The symptoms, including sneezing and watery eyes—and the need for medication—are reduced or disappear.

FDA Consumer, May 1996.

People of any age can develop allergies. Heredity and allergen exposure are important influences in whether allergies develop. Moving from one part of the country to another, especially if the climates, and therefore the native plants, are different, can influence the severity and seasonality of allergic symptoms.

The Food and Drug Administration regulates the biological extracts in allergy shots. The extracts are used both to treat and to test individuals to determine exactly what causes their allergic reactions. (See Standardizing Extracts below.)

In addition to treating pollen allergy from trees, grasses and weeds, immunotherapy is also used to treat allergies to house dust mites, pets, molds found indoors and outside, and stinging insects such as honey bees, yellow jackets, hornets, and wasps.

Who Should Get Shots?

From the time he was 12 months old, Paul was miserable in the spring and, to a lesser degree in the fall, with a runny nose, watery eyes, and itchy skin. By his third birthday, the pollen allergies also triggered asthma attacks. Prescription medications didn't help much to relieve his symptoms, even with constant use.

All this made Paul a good candidate for injections.

"Shots work extremely well in patients that clearly have allergic symptoms, either allergy in their nose like allergic rhinitis or bronchial asthma, where outdoor allergens like tree, weed and grass pollens seem to be a major cause," says Stanley P. Galant, M.D., an allergist in Orange County, CA, and a clinical professor and director of pediatric allergy at the University of California, Irvine.

Patients with allergies to molds, house dust mites (microscopic insects that feed on human skin cells found on furniture, bedding and carpets), and animal dander (tiny skin flakes animals continually shed) don't respond quite as well to shots as those allergic to outdoor allergens, he says. But standardization of extracts for cat dander and dust mites and overall better preparations have increased effectiveness even for these patients, he adds.

Immunotherapy doesn't begin until after skin tests or blood tests have determined the exact culprits.

"You have to show that [the patients] have IgE antibodies to the allergens in question," says John Yunginger, M.D., a member of FDA's Allergenic Products Advisory Committee and a pediatric allergist at the Mayo Clinic, Rochester, MN.

The first time an allergic person is exposed to an allergen, the immune system produces a kind of antibody called immunoglobulin E (IgE for short). But it is rare for a first exposure to cause allergic symptoms. Only on subsequent exposures do typical allergic symptoms, such as sneezing, coughing and rash, appear. Overproduction of IgE is characteristic of allergic reactions.

Deciding which allergens to test "depends very much on the patient's history," says Yunginger. "In somebody who has fairly straight-forward classical seasonal symptoms they may get as few as 15 or 20 [skin] tests. Someone with more extensive perennial disease may get 75 or 80."

Each individual skin test consists of a small amount of the suspect allergen scratched onto the skin, usually on the back. If a hive with surrounding redness appears within 15 minutes, allergy to the substance is probable. The doctor also takes into account the dose of allergen and the size of the response.

Two controls, standards against which experimental observations may be evaluated, are also used to make sure skin-test reactions are caused by the allergens. One of the controls, which should not cause a reaction (no hive), is simply the diluting solution. The other control contains histamine, a naturally occurring substance that causes a hive in almost everyone.

According to Galant, the patient's history is as significant as the testing. "The history is really what tells me whether to put the patient on shots," he says. "Training as a specialist helps me interpret the data from the history and correlate that with the testing and come up with a solution."

While skin tests give quick results and can be done in the doctor's office, there are some cases where a blood test is preferable, says Marshall Plaut, M.D., chief of the allergic mechanisms section in the National Institute of Allergy and Infectious Diseases, National Institutes of Health. Individuals with skin problems or skin diseases are not good candidates for skin tests, he says.

Shot Schedule

Once the problem allergens are identified, the allergist prepares a treatment solution containing those allergens to begin the process of desensitization.

"If the patient is very sensitive to a certain allergen, that allergen should be given separately so local and systemic [whole body] responses can be carefully monitored," says Galant. "For example, some people are astronomically allergic to grass pollen." If the grass pollens are in the treatment solution with other allergens, the desensitization to the other allergens might be delayed if reactions to the grass pollens mean maintaining or reducing the solution dose, he explains. It turned out that Paul was equally and highly sensitive to every tree, weed and grass pollen on the Eastern seaboard as well as dust mites and mold. Only animal dander wasn't a problem. Because he was allergic to so much, he had to get two shots—one containing the pollens, the other with the molds and mites. The amount of allergen in the first solution the allergist prepares is very dilute. The first shot from that solution is usually 0.05 milliliters, resulting in a minute amount of allergen actually being injected. This cautious approach decreases the chance of adverse reactions. The shots are given subcutaneously (under the skin) in the back of the upper arm. The regimen usually starts with shots twice a week, gradually increasing the doses as long as no serious reactions occur.

A little bit of redness, itching or swelling (less than 2 centimeters (cm), or the size of a nickel) around the injection site is all right, and the dose may be increased at the next visit. Cold compresses, oral antihistamines, and topical corticosteroids can relieve these minor reactions.

If the site swells more than 2 cm or allergic symptoms develop, the allergist may decide to repeat the same dose at the next visit or even reduce it, depending on the severity of the previous reaction.

The chances of having an adverse reaction to the injection are more common while the doses are being increased than once a maintenance dose is reached, says Yunginger.

Anaphylaxis—a life-threatening reaction that causes blood pressure to plummet, the throat to swell, and airways in the lungs to constrict—is a slight but real risk with allergy shots. A shot of epinephrine—the same drug used to treat severe allergic reactions to bee stings—is used to treat anaphylaxis. Anaphylactic reactions may result in death, although this is rare.

The American Academy of Allergy and Immunology recommends that patients remain in the doctor's office for 20 minutes after receiving the injection, because reactions usually occur within that time. "High-risk patients may have to wait additional time," says Richard Lockey, M.D., director of the division of allergy and immunology at the University of Southern Florida College of Medicine in Tampa.

If no reactions occur, the amount of allergen in each shot is increased until a maintenance dose is reached. For a very sensitive patient, the maximum dose may be the amount the patient can tolerate without a reaction. Others may be able to reach a predetermined amount that researchers have found to be necessary for optimal allergy relief.

Once the maintenance dose has been reached, the intervals between shots can be gradually increased to two, three and even four weeks apart. Reaching the maintenance dose can take anywhere from six months to three years.

The amount of time needed to reach the maintenance dose can be reduced to as little as a few days with "rush" immunotherapy. Patients receive increasing doses of the allergens several times a day for three or four days. This requires close medical observation because the frequent schedule greatly increases the risk of anaphylaxis. That risk, plus the inconvenience of spending several days all at once at the doctor's office or in a clinic, makes rush immunotherapy unpopular with many patients and physicians, says Yunginger.

Shot Success

"If allergy shots are working, the patient normally feels the benefit within a year, sometimes within six months," writes Stuart H. Young, M.D., and colleagues, in the book *Allergies* (Consumer Reports Books, 1991). "It is usually necessary to continue shots for a couple of years at least, but the idea is to continue only if the treatment is effective, not just in the hope that someday it may help. Fruitless treatment should not drag on for years."

Anywhere from three to five years of treatment is the usual recommendation, says Yunginger.

"The reason for [the three to five years]—and it's not written in concrete—is that the long-term remission of symptoms after the shots stop seems to be better," explains Galant. "If you give a patient shots for a year or two, even if they've had a good year, there's some indication that the relapse rate might be higher."

Galant usually decides to stop shots if the patient has had no symptoms or the degree of symptoms has significantly decreased for about a year. "Generally that's between the second or third year, so when we finish three years, I would seriously consider stopping the shots."

When Yunginger takes his patients off shots, "I have them go through the four seasons to see if the symptoms come back. If the symptoms do come back and can't be completely controlled with medication, then probably the injections should be restarted."

According to Young and colleagues, after stopping shots, one-third of patients will no longer have allergic reactions, one-third will have a partial relapse of symptoms, and one-third will relapse completely.

Lifestyle Changes

"Shots are just one part of this therapy," says Galant. "Good avoidance measures are very important."

Usually outdoor allergens can't be completely avoided. Most people can't stay inside all the time, and, in any case, pollen comes inside through open doors and windows and on people's clothes, hair and shoes. Here are some ways to keep pollen out of the house:

* Keep all windows closed.
* Put a permanent air filter specially designed to keep out pollens and other airborne contaminants in the heating and cooling systems; wash the filter every month.
* Change clothes after coming in from outside, and wash the clothes before wearing them again.
* Keep dirty clothes out of the allergic person's bedroom.
* Wash the allergic person's hair every night to avoid transferring pollen from hair to pillow.

Some indoor allergens are also difficult to avoid, but they can be reduced. When it comes to dust mites, "it's hard to get rid of them," says Galant. Mites like to live in box springs, mattresses, pillows, and carpets. To keep the mite population down, the allergic person's mattress, box spring, and pillows should be encased in special covers available from companies that make allergy-proof products. Washable curtains should be the only window coverings. To kill dust mites in bed linens and curtains, wash water must be at least 130 degrees Fahrenheit (54 degrees Celsius). (But during all other times, keep water temperature at 120 F [49 C] to protect children from accidental scalding.) Carpets should be removed or treated with an anti-allergen spray. (Ask your allergist, or contact organizations listed below for sources of these products.)

For those with allergies to pets, the simple answer, giving up a beloved cat or dog, is often unacceptable. To increase the success of shots, animals should be kept out of the bedroom. Giving pets a weekly bath may help reduce the amount of dander they release into the air.

Whether it means keeping a cat or playing outside in the spring, "my game plan for all patients is to have them live a normal life," says Galant.

That's what I hope will be in store for Paul—time spent outdoors enjoying the sun and spring breezes. For me, it will mean I can finally say, "Yes, it really is a beautiful spring day."

Standardizing Extracts

Biologists and chemists in FDA's Center for Biologics Evaluation and Research are working in their labs to standardize allergenic extracts.

"Without standardization, there is no defined potency for these extracts," says Paul Turkeltaub, M.D., acting director of the center's division of allergenic products and parasitology. "This can reduce the effectiveness of both diagnosis and treatment."

Stanley P. Galant, M.D., an allergist in Orange County, CA, and a clinical professor and director of pediatric allergy at the University of California, Irvine, explains that different lots of nonstandardized extracts may not be the same strength, and allergists have no way to know if there is any variation. He says that to avoid the risk of a bad reaction with these extracts, a patient starting a new vial of treatment solution must get a lower dose than what the patient is on and build up again.

"Standards for extracts improve medical management of allergies and lessen the risk of an adverse reaction," says Turkeltaub. "Standards should reduce the need for retesting of patients who switch physicians, since the physicians will have access to the same extracts."

Currently, FDA scientists have developed standards for cat allergens, dust mites, short ragweed, and several bee venoms. The venoms were among the first to be standardized because life-threatening reactions to them are more common.

FDA has determined, in consultation with industry and medical professionals, the priority for other extracts to be standardized. In most cases, higher priority went to allergens affecting the greatest number of people.

FDA scientists are nearing completion on standards for latex and cockroach extracts, and work is continuing on standardization of a peanut extract and many pollens. (See Chart 50.1.)

"Peanut is the most severe form of food allergy," says Marshall Plaut, M.D., chief of the allergic mechanisms section, in NIH's National

Table 50.1
CBER's Standardization Program for
Allergenic Extracts

STANDARDIZED	IN PROCESS	FUTURE CANDIDATES
Cats	**Grass Pollens**	
Cat Hair	Bermuda Grass	**Dog Epidermals**
Cat Pelt	Red Top Grass	
	June Grass	**Foods**
Mites	Perennial Ryegrass	Shrimp/Seafood
D. farinae	Orchard Grass	Dairy Products
D. pteronyssinus	Timothy Grass	
	Meadow Fescue	**Molds**
Short Ragweed	Sweet Vernal	Aspergillus
		Cladosporium
Venoms	**Latex**	
Honey Bee		**Grass Pollens**
Yellow Hornet	**Cockroaches**	Johnson
Wasp	American	Bahia
White Face Hornet	German	
Yellow Jacket	Oriental	**Weed Pollens**
Mixed Vespid		
	Tree Pollens	**Tree Pollens**
	Birch, White	Cedar
	Box Elder	Olive
	Oak, White	
	Elm, American	**Giant Ragweed**
	Peanuts	**Mites**
		Storage
	Alternaria	
		Fire Ants

Institute of Allergies and Infectious Diseases. "A high proportion of deaths from food allergies are from peanuts, and, unlike most food allergies, which disappear after childhood, peanut allergies tend to last a lifetime."

The agency plans to standardize other food allergens, pollens and insect venoms in the future.

—by Isadora B. Stehlin

Isadora B. Stehlin is a member of FDA's public affairs staff.

More Information

The following organizations have more information on allergy shots and products to reduce allergens in the home:

Asthma and Allergy Foundation of America
1125 15th St., N.W.
Suite 502
Washington, DC 20005
1-800-727-8462

Allergy and Asthma Network
3554 Chain Bridge Road
Suite 200
Fairfax, VA 22030
1-800-878-4403
E-mail: aanma@aol.com
Internet: http://www.podi.com/health/aanma/

Chapter 51

Adverse Effects from Asthma and Allergy Medications

In most instances, your particular asthma and allergic disease can be successfully treated with only slight, if indeed any, adverse, or unwanted, effects. Your physician always weighs the pattern of the untreated disease against any possible adverse effects of medications prescribed for it.

Nevertheless, it is important for the patient to be aware of potential unwanted effects. If or when noted, they should be promptly reported to the physician who can then modify the treatment being given.

In this chapter, adverse drug effects are listed according to the drug's classification. Their general uses are noted, as are possible unwanted effects. The effects listed below are those that have been observed and reported. However, the list is not all inclusive.

Adrenergics

These adrenaline-like drugs are used to rapidly open airways (bronchodilation). They are mainstays for acute and/or chronic asthma therapy. This class includes albuterol (Ventolin, Proventil), metaproterenol (Alupent, Metaprel), terbutaline (Bricanyl, Brethine), pirbuterol (Maxaire), epinephrine (Adrenaline), and isoproterenol (Isuprel).

Adrenergic drugs are among the safest medications known for treating asthma. By and large, their adverse effects are related to dose. That is, the higher the dose being taken, the more likely may be the adverse effect. For this reason, many physicians prefer to prescribe aerosol forms of the drug rather than an oral form, since the dose by aerosol is many times less, and therefore the adverse effects are less. Most often, the adverse effects are trivial and become less bothersome with continued use of the drug. For example, patients may become "tolerant" or less bothered by hand tremors after a few weeks of taking adrenergic medication.

Possible adverse effects. Adrenergics can have the following negative side-effects:

neuromuscular

* tremor;

cardiovascular system

* rapid heart beat,
* palpitations,
* abnormal heart rhythm,
* hypertension;

nervous system

* restlessness,
* nervousness,
* wakefulness (insomnia),
* headache;

gastrointestinal system

* nausea,
* vomiting.

Theophylline

A derivative of caffeine, theophylline has been used to treat asthma for over 40 years. As effective as it is, it also has the potential to cause severe and even life threatening adverse reactions. Fortunately, serious reactions are rare. Theophylline, more so than any other drug, requires careful attention to dosing since it has a narrow "therapeutic window." That is, the range of doses that provides good asthma control and that which produces adverse effects is very narrow.

Since different individuals, children or adults, have different dose requirements, the amount of theophylline taken has to be tailored to the individual. There are a number of factors that can influence the amount of theophylline in the blood, causing it to either increase or decrease. For example, the existence of a respiratory viral infection, or other drugs being taken, may affect the blood level of theophylline and cause it to rise, producing one or more of the adverse effects listed below. Probably more so with theophylline than with any other drug used to treat asthma, the patient needs to recognize the signs and symptoms of theophylline toxicity and discontinue the drug promptly thereafter. Severe theophylline toxicity is a major concern. Not only could theophylline toxicity lead to death, but survivors—particularly children—may suffer severe, irreversible brain damage.

Fortunately, awareness of the early signs and symptoms of theophylline toxicity—nausea, vomiting, restlessness and agitation—and discontinuation of further dosing can avoid the most severe adverse effects. Notwithstanding the need for vigilance, theophylline remains an effective drug for asthma treatment and can be used safely by patients under knowledgeable professional care.

Possible adverse effects. Theophylline can have the following negative side-effects:

gastrointestinal system

- nausea,
- vomiting;

nervous system

- dizziness,
- restlessness,
- wakefulness (insomnia),
- headache,
- seizures (convulsions);

cardiovascular system

- rapid heartbeat,
- abnormal heart rhythm;

urinary tract

- excessive urination,
- bed-wetting in children,
- difficult urination (in older men only).

Corticosteroids

Very effective drugs available for the treatment of asthma and allergies, corticosteroids also carry a substantial risk of possible adverse effects. All unwanted effects associated with this family of drugs appear to be related to dose and duration of therapy. Physicians try to limit the use of systemically administered (oral) corticosteroids to a brief period of time. For patients who require long term steroids, the use of alternate day doses (single dose given every 48 hours early in the morning), and prescription of one of the newer generation of inhaled (topical) steroids greatly reduces the frequency of adverse effects.

Possible adverse effects. Corticosteroids can have the following negative side-effects:

general

- Cushing syndrome (rounding of the face, accumulation of fat at the base of the back of the neck and weight gain);

skin

- thinning of the skin,
- easy bruising,
- acne,
- increased hair growth;

cardiovascular system

- hypertension;

gastrointestinal system

- peptic ulcer (a controversial effect),
- pancreatitis,
- perforation of the bowel;

nervous system

- mood changes (euphoria, depression),
- increase in spinal fluid pressure;

eyes

- glaucoma,
- cataracts;

endocrine-metabolic system

- suppression of the patient's own steroid production,
- growth retardation,
- diabetes,
- delayed sexual maturity;

immune system

- decrease resistance to certain fungi and viruses,
- depression of certain immune functions;

musculoskeletal system

- osteoporosis,
- vertebral collapse,
- disintegration of the head of the femur,
- delayed skeletal maturity,
- muscle weakness (generalized with systemic steroids,
- weakness of larynx muscles leading to hoarseness following inhaled steroids).

Cromolyn Sodium

Cromolyn (Intal) is a very safe medication used to treat asthma and nasal and eye allergies. Patients will rarely experience adverse effects with cromolyn of such a degree that would require its discontinuation.

Possible adverse effects. Cromolyn Sodium can have the following negative side-effects:

skin

- skin eruptions,
- hives,
- localized swelling of tissue;

respiratory system

- nasal congestion,
- sore throat,
- hoarseness,
- cough,
- bronchospasm;

gastrointestinal system

- nausea,
- vomiting.

Antihistamines

A widely used class of medication used to reduce the symptoms of allergic rhinitis (hay fever), their most bothersome adverse effect is sleepiness (sedation). However, only about 20 percent of the adult population experiences this effect. The sedative effects can be reduced further by the use of one of a new generation of so-called non-sedating antihistamines.

Possible adverse effects. Antihistamines can have the following negative side-effects:

general

- dry nose,
- mouth and throat;

nervous system

- sedation,
- sleepiness,
- dizziness,
- disturbed coordination,
- excitation and irritability in children;

urinary tract

- difficult urination and urinary retention (in older men).

This information should not substitute for seeking responsible, professional medical care.

—by Elliot F. Ellis. M.D.

Elliot F. Ellis, M.D., is an allergist at the Nemours Children's Clinic in Jacksonville, FL, and a past president of the American Academy of Allergy and Immunology.

Part Eight

Glossary of
Common Medical Terms

Chapter 52

Glossary of Medical Terms

Acquired immunodeficiency syndrome (AIDS): A life-threatening disease caused by a virus and characterized by breakdown of the body's immune defenses. A disorder resulting from infection by the human immunodeficiency virus (HIV), which greatly depletes the helper T cell population, causing various infections and/or tumors.

Active immunity: Immunity produced by the body as a result of previous exposure to an antigen, an allergen, or vaccination.

Acute phase proteins: Serum proteins whose levels increase during infection or inflammatory reactions.

Adjuvant: A substance that non-specifically enhances the immune response to an antigen.

Agammaglobulinemia: An almost total lack of immunoglobulins, or antibodies.

AIDS: See Acquired immunodeficiency syndrome.

Airway obstruction: A narrowing, clogging, or blocking of the airways that carry air to the lungs; a major problem in an acute asthma attack.

Allergen: A substance capable of causing an allergic reaction. Plant pollens, fungi spores, and animal danders are some of the common allergens.

Allergic contact dermatitis: A type of rash caused by an allergic reaction to some substance that comes in contact with the skin.

Allergic reaction: An adverse immune response following repeat contact with otherwise harmless substances such as pollens, molds, foods, cosmetics and drugs.

Allergic bronchopulmonary aspergillosis (ABPA): An unusual lung disease found in allergic asthmatics and caused by an allergic reaction to a fungus growing in the lungs.

Allergic rhinitis: An inflammation of the membranes in the nose caused by an allergic reaction; seasonal allergic rhinitis is known as hay fever.

Allergy: An inappropriate and harmful response of the immune system to normally harmless substances. A specific IgE antibody response to a specific antigen.

Altered self: The concept that the combination of antigen and a self-MHC molecule interacts with the immune system in the same way as an allogeneic MHC molecule.

Alveoli: The lung's tiny air sacs.

Anaphylactic shock: life-threatening allergic reaction characterized by a swelling of body tissues including the throat, difficulty in breathing, and a sudden fall in blood pressure.

Anaphylactoid reaction: A severe response with the same symptoms as anaphylaxis; however, an anaphylactoid reaction is not IgE-mediated.

Anaphylatoxin: Complement peptides (C3a and C5a) that cause mast cell degranulation and smooth muscle contraction.

Anaphylaxis: An antigen-specific immune reaction mediated primarily by IgE, which results in vasodilation and constriction of smooth muscles, including those of the bronchus, and which may result in death.

Anergy: A state of unresponsiveness, induced when the T cell's antigen receptor is stimulated, that effectively freezes T cell responses pending a "second signal" from the antigen-presenting cell (see costimulation).

Angioedema: A reaction in the skin and underlying tissue marked by swelling and red blotches (see also hereditary angioedema).

Antibody: A protein in the bloodstream or other body fluids that is produced in response to foreign materials that enter the body; antibodies, also known as immunoglobulins, usually protect us.

Antibody-dependent cell-mediated cytotoxicity (ADCC): An immune response in which antibody, by coating target cells, makes them vulnerable to attack by immune cells.

Antigen presentation: The process by which certain cells in the body (antigen-presenting cells) express an antigen on their cell surface in a form recognizable by lymphocytes.

Antigen processing: The actions that a cell makes to convert antigen into a form in which it can be recognized by lymphocytes.

Antigen: Any substance that, when introduced into the body, is recognized and elicits a response by the immune system.

Antigen-presenting cells: B cells, cells of the monocyte lineage (including macrophages as well as dendritic cells), and various other body cells that present antigen in a form that T cells can recognize.

Antihistamine: A drug that blocks the effects of histamine, a chemical which is responsible for many of the symptoms of allergy when released by the body's mast cells during an allergic reaction.

Antinuclear antibody (ANA): An autoantibody directed against a substance in the cell's nucleus.

Antiserum: Serum that contains antibodies.

Antitoxins: Antibodies that interlock with and inactivate toxins produced by certain bacteria.

Antiviral proteins: Proteins induced by interferons that render a cell resistant to viral replication.

Appendix: Lymphoid organ in the intestine.

Asbestosis: A chronic inflammation of the lung caused by inhaled asbestos fibers.

Asthma: A genetically linked problem, believed to cause airway obstruction, that is associated with narrowing of air passages, airway inflammation, and airway hypersensitivity to multiple stimuli.

Atopic dermatitis: A chronic, itching, inflammation of the skin; also referred to as eczema.

Atopic/Atopy: A genetically determined clinical manifestation of type I hypersensitivity, which includes reactions such as eczema, asthma, and rhinitis.

Attenuated: Weakened; no longer infectious.

Autoantibody: An antibody that reacts against a person's own tissue.

Autocrine: Acting on self; e.g., describes hormones that are produced and utilized by the same cell or organ.

Autoimmune disease: A disease that results when the immune system mistakenly attacks the body's own tissues. Rheumatoid arthritis and systemic lupus erythematosus are autoimmune diseases.

Avoidance: Measures taken to avoid contact with allergy-producing substances.

B cells: Small white blood cells crucial to the immune defenses. Also known as B lymphocytes, they are derived from bone marrow and develop into plasma cells that are the source of antibodies.

B cell growth factor (BCGF): A factor that is involved in B cell proliferation.

B cell differentiation factor (BCDF): A factor that is involved in the induction of antibody secretion by B cells.

Bacterium: A microscopic organism composed of a single cell; many, but not all, bacteria cause disease.

Bagassosis: A form of allergic lung disorder caused by exposure to moldy sugar cane.

Basement membrane: A delicate layer of connective tissue lying beneath the epithelial cells which cover the internal and external surfaces of the body.

Basophil: A white blood cell that contributes to inflammatory reactions. Along with mast cells, basophils are responsible for the symptoms of allergy. They contain numerous lysosomes and granules (secretory vesicles), which release histamine and serotonin in certain immune reactions. Although basophils and mast cells are not identical, they are very similar and the terms are often used interchangeably.

Berylliosis: A lung inflammation caused by inhaling fumes or dust of the metal beryllium.

Biological response modifiers: Substances, either natural or synthesized, that boost, direct, or restore normal immune defenses. BRMs include interferons, interleukins, thymus hormones, and monoclonal antibodies.

Biotechnology: The use of living organisms or their products to make or modify a substance; biotechnology includes recombinant DNA techniques (genetic engineering) and hybridoma technology.

Blocking antibody: Antibody of one class that combines with an antigen, thus preventing the antigen from reacting with an antibody of another class.

Blood groups: Categories of blood determined by inherited antigens present on red blood cell surfaces. The most important human blood groups are A, B, O, and Rh.

531

Bone marrow: Soft tissue located in the cavities of the bones; consists, in varying proportions, of fat cells and maturing blood cells. The bone marrow is the source of all blood cells.

Bradykinin: One member of the family of body chemicals known as kinins. Bradykinin contracts smooth muscle, lowers blood pressure, and stimulates secretion of the mucous glands.

Bronchi: The tubes that branch from the windpipe, one to each lung, through which air enters and leaves the lungs.

Bronchial asthma: See asthma.

Bronchiole: One of the thousands of tiny airways into which the bronchi split, forming a tree-like network inside each lung.

Bronchodilator: A drug that relaxes the smooth muscles in constricted airways; often used in acute asthma.

Bronchospasm: Tightening of the muscles surrounding the bronchial tubes.

Bullous pemphigoid: A blistering disorder found mostly in the middle-aged and elderly that is disabling but rarely fatal.

C1-C9 complement: The components of the complement classical and lytic pathways, which are responsible for mediating inflammatory reactions, opsonization of particles, and lysis of cell membranes.

Cascade reaction: A series of reactions, such as that of the serum complement system, in which the reaction of the first component triggers the reaction of the next component, etc., until all components of the system have reacted in a given order.

CD markers: Cell surface molecules of lymphocytes, including

- **CD1:** A cortical thymocyte differentiation marker
- **CD2:** A receptor involved in antigen; nonspecific T cell activation (E receptor)
- **CD3:** A constant portion of the T cell antigen receptor
- **CD4:** A marker of T helper cells involved in MHC class II recognition

- **CD5:** A T cell marker also present on a sub-population of B cells
- **CD8:** A marker of T cytotoxic cells involved in MHC class I recognition
- **CD25:** The IL-2 receptor present on activated T cells and on some activated B cells.

Cell-mediated immunity: That portion of the immune system mediated by the small white blood cells called T cells or T lymphocytes.

Cellular immunity: Immune protection provided by the direct action of immune cells (as distinct from soluble molecules such as antibodies).

Challenge test: A medical procedure also known as provocative testing used to identify those substances to which a person is sensitive by deliberately exposing a patient to dilute amounts of those substances until allergic symptoms are provoked.

Chemotaxis: Increased directional migration of cells, particularly in response to concentration gradients of certain chemotactic factors.

Chimera: An organism whose body contains different cell populations of the same or different species.

Chromosomes: Physical structures in the cell's nucleus that house the genes; each human cell has 23 pairs of chromosomes.

Class I, II, and III molecules: Three major classes of molecules coded within the MHC:

- **Class I molecules:** Expressed on virtually all cell types, consisting of a heavy alpha chain associated with a light beta chain (ß2 microglobulin) not encoded by the MHC
- **Class II molecules:** Tend to be expressed on B cells, macrophages, and activated T cells; consisting of two noncovalently linked alpha and beta chains, which are thought also to interact to form a common binding site
- **Class III molecules:** Predominantly plasma proteins that act as complement proteins; thought to involve the induction of the immune response.

533

Class I/II restriction: The observation that immunologically active cells will cooperate effectively only when they share MHC haplotypes at either the class I or class II loci.

Clone: A group of genetically identical cells or organisms descended from a single common ancestor, or, to reproduce multiple identical copies.

Co-stimulation: The delivery of a second signal from an antigen-presenting cell to a T cell. The second signal rescues the activated T cell from anergy, allowing it to produce the lymphokines necessary for the growth of additional T cells.

Cold-induced urticaria: Hives produced in response to cold temperatures.

Complement: A complex series of blood proteins whose action "complements" the work of antibodies. Complement destroys bacteria, produces inflammation, and regulates immune reactions.

Complement system: A series of interacting serum proteins that are activated by antigen-antibody reactions. These proteins play a role in important body responses, such as the engulfment of foreign material by segments of the immune system. See C1-C9 complement.

Complement cascade: A precise sequence of events usually triggered by an antigen-antibody complex, in which each component of the complement system is activated in turn.

Constant region: That part of an antibody's structure that is characteristic for each antibody class.

Corticosteroids: A group of hormones produced by the adrenal glands that play key roles in many body functions, such as metabolism, muscle function and resistance to stress. Man-made corticosteroids are used as powerful anti-inflammatory drugs.

Crohn's disease: A chronic inflammation of the ileum, a section of the small intestine; also, regional ileitis.

Cross-reactivity: When the body mistakes one compound for another of similar chemical composition.

Cutaneous necrotizing angiitis: A chronic inflammation of blood vessels that produces small, solid, reddish elevations on the skin. Apparently it results from an allergic reaction involving immune complexes.

Cyclosporine (cyclosporin A): A drug derived from fungal extracts; used to suppress immune reactions and to prevent rejection of transplanted organs and tissues.

Cytokines: Powerful chemical substances secreted by cells. Cytokines include lymphokines produced by lymphocytes and monokines produced by monocytes and macrophages.

Cytotoxic T cells: A subset of T lymphocytes that carry the T8 marker and can kill body cells infected by viruses or transformed by cancer.

Cytotoxic: Having the ability to kill cells.

Dander: Small scales from animal skin. Dander is a common allergen.

Degranulation: Exocytosis of granules from cells such as mast cells and basophils.

Dendritic cells: White blood cells found in the spleen and other lymphoid organs. Dendritic cells typically use thread-like tentacles to enmesh antigen, which they present to T cells.

Dermatitis herpetiformis: A chronic, debilitating skin disorder characterized by firm blisters with reddened bases.

Desensitization: See immunotherapy.

DNA (deoxyribonucleic acid): A nucleic acid that is found in the cell nucleus and is the carrier of genetic information.

ECF (eosinophil chemotactic factor): A factor produced at sites of inflammation by T cells that attracts eosinophil; other ECFs are produced by triggered mast cells.

Eczema: See atopic dermatitis.

Edema: Swelling of tissue due to injury or disease.

Effector cells: Generally denotes T cells that are capable of suppressing cytotoxicity (helper T cell function).

Elimination diet: A restricted diet in which foods suspected of causing allergic reactions are introduced one at a time so that the blameworthy ones can be identified.

Endotoxin: Lipopolysaccharide component of the cell wall of several species of gram-negative bacteria; a potent immunostimulant.

Enzyme: A protein, produced by living cells, that promotes the chemical processes of life without itself being altered.

Eosinophil chemotactic factor of anaphylaxis (ECF-A): A chemical mediator, released by mast cells, that attracts a type of cell called an eosinophil.

Eosinophil: A white blood cell that contains granules filled with chemicals damaging to parasites and enzymes that damp down inflammatory reactions.

Epinephrine: A powerful drug used to counter anaphylaxis. It is a heart-muscle stimulant and is also used to relax bronchial smooth muscle. Another name for it is adrenaline.

Epitope: A unique shape or marker carried on an antigen's surface, which triggers a corresponding antibody response.

Erythroblastosis fetalis: The medical term for Rh incompatibility disease of newborn infants.

Eustachian tubes: Two tubes in the back of the throat, one leading to each ear.

Extrinsic asthma: Asthma caused by external sources, e.g., allergens.

Farmer's lung: A form of allergic lung disorder caused by exposure to moldy hay.

Fc receptor: A protein on the surface of a cell that recognizes and binds Fc portions of antibody molecules.

Fc: The portion of an antibody that is bound by specific receptors on cells and the C1a component of complement.

Food allergy or hypersensitivity: An abnormal reaction to certain foods, which may be manifested as severe indigestion, diarrhea, vomiting, rash, trouble breathing, etc., which is triggered by the immune system.

Food intolerance: An unpleasant reaction to specific foods, not triggered by the immune system and therefore not an allergic reaction.

Forced-air system's lung: An allergic lung disorder caused by exposure to molds growing in air conditioners, heating systems, or humidifiers.

Fungus: Member of a class of relatively primitive vegetable organisms. Fungi include mushrooms, yeasts, rusts, molds, and smuts.

Gastrointestinal (GI) tract: The stomach and intestines.

Gene: A unit of genetic material (DNA) that occupies a definite locus on a chromosome and contains the plan a cell uses to perform a specific function (e.g., making a given protein).

Genetic markers: Inherited features that scientists are identifying which may enable them to understand the genetic aspects of many normal and abnormal processes in the body. Some markers for which tests now exist can predict who is at high risk of inheriting or developing specific diseases.

Genetic association: A term used to describe the condition in which particular genotypes are associated with other phenomena such as particular diseases.

Glomerulonephritis: An inflammation of capillaries in the kidney. The disease accounts for over half the 42,000 annual kidney-deaths in the United States.

Glycoproteins: Proteins combined with a carbohydrate; frequently on cell surfaces.

Granulocytes: Phagocytic white blood cells filled with granules containing potent chemicals that allow the cells to digest microorganisms; neutrophils, eosinophils, basophils, and mast cells are examples of granulocytes.

Guillain-Barré syndrome: An illness consisting of muscle weakness which may progress to complete paralysis; it is thought to be due to an autoimmune mechanism.

Hageman factor systems: The three enzyme systems in the body responsible for blood clotting, dissolving blood clots, and the formation of powerful blood-vessel dilators called kinins.

Haplotype: A set of genetic determinants located on a single chromosome.

Hay fever: See allergic rhinitis.

Helper T cells: A subset of T cells that typically carry the T4 marker and are essential for turning on antibody production, activating cytotoxic T cells, and initiating many other immune responses.

Helper factors: Molecules that can deliver T-cell help to other lymphocytes; the term is usually reserved for antigen-specific interferons and interleukins.

Hematopoiesis: The formation and development of blood cells, usually taking place in the bone marrow.

Hereditary angioedema: A rare inherited disorder that produces recurrent abdominal pain and episodes of swelling, mostly in the face and extremities or airway passages. It may prove fatal if swelling, which occurs in the tongue, throat, or larynx, shuts off air to the lungs.

Heterologous: Refers to interspecies antigenic differences.

Histamine-release test: A method of measuring the amount of histamine released by certain cells in a sample of blood from an allergic patient when the cells are exposed to an allergen. It is used to gain some idea of a patient's reactivity to specific substances.

Histamine: A chemical released by mast cells and considered responsible for much of the swelling and itching characteristic of hay fever and other allergies.

HIV (human immunodeficiency virus): The virus that causes AIDS.

HLA histocompatibility antigens: Molecules on the surface of human cells which the immune system reads to determine if the cells are "self" or "nonself."

HLA (human leukocyte antigen): The major histocompatibility genetic region in humans; protein markers of "self."

Homologous: Of the same species.

Human leukocyte antigens (HLA): protein in markers of "self" used in histocompatibility testing. Some HLA types also correlate with certain autoimmune diseases.

Humoral immunity: Immune protection provided by soluble factors such as antibodies, which circulate in the body's fluids or "humors," primarily serum and lymph.

Humoral: Pertaining to the extracellular fluids, including the plasma and lymph.

Hybridoma: A hybrid cell created in vitro by fusing a B lymphocyte with a long-lived neoplastic plasma cell, or a T lymphocyte with a lymphoma cell. A B-cell hybridoma secretes a single specific antibody.

Hypersensitivity pneumonitis: A group of allergic lung disorders that result from inhaling a wide variety of substances, such as dusts and molds.

Hypersensitivity: The condition—existing in a person previously exposed to an antigen—in which tissue damage results from an immune reaction to a further dose of the antigen. Classically, four different types of hypersensitivity are recognized, but the term is often used to mean the type of allergy associated with hay fever and asthma.

Hypogammaglobulinemia: Abnormally low levels of immunoglobulins.

Hyposensitization: Term previously used to describe allergy treatments commonly called "allergy shots." Immunotherapy is the term presently in use.

Idiotypes: The unique and characteristic parts of an antibody's variable region, which can themselves serve as antigens.

IFN: See interferon.

Immune complexes: Large molecules formed when antigen and antibody bind together.

Immune system: The complex system of cells and chemicals that reacts against foreign substances entering the body.

Immune reaction or response: The activity of various specialized body cells and chemicals against foreign substances.

Immunity: The overall capability of an individual to resist or overcome an infection.

Immunoassay: A test using antibodies to identify and quantify substances. Often the antibody is linked to a marker such as a fluorescent molecule, a radioactive molecule, or an enzyme.

Immunocompetent: Capable of developing an immune response.

Immunodeficiency: A condition that results from a defect in the immune system.

Immunoglobulins: A family of large protein molecules, also known as antibodies (e.g., IgA or IgG).

- **Immunoglobulin A (IgA):** A class of antibody found in such body secretions as saliva, tears, and intestinal and bronchial fluids. It serves as the first line of defense against organisms invading the respiratory and gastrointestinal systems.

- **Immunoglobulin D (IgD):** A class of antibody present in very low concentrations. Its exact role remains unknown.

- **Immunoglobulin E (IgE):** A class of antibody normally present in very low levels in humans, but found in larger quantities in people with allergies and certain infections. Its protective role is unknown, but evidence suggests it is the only antibody responsible for the classic allergy symptoms.

- **Immunoglobulin G (IgG):** The most abundant class of antibody in human serum. The major immunoglobulin to be made by the body in a secondary immune response against invading organisms.

- **Immunoglobulin M (IgM):** A class of antibody produced in early immune responses. IgM is effective as the first line of defense against bacteria.

Immunosuppression: Reduction of the immune responses, for instance, by giving drugs to prevent transplant rejection.

Immunotherapy: Injections of gradually increasing amounts of allergens known to trigger a patient's allergic response. Also called desensitization, hyposensitization, injection therapy, and "allergy shots."

Immunotoxin: A monoclonal antibody linked to a toxic drug or a radioactive substance.

In vitro: Referring to studies performed on tissues removed from the living organism under artificial conditions in the laboratory.

In vivo: Referring to studies performed on tissues not removed from the living organism, or in the organism itself.

Inflammation: A basic response of the body to injury, usually characterized by redness of the skin, warmth, swelling, and pain.

Inflammatory response: Redness, warmth, swelling, pain, and loss of function produced in response to infection, as the result of increased blood flow and an influx of immune cells and secretions.

Injection therapy: See immunotherapy.

Intercellular: Between cells.

Interferon (IFN): A group of mediators that increase the resistance of cells to viral infection, by altering the activities of the cells' metabolic machinery; also has numerous other effects in modulating immune responses; group includes.

- **IFN-α:** Produced by leukocytes
- **IFN-γ:** Produced by T cells
- **IFN-ß:** Produced by fibroblasts

Interleukins (IL): A group of molecules involved in signaling between cells of the immune system

- **IL-1:** Released by numerous cells in the body, including macrophages; it has a wide variety of effects, including activation of T cells to express IL-2 receptors
- **IL-2:** Released by activated T cells and is required for T cell proliferation
- **IL-3:** Released by activated T cells and acts as a panspecific hemopoietin
- **IL-4:** Provisionally allocated to the B cell growth factor (BCGF).

Intracellular: Within a cell

Intrinsic asthma: Asthma without external cause.

Kupffer cells: Specialized macrophages in the liver.

LAK cells: Lymphocytes transformed in the laboratory into lymphokine-activated killer cells, which attack tumor cells.

Langerhans cells: Dendritic cells in the skin that pick up antigen and transport it to lymph nodes.

Leukocytes: All white blood cells; see lymphocytes.

Leukotrienes: Signaling compound chemically related to prostaglandins.

Line: A collection of cells produced by continuously growing a particular cell culture *in vitro*; such cell lines will usually contain a number of individual clones.

Lupus erythematosus of the skin: An inflammatory disease that may involve the skin only or, the skin in addition to several organs, primarily the brain and kidneys.

Lymph nodes: Small bean-shaped organs of the immune system, distributed widely throughout the body and linked by lymphatic vessels; lymph nodes are garrisons of B, T, and other immune cells.

Lymph: A transparent, slightly yellow fluid that carries lymphocytes, bathes the body tissues, and drains into the lymphatic vessels.

Lymphatic vessels: A body-wide network of channels, similar to the blood vessels, which transport lymph to the immune organs and into the bloodstream.

Lymphocyte: A white blood cell important in immunity. There are two major types. T lymphocytes are processed by the thymus and are involved in cell-mediated immunity; B lymphocytes are derived from the bone marrow and are the precursors of those cells (plasma cells) that produce antibody. However, both types of lymphocytes have subclasses of cells.

Lymphoid organs: The organs of the immune system, where lymphocytes develop and congregate. They include the bone marrow, thymus, lymph nodes, spleen, and various other clusters of lymphoid tissue. The blood vessels and lymphatic vessels can also be considered lymphoid organs.

Lymphokines tolerance: A state of specific immunological unresponsiveness.

Lymphokines: Powerful chemical substances secreted by lymphocytes. These soluble molecules help direct and regulate the immune responses.

Macrophage: A large and versatile immune cell that acts as a microbe-devouring phagocyte, an antigen-presenting cell, and an important source of regulatory proteins—immune secretions.

Major histocompatibility complex: see **MHC**

Maple bark stripper's disease: An allergic lung disorder caused by exposure to a mold that grows beneath the bark of maple logs.

Mast cells: Tissue cells which contain packets of chemicals responsible for the symptoms of allergy. When allergens attach to IgE antibodies sitting on the surface of these cells, a signal is sent, causing them to release these chemical mediators of allergy.

Mediators: chemical substances that attract or activate other parts of the immune system; the best known mediator is histamine.

MHC restriction: A characteristic of many immune reactions, in which cells cooperate most effectively with other cells sharing an MHC haplotype.

MHC (major histocompatibility complex): A genetic region, found in all mammals, whose products are primarily responsible for the rapid rejection of grafts between individuals and which functions in signaling between lymphocytes and cells expressing antigen.

Microbes: Minute living organisms, including bacteria, viruses, fungi, and protozoa.

Micro-organisms: Microscopic plants or animals.

Molecule: The smallest amount of a specific chemical substance that can exist alone. (To break a molecule down into its constituent atoms is to change its character. A molecule of water, for instance, reverts to oxygen and hydrogen.)

Monoclonal antibodies: Antibodies produced by a single cell or its identical progeny, specific for a given antigen. As a tool for binding to specific protein molecules, monoclonal antibodies are invaluable in research, medicine, and industry.

Monoclonal: Derived from a single clone, e.g., monoclonal antibodies that are produced by a single clone and are homogeneous.

Monocyte: A large phagocytic white blood cell which, when it enters tissue, develops into a macrophage.

Monokines: Powerful chemical substances secreted by monocytes and macrophages. These soluble molecules help direct and regulate the immune responses.

Mucous membranes: Thin layers of tissue that are kept moist by a sticky substance called mucus. These membranes line the nose and other parts of the respiratory tract, and are found in other parts of the body which have communication with air.

Multiple sclerosis: A disorder of the central nervous system that results in the degeneration of the protective coating on nerve fibers and a decline in muscle coordination.

Murine: Pertaining to the genus that includes mice and rats.

Myasthenia gravis (MG): A disorder that causes muscular weakness and fatigue, and may lead to a life-threatening interference with breathing. New evidence implicates MG as an autoimmune disease.

NADPH: The reduced form of NADP (nicotinamide-adenine dinucleotide phosphate).

Natural killer (NK) cells: Large granule-filled lymphocytes that take on tumor cells and infected body cells. They are known as "natural" killers because they attack without first having to recognize specific antigens.

Neoplasm: A new and abnormal growth; used as a synonym for cancerous tissue.

Neutrophil: A large white blood cell that an abundant and important phagocyte.

Nucleic acids: Large, naturally occurring molecules composed of chemical building blocks known as nucleotides. There are two kinds of nucleic acids, DNA and RNA.

OKT3: A monoclonal antibody that targets mature T cells.

Opportunistic infection: An infection in an immunosuppressed person caused by an organism that does not usually trouble people with healthy immune systems.

Opsonize: To coat an organism with antibodies or a complement protein so as to make it palatable to phagocytes.

Organism: An individual living thing.

Paracrine: Produced by one cell/organ and acting on another.

Parasite: A plant or animal that lives, grows, and feeds on or within another living organism.

Parasympathetic nervous system: A part of the body's involuntary nervous system which helps regulate body functions like heart rate and respiration; also known as the cholinergic nervous system.

Passive immunity: Immunity resulting from the transfer of antibodies or antiserum produced by another individual.

Patch tests: A form of skin testing in which suspected allergens are applied to the skin, covered, and observed for several days to see if a reaction occurs. This is often used in identifying the possible causes of allergic contact dermatitis.

Pathogen: An organism that causes disease, e.g., streptococcus, HIV.

Pemphigus vulgaris: A rare, chronic, blistering disease that involves an allergic reaction to immune complexes. Once fatal in nearly 50 percent of the patients within the first 2 years of onset, this disease can now usually be controlled with steroids.

546

Peptide: A compound of two or more amino acids in which the alpha carboxyl group of one is united with the alpha amino group of another, forming a peptide bond.

Peyer's patches: A collection of lymphoid tissues in the intestinal tract.

Phagocytes: Large white blood cells that contribute to immune defenses by ingesting foreign material, e.g., macrophages, neutrophils.

Phagocytosis: The process by which cells engulf material and enclose it within a vacuole (phagosome) in the cytoplasm.

Plasma cells: Large antibody-producing cells that develop from B cells.

Platelets: Granule-containing cellular fragments critical for blood clotting and sealing off wounds. Platelets also contribute to the immune response.

Pleiotropic: Refers to the ability of a gene to manifest itself in many ways.

Pluripotent: Able to act or to develop in any one of several different ways.

Pollen: The tiny spores of flowering plants. Airborne pollen is a major allergen responsible for hay fever.

Polyclonal activators: Agents that stimulate the activation/proliferation of many cell types; nonspecific activators.

Polymorph: Short for polymorphonuclear leukocyte or granulocyte.

Polymyositis: A painful inflammation of several muscles at once. It is thought to be an autoimmune disorder. It may occur in conjunction with other presumably autoimmune diseases or in some cancer patients.

Polyp: A protrusion growing outward from a mucous membrane.

Proliferate: To reproduce.

Prostaglandins: A family of fatty acid derivatives producing a variety of biological effects, including inflammatory responses.

Proteins: Organic compounds made up of amino acids; proteins are one of the major constituents of plant and animal cells.

Protozoa: A group of one-celled animals, a few of which cause human disease (including malaria and sleeping sickness).

Pulmonary mycotoxicosis: An unusual disease similar to farmer's lung that results from inhaled fungi and bacteria associated with silos.

Pyrogenic: Causing fever.

Radioallergosorbent test (RAST): A test for measuring the amount of specific IgE antibodies in a patient's blood. Along with a medical history, this test can help identify some allergens to which a person is allergic.

Receptor: A cell surface molecule that binds specifically to particular proteins or peptides in the fluid phase. Sites on cell's surfaces where drugs and other chemicals either attach or enter.

Recessive trait: An inherited characteristic usually masked or hidden by the presence of a "stronger" so-called dominant trait. It shows itself only when two pieces of genetic material carrying the same recessive characteristic are inherited by one individual.

Rejection: Destruction of transplanted foreign tissues or cells by immune reactions of the recipient; also referred to as graft rejection.

Rh antigen: Rhesus antigen; a red blood cell surface antigen.

Rheumatoid arthritis: A chronic inflammatory disease primarily of the joints, but which may affect other systems or tissues in the body.

Rheumatoid-factor: An autoantibody found in the serum of most persons with rheumatoid arthritis.

Rhinitis medicamentosa: A form of rhinitis caused by the prolonged use of decongestant nose drops and sprays.

Rhinitis: An inflammation of the membrane lining the nose. Allergic rhinitis (misnamed hay fever) is an IgE-mediated reaction. Nonallergic forms of rhinitis may result from infections, hormonal changes, or certain drugs.

RNA (ribonucleic acid): A nucleic acid that is found in the cytoplasm and also in the nucleus of some cells. One function of RNA is to direct the synthesis of proteins.

Scavenger cells: Any of a diverse group of cells that have the capacity to engulf and destroy foreign material, dead tissues, or other cells.

Schistosomiasis: A disease caused by flatworms. It occurs mainly in Africa and Asia, but is also found in Puerto Rico and Venezuela, and is considered second only to malaria in worldwide importance as a parasitic disease.

SCID mouse: A laboratory animal that, lacking an enzyme necessary to fashion an immune system of its own, can be turned into a model of the human immune system when injected with human cells or tissues.

Second messengers: Intracellular signaling mediators that, when activated, in turn alter the behavior of other target proteins within a cell, ultimately resulting in a cellular response such as activation.

Sensitize: Synonymous with immunize; to administer or expose to an antigen provoking an immune response so that, on later exposure to that antigen, a more vigorous secondary response will occur.

Serotonin: A body chemical that causes a variety of effects such as contraction of smooth muscle. It plays a role in anaphylactic reactions in several species of animals but its role in allergic reactions in humans is not yet known.

Serous otitis media: An inflammation of the middle ear, commonly found in infants and children with allergic rhinitis.

Serum sickness: A disease characterized by fever, joint swelling, and enlarged lymph nodes that occurs in humans after repeated injections of rather large quantities of foreign antigens, particularly animal serum.

Serum: The clear liquid that separates from the blood when it is allowed to clot. This fluid retains any antibodies that were present in the whole blood.

Silicosis: A severe lung disease that results from inhaling dust containing silica; also, sandblaster's silicosis and grinder's disease.

Sinusitis: An inflammation of the air spaces around the nose.

Site-associated idiotopes: Idiotopes present in the antibody-combining site; this is usually defined functionally by inhibiting antigen binding with anti-idiotype or vice versa.

Skin tests: The injection of a small, dilute amount of allergen under the skin or its application to a scratch on the patient 's arm or back. If the patient is allergic to that substance, a small raised area surrounded by redness will appear at the test site within 15 minutes.

SLE (systemic lupus erythematosus): An autoimmune disease of humans.

Slow reacting substance of anaphylaxis (SRS-A): A chemical mediator which is the most powerful known direct constrictor of human bronchial smooth muscle.

Specificity: The characteristic of antibodies and white blood cells that enables them to recognize and interact only with the specific antigen that they were produced to battle.

Spirometer: A device that measures the amount of air inhaled and exhaled. It is used by physicians to measure the amount of airway obstruction in patients with asthma.

Spleen: A lymphoid organ in the abdominal cavity that is an important center for immune system activities.

Spores: The reproductive cells of certain organisms and plants.

Sputum: Material often containing mucus, pus, and micro-organisms which is expelled from the chest by coughing or clearing the throat.

Stem cells: Cells from which all blood cells derive. The bone marrow is rich in stem cells.

Steroids: See corticosteroids.

Subunit vaccine: A vaccine that uses merely one component of an infectious agent, rather than the whole, to stimulate an immune response.

Superantigens: A class of antigens, including certain bacterial toxins, that unleash a massive and damaging immune response.

Superoxide radical: An unstable form of oxygen generated by mast cells in human lungs in response to immunologic and nonimmunologic stimulation. Its exact role in human asthma is not yet defined.

Suppressor T cells: A subset of T cells that turn off antibody production and other immune responses.

Sympathetic nervous system: Part of the body's involuntary nervous system. These nerves stimulate the body in times of crisis; another name for it is the adrenergic nervous system.

Sympathomimetic: An agent or drug which mimics the sympathetic nervous system.

Systemic lupus erythematosus (SLE): A serious disease of the connective tissue which predominantly strikes women of childbearing age. Its most serious damage involves the kidney and brain. Genetic, immunologic, and viral factors may all play roles in SLE.

T cells: White blood cells that are processed in the thymus and are responsible for cell-mediated immunity; they are also called T lymphocytes.

T lymphocytes (T cells): Lymphocytes that are processed in the thymus (thus T cell); they directly participate in immune responses and produce lymphokines.

Thymic epithelial cells: Thymic antigen presenting cells, expressing high levels of class II MHC antigens, thought to be important in the development of T cell immune recognition.

Thymus: A primary lymphoid organ, high in the chest, where T cells proliferate and mature.

Tolerance: A state of nonresponsiveness to a particular antigen or group of antigens.

Tonsils and adenoids: Prominent oval masses of lymphoid tissues on either side of the throat.

Toxins: Agents produced by plants and bacteria, normally very damaging to mammalian cells, that can be delivered directly to target cells by linking them to monoclonal antibodies or lymphokines.

Transgenes: Genes from one organism that have been transferred to another organism; these genes are inserted into the host DNA.

Transgenic mice: Mice that have had specific genes, usually human, inserted into their genomes.

Triggering of mast cells: Stimulation of mast cell degranulation, effected by cross-linking of surface-bound IgE, direct triggering by C3a and C5a, or by drugs.

TSH: Thyroid-stimulating hormone.

Types of allergic reactions: Four groups of allergic mechanisms which generally cover all allergic reactions.

- **Type I:** The most common type of allergic reaction. Immediate hypersensitivity or anaphalaxis. Occurs with hay fever, insect stings, or other allergic shocks.
- **Type II:** Cytotoxic or reaction with cell membrane. Occurs with incompatible blood transfusions.

- **Type III:** Arthus or deposition of immune complexes in walls of blood vessels or kidneys. Occurs in serum sickness and some drug reactions.
- **Type IV:** Delayed hypersensitivity or cell-mediated response. Occurs with poison ivy and graft rejections.

Ulcerative colitis: A chronic, recurrent ulceration of the colon.

Urticaria: Hives; a reaction in the skin marked by swelling, redness, and itching.

Vaccination: Administration of specific weakened or killed antigens to stimulate the immune system so that the body will be protected against further exposure to the antigen.

Vaccine: A substance that contains antigenic components from an infectious organism; by stimulating an immune response (but not disease), it protects against subsequent infection by that organism.

Variable region: That part of an antibody's structure that differs from one antibody to another.

Vesiculobullous diseases: A variety of disorders in which blistering is a major symptom.

Virus: Submicroscopic microbe that consists of a protein coat and a nucleic acid core; viruses' inability to grow or reproduce outside of living cells makes them the cause of many infectious diseases.

Xenografts: Tissue grafts between species.

Index

Index

A page number in *italics* indicates an illustration; a t following a page number represents a table.

A

AAIDCRCs
    see Asthma, Allergy, and Immunologic Diseases Cooperative Research Centers (AAIDCRCs)
ABPA
    see allergic bronchopulmonary aspergillosis (ABPA)
ACD
    see allergic contact dermatitis
acetylcholine, in myasthenia gravis 183
acetylsalicylic acid
    see aspirin
acid anhydrides 392
acne medications, and contact dermatitis 399
acquired immunodeficiency syndrome (AIDS)
    defined 527
    hospitalizations (U.S.) for *46*
    latex gloves as protection against 417
    T-cell deficiency in 485

actinomycetes 317
active immunity, defined 527
acute phase proteins, defined 527
Adams, Robert M. 426
additives
    color
        see color additives
    in drugs, allergic reaction to 118
adenoids, defined 552
adenoviruses 99, 158
adhesion molecules 471
adjuvant, defined 527
adolescents
    see young adults
adrenal steroids (cortisones), for insect sting 360
adrenaline 88, 203
    see also epinephrine
Adrenaline (epinephrine) 517
adrenergic agents 73
    adverse effects from 517-18
adults
    asthma in 23, 452
    with contact dermatitis 402
    food allergy in 197
    immunotherapy for 365
    and poison ivy/oak/sumac 369-70
    theophylline and 519
adverse drug reaction, defined 115

Adverse Reaction Monitoring System (ARMS) 213, 214, 225
  address 214, 225
Advil (ibuprofen), photoallergic reaction to 135
Advisory Review Panel on OTC Topical Analgesic, Antirheumatic, Otic, Burn, and Sunburn Prevention and Treatment Drug Products 476
aeroallergens
  see airborne allergens
African-American children, asthma in 53, 470
African-Americans
  asthma in 327, 439, 444, *444,* 445, 446, 466
  lactose intolerance in 234
Afrin (oxymetholone) 495
aftershave lotion, and contact dermatitis 399
agammaglobulinemia, defined 527
age
  and allergic drug reactions 126-27
  and asthma *440, 442*
aged
  see elderly
agricultural (harvester) ant 352
AIDS
  see acquired immunodeficiency syndrome (AIDS)
air cleaners, portable 175
air conditioner lung 148t, 151, 317
air conditioning 21, 69, 322-23, 328
  for sinusitis 101
air filters
  in treatment of allergic disease 322-23, 487, 512
  in treatment of allergy-induced asthma 87
air fresheners 176
air pollutants (air pollution) 322, 341-44, 343t
  and asthma 24, 141
  effect of on respiratory system 344
  indoor *70,* 328
  particulate, populations at risk from 341-44
  and sinusitis 101
  types of 393-94

air travel, and sinusitis 101
airborne allergens 63-69, 309-25
  affect of on children's allergies 159
  air conditioning and 21
  in allergic rhinitis 18, 63-64, 69
    at home 20, 64, 69
    naturally occurring 20, 64
    smoke and fumes as 69
    at work 69
  from animals 336
  avoidance of 487
  indoor 20, 64, 327-29
  information resources on 325
  molds as 314-17
  outdoor 19-20, 64
  pollen as 312-14
  reaction to, symptoms of 19, 311
  in sinusitis 100
  size of 64
  types of 310
air-cleaning devices 322, 325
air-filtering devices 322-23
  for asthma sufferers 87
airway closure, in insect sting 360
airway hyper-reactivity 25
airway obstruction, defined 527
airway responsiveness, nonspecific 25
airways
  asthmatic 22-23
    inhaled irritants and 141t, 142
  of infants 158
  inflammation of, in asthma 78, 79
Alabama, pollen calendar for *65*
albuterol (Ventolin, Proventil) 517
  for cat-induced asthma 340
alcohol(s) 477
  and sinusitis 101
Aleve (naproxen sodium), photoallergic reaction to 135
alkylamines 503-4
allergen(s) 6, *8,* 16-17, 32
  airborne 63-69, 309-25
    see also airborne allergen
  in allergy diagnosis and treatment, anaphylactic reactions to 166
  avoidance of
    see avoidance of allergens
  defined 528
  food 107, 197, 202, 207

allergen(s), continued
  indoor 327-29, 399
  major
    in United States 15
    worldwide 15
  skin test for
    see skin test
  see also specific allergen, e.g., saliva
allergen immunotherapy
  see immunotherapy (allergy shots)
allergenic extracts 482-84
  for immunotherapy 513-15, *514*
Allergenic Products Advisory Committee (FDA) 508
allergens, outdoor 512
allergic bronchopulmonary
  aspergillosis (ABPA) 91, 153, 316
  defined 528
allergic contact dermatitis 107-9,
  397-98, 407
  bathing and 107
  defined 528
  from poison ivy 107, 369
  prevention of 404-5
  "spread" of 107
  symptoms of 107
  testing for 400
allergic disease(s) 3-29, 37-42, 45-54
  basic mechanisms of 3-26, 33-35, *34*
    research on 39-40
  in children 52-53
  diagnosis of 319-20
  eczema and 106
  immune system and 33-35
  prevalence of 48-50, 49t
  research on 37-42
  secretory process in, research on 40
  socioeconomic impact of 45-54
    see also specific condition, e.g.,
      asthma
  treatment of 320-24
    air conditioners and filters in 322-23
    antihistamines in 323
    avoidance of allergen in 20-21,
      320-22
    cromolyn sodium in 323
    immunotherapy in 324
    medication in 322-23

allergic disease(s), continued
  treatment of, continued
    research on 41
    topical nasal steroids in 323
  in young adults 52-53
allergic drug reactions 5, 115-31, 117t
  anaphylactic 119
  and angioedema (giant hives) 119
  to antibiotics 123
  basic mechanisms of 125-27
  breakdown products of drugs and 127
  causes of 123-24
  to chloramphenicol 123
  desensitization to 131
  diagnosis of 127-29
  and drug fever 120
  environmental factors and 127
  identification of drug in 129-30
  to insulin 124
  and lung involvement 120-21
  medical history of patient and 128,
    129
  to neomycin 123
  to penicillin 123
  photosensitivity and 135-36
  prevention of 127-29
  pseudoallergic 121-23
  research on 42
  and serum sickness 119
  severe 130
  and skin reactions 120
  socioeconomic impact of 115-16
  to streptomycin 123
  to sulfonamides 123-24
  symptoms of 118
  treatment of 129-31
  types of 118-23
  vs. overdosage 124-25
allergic emergencies 163-71
  aspirin and 169-70
  cold-induced urticaria and 168-69
  diagnostic allergens (skin test) and
    166
  drug-induced 164
  foods and 167-68
  hereditary angioedema attack and
    170-71
  injected dyes and 168
  insect stings and 166-67

allergic emergencies, continued
  therapeutic allergens (immuno-
    therapy) and 166
  transfusion reactions as 169
  vaccines and 165-66
  see also anaphylaxis (anaphylactic
    reaction)
allergic gastroenteropathy 161
allergic lung reactions, eosinophils in
  459-62
allergic patients, sinusitis in 100
allergic pneumonia (hypersensitivity
  pneumonitis) 147-51, 148t
  forms of 148-49
  socioeconomic impact of 148
allergic reaction(s) 4-6, 5t, *8-12, 38*
  to airborne substances 311
  anaphylactic (immediate hypersen-
    sitivity) 4, 5t
  arthus 5, 5t
  in asthma 80-81
  to cats and dogs 335-37
    see also under animal; cat; dog;
      pet
  cell-mediated (delayed hypersensi-
    tivity) 5, 5t
  cytotoxic 5, 5t
  defined 310-11, 528
  frequency of occurrence, by body
    site 7
  how it works 80-81
  to insect stings 355-56
  mechanism of 6, *8-10, 34, 38, 39,*
    310-11
  mediators orchestrate 17, 35
  most common 6
  to occupational chemicals 142
  prevalence of 49t
  prevention of 486-87
  research on 69
  role of immune system in 31-35, *34,*
    246
  and sinusitis 101
  speed of 17
  types of 4-6, 5t, 552-53
  see also allergy(ies)
allergic respiratory disease, history of
  139
  see also occupational asthma

allergic response
  see allergic reaction(s)
allergic rhinitis (hay fever) 18-22, 61-
  75, 489-99
  airborne allergens and 63-64, 69,
    311, 312
    at home 64
    naturally occurring 64
    smoke and fumes as 69
    at work 69
  cause(s) of 18, 62
  in child 159-60
  common features of 19
  complications of 505
  course, prognosis, and complica-
    tions of 71-72
  decongestants for 481
  defined 61, 528
  and development of asthma 71-72,
    75
  diagnosis of 73-74, 480
  "hay fever" as term for 61, 479
  immunologic response in 69-71
  immunotherapy for 482, 484
  information resources on 325
  nasal physiology of 62-63
  pathophysiology of 491
  perennial (year-round) 19, 20, 62
  prevalence of 18, 49t
  prevention of 486-87
  priming effect in 491
  "priming" effect in 491
  seasonal 19-20, 62
    treatment of 19-20, 503-5
  severity of 71
  socioeconomic impact of 48-49, 62
  symptoms of 61, 71, 503
  treatment of 22, 481-82, 484, 489-99
    allergen avoidance in 20-21, 496
    antihistamines and decongestants
      in 496-97
    antihistamines in 22, 73, 481,
      490, 496-97
    cromolyn sodium in 22
    drug 22, 72-73
    immunotherapy 21, 74-75
    immunotherapy/immune modula-
      tion in 497-99
    over-the-counter drugs in 503-5

allergic rhinitis (hay fever), continued
  treatment of, continued
    topical nasal sprays in 489-99,
      490t, 493t, 497
    topical nasal steroids in 22
  vs. cold 480-81
"allergic salute" 62, 311
allergic shiners 311
allergic skin diseases
  see dermatologic allergy(ies)
allergic skin reactions, prevalence of
  49t
allergic tension fatigue syndrome
  204-5
Allergies and Your Family (Rapp) 177
allergist
  in diagnosis of asthma 24-25
  skin testing by 18
allergy(ies)
  to airborne substances 309-25
  asthma mechanisms in 445-49
  as cause of asthma 23, 79-81, 311
  causes of 14-15
  components of 15-17
  cosmetic 425-33
  defined 3, 310, 349-50, 528
  dermatologic 105-13
    see also dermatologic allergy(ies)
  diagnosis of 17-18
    anaphylaxis and 166
  economic impact of 50
  food
    see food allergy(ies)
  genetics and 13
  holiday 173-78
  industrial materials causing 140t,
    143t
  information resources on 325
  latex
    see latex allergies
  lifestyle and 512-13
  mechanism of 15-17
  medications for
    adverse effects from 517-23
    nonprescription 483t
    over-the-counter 503-5
    side effects of 27-28
  patient history and 509
  prevalence of 14-15

allergy(ies), continued
  propensity for 310
  research on 324-25, 467-68, 471-72
  skin 397-98
  socioeconomics of 467-68
  symptoms of, causes of 6, *10,* 17, 35
  vs. cold 309-11, 319, 480-81
  see also allergic reaction(s); allergic
    rhinitis (hay fever)
allergy action plan 176
Allergy and Asthma Network 325
  address 472, 515
allergy immunotherapy
  see immunotherapy (allergy shots)
allergy shots
  see immunotherapy (allergy shots)
Allura Red AC, defined 224
almond flavoring 177
alpha-1-antitrypsin deficiency 91
altered self, defined 528
Alternaria 315
alternaria, extract for 514t
aluminum acetate (Burow's solution),
  for poison ivy exposure 371, 476
aluminum hydroxide gel, for poison
  ivy blisters 476
Alupent (metaproterenol) 517
alveoli
  defined 528
  in hypersensitivity pneumonitis (al-
    lergic pneumonia) 150
American Academy of Allergy & Immunology 93, 325, 350, 423
  address 472
American Academy of Dermatology
  425, 431
American College of Allergy & Immunology 93
  address 472
American College of Chest Physicians, address 472
American Lung Association (ALA) 93,
  341
  address 472
aminophylline, allergic reaction to
  116
amiodarone (Cordarone)
  as photosensitizer 137t
  and phototoxicity 136

ampicillin
  allergic reaction to 116, 123
  for elderly asthmatic 456
  and pseudoallergic reactions 121
amyotrophic lateral sclerosis (Lou
  Gehrig's disease) 184
anabolic steroids 323
Ana-Kit, Ana-Guard 366
analgesics, external 477
anaphylactic shock 228
  defined 35, 528
anaphylactic-hypersensitivity reaction (immediate hypersensitivity) 4
anaphylactic-hypersensitivity reaction (immediate hypersensitivity;
  Type I allergic reaction) 4
anaphylactoid reaction
  defined 528
  vs. anaphylaxis 164, 229
anaphylatoxin, defined 528
anaphylaxis (anaphylactic reaction)
  227-32, 529
  deaths from 163, 164, 196, 228, 349,
    363, 467
  diagnostic allergens (skin test) and
    166
  drugs and 119, 164
  exercise and 229-30
  foods and 167-68, 196, 203, 227-32,
    468
    skin testing and 201
  history of 228
  hospitalizations (U.S.) for *46*
  idiopathic 230
  injected dyes and 168
  insect stings and 166-67, 349, 356,
    363, 468
  latex and 416-17, 422
  penicillin and 164, 228, 229, 467
  predisposition to 232
  prevalence of 49t
  socioeconomic impact of 49
  symptoms of 228
  therapeutic allergens (immuno-
    therapy) and 166
  treatment of 163
  triggers of 230
  vaccines and 165-66

anemia
  aplastic 123
  drug-induced 121
anergy, defined 529
anesthesia equipment, latex in 415
angiitis, necrotizing, cutaneous 112
angioedema (giant hives) 207-8
  defined 529
  drug-induced 119
  hereditary 110
    defined 538
  idiopathic 207
anhydrides, acid 392
aniline 135
  in synthetic colors 222
animal(s) 333
  allergen control for 322
  avoiding 326
  and occupational asthma 141
animal allergy(ies) 318, 335-40
  avoidance of allergens in 336
  medications for 337
  see also pet(s)
animal cell cultures, anaphylactic reaction to 165
animal dander 337, 438, 512, 535
animal protein, in insulin 124
animal serum, and serum sickness 119
ankylosing spondylitis 14
ant
  behavior of 352-53
  venom of 356
anthranilates, in sunscreens 138
antibacterial soaps 134
antibacterials, quinolone 135
antibiotics
  and allergic contact dermatitis 107
  and allergic drug reactions 123, 130
  and contact dermatitis 400.
  and drug-induced photosensitivity
    120
  macrolide, second-generation anti-
    histamines contraindicated with
    497
  and phototoxicity 136
antibody(ies) 4, 15, 16-17
  blocking, defined 531
  defined 529

antibiotics, continued
  duration of in body 16
  see also specific antibody, e.g., im-
    munoglobulin E (IgE)
antibody-deficiency syndromes 182
antibody-dependent cell-mediated cytotoxicity (ADCC), defined 529
anti-cat IgE 338
anti-cholinergic agents 73, 74
  for asthma 26, 87-88
  in topical nasal sprays 494t
  see also specific agent, e.g.,
    ipratropium
antifungal agents
  and drug-induced photosensitivity
    120
  second-generation antihistamines
    contraindicated with 497
anti-GBM disease
  see antiglomerular basement mem-
    brane antibody disease (anti-
    GBM disease)
antigen (allergen)
  defined 6, 32, 529
  MHC, classes of 33
  type I response to 4
  see also allergen(s)
antigen presentation, defined 529
antigen processing, defined 529
antigenic cross-reactivity, defined 126
antigen-presenting cells, defined 529
antiglomerular basement membrane
  antibody disease (anti-GBM disease) 187
antihistamines 477
  adverse effects from 522-23
  for allergic rhinitis (hay fever) 22,
    71, 496-97
  amount prescribed 48-49
  for atopic dermatitis 409
  for cold-induced urticaria 169
  and contact dermatitis 400
  defined 529
  for eczema 107
  for food allergy 203
  for hives 110
  ineffective for anaphylaxis 231
  for insect sting 358, 361

antihistamines, continued
  non-sedating 22, 323, 504, 522
  over-the-counter 29, 503-4
  second-generation 497
  side effects of 73
  in treatment of allergic disease 323
  use of for asthmatic child 28-29
anti-inflammatory drugs 73, 74
anti-inflammatory steroids, for allergic rhinitis 22
antimicrobials
  food preservatives as 209-10
  nitrites as 211
antinuclear antibody (ANA), defined
  529
antioxidants
  food preservatives as 209-10
  synthetic, substitutes for 214
antiperspirants, and contact
  dermatitis 399
antiserum, defined 530
antitoxins, defined 530
antiviral proteins, defined 530
ants 167, 351, 359
  anaphylactic reaction to 167
aplastic anemia 123
appendix, defined 530
apple(s)
  candied 177
  dried
    sulfites and 213
    sulfites in 83
  peel of 198
Apple Crisp *280*
Apple Juice Rice Pudding *287*
Applesauce Drop Cookies *281*
Apricot Bread *277*
Apricot Dessert Sauce *292*
Apricot-Pineapple Pie *282*
Archives of Internal Medicine 230
Arizona, pollen calendar for *65*
Arkansas, pollen calendar for *65*
armpits, and contact dermatitis 399
ARMS
  see Adverse Reaction Monitoring
    System (ARMS)
arrowroot starch 262
  contains no gluten 258

Arrowsmith-Lowe, Thomas 423
artificial Christmas trees 176
artificial sweeteners 134
asbestosis 146-47
   defined 530
ash 313
Asian-Americans, lactose intolerance
   in 234
aspergillosis, bronchopulmonary, allergic 153
Aspergillus 315, 316
aspirin
   allergic reaction to 116
   anaphylactic reaction to 169-70
   in combination drugs 122, *122*, 505
   and pseudoallergic reactions 121-
      22, *122*, 130-31
aspirin intolerance 121-22, *122*
aspirin reactions 169-70
aspirin/aspirin-like drugs
   and asthma 24, 82, 169-70
   and sinusitis 100
astemizole 497
asters, and contact dermatitis 403
asthma 22-26, 77-92, 437-39, 445-49,
   451-57, 459-62, 465-72
   by age group 451-57
      adults 452
      children 451-52
      elderly 453-57
   and air pollution 141
   airflow obstruction in, causes of 22
   and aspirin 24, 82, 122t, 169-70
   breast-feeding and, myths about 91
   breathing out in 23, 78, 85-86
   cat-induced 337-40
   cause(s) of 23-24, 79-85
      allergy as 79-81, 311, 327
      chemical 81-83
      exercise as 83
      idiopathic (unknown) 84
      infection as 81
      myths about 90
      vasculitis as 84
   and chicken pox 176
   in children 53, 161, 469-70
   and climate 141
   cold and 174

asthma, continued
   cost of 78, 328, 465, 466
   in cystic fibrosis 162
   death from 327, 437, 444, *444,* 445,
      446
   defined 447, 530
   demonstration and education
      projects on 470
   development of, and allergic
      rhinitis (hay fever) 71-72, 75
   diagnosis of 24-25, 85-86
   dismissing seriousness of 437
   doctor office visits for 442, *442*
   drug-induced 121
   economic costs of 51, 52t
   in elderly 453-57
   emphysema and, myths about 91
   epidemiology of 466
   exercise and 26, 174
      myths about 91
   extrinsic 446
      defined 537
   and flu shot 176
   folk "cures" for 438
   foods and, myths about 92
   and geographic location 438
   heredity and 156
   hospitalizations for *46,* 50, 344, 443,
      443, 446, 466, 467
   household items and 141, 141t
   idiopathic 84
   immunological basis of 445, 446-47
   incidence of 446
   indoor allergens and 327-28, 467
   infantile 161
   inflammation in, *in vivo* analysis of
      448
   information resources for 93, 472
   intrinsic 446
      defined 542
   mechanism of 78-79, 445-49
      in allergy 445-49
   medical attention unnecessary for,
      myth of 438
   medications for, adverse effects
      from 517-23
   mortality rates for 444, *444*
   myths about 90-92

asthma, continued
myths of 437-39
night-time 84, 144, 454
over-the-counter antihistamines
contraindicated in 504
over-the-counter drugs and 92, 505
pathogenesis of 448
prelavence of 22, 77-78, 439-41,
440, 441
prevalence of 22, 49t, 77-78, 439-41,
440, 441, 446-47, 448
psychological aspect of 437-38
psychological aspects of 28
relocation for 438-39
research on 92, 446-49, 459-62, 465-
72
role of eosinophils in, research on
459-62
self-induced 438
short-haired pets and 438
simulating feeling of 78
smoking and, myths about 92
socioeconomic impact of 22, 50-52,
52t, 54t, 78, 452, 466-67
sporadic 81
statistics on 439
toluene di-isocyanate (TDI)-induced
142
treatment of 25-26, 86-90
avoidance of allergen in 86-87
medications in 87-89
peak flow meters in 89-90
research on 449
symptomatic 25
trigger(s) of 84-86
emotions as 85
gastroesophageal reflux as 84
hyperthyroidism as 85
pregnancy as 85
sinusitis as 84
in vivo analysis of inflammation in
448
wheezing in 79
in young adults 53
Asthma, Allergy, and Immunologic
Diseases Cooperative Research
Centers (AAIDCRCs) 324, 470
Asthma & Allergy Foundation of
America 93

asthma action plan 176
Asthma and Allergy Foundation of
America 325
address 472, 515
asthmatic child 161
birthdays and 178
outgrowing asthma 90
peak flow monitoring for 89-90
relationship with mother 438
asthmatics
air pollution and 342, 343t
exercise recommended for 26
atopic, defined 407
atopic dermatitis (eczema) 105-7,
407-10
in allergic child 160-61
allergy shots and 107, 409
avoidance of allergens in 107
of childhood, food allergy and 160-
61, 196, 245-51
defined 530
environmental causes of 409
food allergies and 196, 408-9
physiologic features of 106-7
recognizing 408
skin tests and 106, 409
treatment of 107, 409-10
atopic/atopy, defined 530
Atrovent (ipratropium) 490t, 493t,
495
attenuated, defined 530
Aureobasidium (Pullularia) 316
autoantibody
in anti-GBM disease 187
defined 180, 530
autocrine, defined 530
autoimmune disease(s) 13, 32
defined 530
automobile air conditioning 21
Aveeno
for cosmetic allergic reaction 426
for poison ivy blisters 476
avoidance of allergens 20-21, 320-22,
328
for allergic rhinitis 20-21, 486-87,
496
in asthma treatment 86-87
cat and dog 326, 329

avoidance of allergens, continued
  defined 530
  and immunotherapy 512-13
  occupational asthma and 145
  in treatment of allergic disease 20-
    21, 320-22
  see also specific allergen, e.g., pollen
avoidance of foods 197, 202
  for eczema 107
  during pregnancy 207
  see also under specific food, e.g.,
    chocolate
azithromycin (Zithromax), second-
  generation antihistamines
  contraindicated with 497
Azulfidine (sulfasalazine), as photosensitizer 133, 134

B

B. subtilis 142, 145
B cell(s), defined 530
B cell differentiation factor (BCDF),
  defined 531
B cell growth factor (BCGF), defined
  531
babies
  see infant(s)
"baboon syndrome" 400
bacterial enzymes 69
bacterial infections 405
  secondary, to allergic drug reactions
    130
  and sinusitis 99
bacterium, defined 531
Bactrim (trimethoprim), as photosensitizer 137t
Baer, Harold 476
bagassosis 148, 148t
  defined 531
Bailey, John E. 217-18, 219, 221
baked goods
  color additives in 220
  maximum sulfite levels for 215
  nonwheat, storage of 265
  with nonwheat flours 264-65
bakers, and contact dermatitis 401

baking
  holiday 176
  with nonwheat flours 264-65
  omitting basic ingredient during
    263-65
  without eggs 263-64
  without milk 264
baking powder, cereal-free 267, 269
baking soda, for poison ivy exposure
  371
balanced nutrition, and lactose intolerance 236-37
balloons, latex in 416
Bard, John 431
Bardana, Emil J., Jr.
barium enema tips, latex in 416
barley
  anaphylactic reaction to 167
  gluten in 258
Barton, Charles R. 419
basement membrane
  in asthma 79
  in blistering disorders 111
  defined 531
basophils 6, *8-11,* 35
  defined 531
  in late-phase response 246, 247
bathing, for allergic contact
  dermatitis 107
beauty products, color additives in
  217
beclomethasone (Vancenase AQ,
  Vancenase Pockethaler; Beconase
  AQ, Beconase aerosol) 492, 493t
Beconase aerosol (beclomethasone)
  493t
Beconase AQ (beclomethasone) 492,
  493t
bed 331
bed springs 331
bedding 21, 86, 321, 512
  and contact dermatitis 404
bedroom 322, 328
  creating dust-free 21, 321, 331-33
bee(s)
  anaphylactic reaction to 167
  behavior of 352
bee stings 167

bee venom, extract for 513
beef dishes, for person with food allergy *272, 273*
beer
  maximum sulfite levels for 215
  sulfites in 83
beetle 354
Benadryl (diphenhydramine) 497
  use of for asthmatic child 28-29
benzoate preservatives 82
benzocaine 405, 477
  and contact dermatitis 400
benzophenones, in sunscreens 138
benzopyrene 394
benzyl alcohol 477
bergamot oil 134, 135
  in sunscreens 138
Bermuda (grass) 313
berylliosis 147
  defined 531
beryllium, and allergic contact
  dermatitis 107
beta blockers (beta adrenergic agonists, beta adrenergic blocking
  agents)
  for asthma 25-26, 83, 88-89
  as cause of asthma 24
betamethasone, in older nasal sprays
  491
BHA
  see butylated hydroxyanisole (BHA)
BHT
  see butylated hydroxytoluene (BHT)
Biaxin (clarithromycin), second-generation antihistamines
  contraindicated with 497
biking, and asthma 26, 83
biochemical cascades, research on 40
biological response modifiers, defined
  531
biotechnology, defined 531
birch pollen 198
  and contact dermatitis 403
bird(s) 86
bird fancier's disease 147, 148t, 150
birth control pills, lactose in 238
birthday parties, allergies and 178
biting insects, allergy-causing 353-54

biting midge 353
Black Americans
  see African Americans
black fly 353
black lacquer 384
blankets 21, 321, 332
Blankingship, Page 432
blistering disorders 110-12
blisters
  of contact dermatitis 398
  of poison ivy 371-72, 374, 385, 476
blocking antibody, defined 531
blood, complement system of 11
blood cells, and allergic drug reaction
  121
blood disorders 184-86, *185*
blood groups
  defined 531
  transfusions and 184-86
blood pressure
  and decongestants 504
  and food allergy 197
  and insect sting 356
blood test(s) 319-20
  in allergy diagnosis 18, 19
    see also radioallergosorbent test
      (RAST)
  in diagnosis of allergic rhinitis 72
  in diagnosis of food allergy 201
  for histocompatibility antigens 189
  before immunotherapy 508-9
  for insect sting 357
  for latex allergy 418
Blueberry Muffins *278*
blusher, allergic reaction to 426
Boehringer Ingelheim Pharmaceuticals 459
bogs, poison sumac in 382
bologna, hidden milk proteins in 241
bone marrow, defined 532
Boston Collaborative Drug Surveillance Program 116, 164
Boston ivy, *vs.* poison ivy 377
botulism 211
bouillon 303
bowel disease, special diet for 303
bowel disorders, in dermatitis
  herpetiformis 111

bowel obstruction, fiber and 303
box elder 313
box springs 331
bradykinin 11
   defined 532
breads and crackers, recipes for 277-80
breakfast cereal, nonwheat, as baked-good ingredient 267
breast milk, transmission of allergens through 204, 250
breast-feeding
   antigen transference and 157
   asthma and, myths about 91
   recommendations for 27, 204
Brethine (terbutaline) 517
Bricanyl (terbutaline) 517
brompheniramine (Dimetapp, Dristan Allergy) 496
bronchi, defined 532
bronchial asthma 77
   see also asthma
bronchiole, defined 532
bronchiolitis, as cause of asthma 23, 81
bronchitis 81
   chronic
      in elderly 454
      over-the-counter antihistamines contraindicated in 504
   chronic progressive, *vs.* farmer's lung 149
bronchodilator(s)
   for asthma 87
      in elderly 454, 455
      and peak flow rate 24
   for cat-induced asthma 339-40
   defined 532
   for food allergy 203
   inhaled 88
   see also specific bronchodilator, e.g., theophylline
bronchopulmonary aspergillosis, allergic 153
bronchospasm
   defined 532
   sulfite-induced 199
brother, of asthmatic child 452
bubble gum 220

buckwheat, gluten in 258-59
budesonide 489, 492
building products, and chemical sensitivity 394
"building-related illness" 394
bullous pemphigoid 111
   defined 532
bumblebee 229, 352
Burow's solution (aluminum acetate), for poison ivy exposure 371, 476
"butterfly rash" 113
butylated hydroxyanisole (BHA) 211-12
butylated hydroxytoluene (BHT) 211
byssinosis 139

C

C1 enzyme 13
C9 enzyme 13
caddis fly 354
cadmium sulfide 134
caffeine 88
-*caine* medications, and contact dermatitis 400
cake, for person with food allergy *284, 289-90*
cake mix 264
calamine
   for insect sting 358
   for poison ivy blisters 476
   for poison ivy exposure 371
calcium
   and lactose intolerance 236-37, 258
   nutrition claims for 304
   and osteoporosis 303
calcium propionate 209
calcium requirements, and lactose intolerance 236-37
California
   air quality standard in 341
   pollen calendar for *65*
calorie information, on nutrition facts panel 299
cancer
   gastrointestinal, *vs.* food allergy 199
   immune system and 191
   special diet for 303

"Candida hypersensitivity" 392
candidiasis 405
candies
 at Easter 177
 at Halloween 177
candle smoke 178
candy, color additives in 217, 220
canned vegetables
 maximum sulfite levels for 216
 sulfites in 83
cantaloupe, and ragweed allergy 198
car air conditioning 21, 322
carbohydrates
 allergic reactions to 126
 on nutrition facts panel 299
carbon monoxide 394
cardiac
 see also under heart
cardiac arrhythmias, second-
 generation antihistamines
 contraindicated in 497
cardiovascular system
 adrenergics and 518
 corticosteroids and 520
 theophylline and 520
cardroom (cotton) workers 139
carob 267
carpet backing, latex in 416
carpeting 331, 512
 and pet allergens 318
 wall-to-wall 86, 321, 328
Carrot-Raisin Cookies *283*
carrots, and contact dermatitis 403,
 405
cascade reaction
 in allergic reaction *12,* 40-41, 471
 defined 532
caseinate, on ingredient list 300
cashew nuts 403
cassava plant 262
casseroles, for person with food allergy *271*
castor beans 69, 142
 and contact dermatitis 403
cat(s) 321, 335-40, 481
 allergen control for 322
 and asthma
 see cat-induced asthma

cat(s), continued
 avoiding 326, 339
 saliva of 20, 318, 335-40
 skin glands of 336
cat allergens
 allergenic extract for 513, 514t
 in cat-free house 339
cataracts 107
caterpillar 353-54
catheters, latex in 415
cat-induced asthma 86, 337-40
 diagnosis of 338
 prevention of 339
 treatment of 339-40
C1-C9 complement, defined 532
CD1, defined 532
CD2, defined 532
CD3, defined 532
CD4, defined 532
CD5, defined 533
CD8, defined 533
CD25, defined 533
CD markers, defined 532
celiac disease (gluten-sensitive
 enteropathy) 208
 special diet for 303
cell cultures, anaphylactic reaction to
 165
cell membrane, IgG reacts against 5
cell-mediated immunity 5, 5t, 106,
 108, 149, 191
 defined 533
cells, biological communication
 among, research on 40-41
cellular immunity, defined 533
Center for Biologics Evaluation and
 Research (FDA) 480-81
Center for Biologics Evaluation
 (FDA) 513
Center for Food Safety and Applied
 Nutrition 211
central air conditioning
 see air conditioning
cereal-free baking powder 267, 269
cereals, BHA in 212
cerebral allergy 204-5
"cerebrovascular accident," *vs.* anaphylaxis 363

certifiable color additives, defined
224
Chagas' disease 190
challenge chamber 144
challenge test, defined 533
Chanukah, allergies at 178
chapped lip medications, and contact
dermatitis 399
Charous, B. Lauren 415, 423
cheeks, and contact dermatitis 402
cheese
mold allergy and 315
natural histamines in 198
Cheese Pizza with Rice Crust *270*
cheesewasher's disease 148t
"chemical AIDS" 392
chemical mediators
see mediators
chemical photosensitivity 133-38
see also photosensitivity
chemical sensitivity(ies) 318, *391-96*
classification of 392-93
current interest in 391-92
diagnosis of 395-96
pollutants causing 393-94
chemicals 322
and allergic contact dermatitis 107
as cause of asthma 81-83
in home and office 141, 141t
chemotaxis, defined 533
cherries, maraschino, maximum
sulfite levels for 216
Cherry Dessert Sauce *292*
chestnuts 178
chicken 178
chicken pox, and asthma 176
Chicken-Rice Casserole *271*
chickpeas (garbanzo beans) 258
Chiffon Cake *284*
child(children)
air pollution and 342, 343t
allergic diseases in 52-53, 155-56,
393
allergic rhinitis in 62, 71, 155
asthma in 23, 52-53, 54t, 90, 155,
438
asthmatic, birthdays and 178
atopic dermatitis in 407-8

child(children), continued
common food allergens in 197
contact dermatitis in 401-2
cow's milk allergy in 241-43
dust-sensitive 332-33
eczema (atopic dermatitis) in 106,
155, 160-61, 245-51, 408, 451-52
food allergies in 155, 161-62, 196,
197, 203-4, 241-43, 245-51, 467
introduction of foods and 27
gastrointestinal disorders, from
food allergy 161-62
immunotherapy for 365
inner-city, asthma in 469-70
insect sting allergy in 363, 365
lactose intolerance in 235, 236
latex allergy in 416-17, 420-21
outgrowing allergies 198
peak flow monitoring for 89-90
and poison ivy/oak/sumac 369, 385
serous otitis media in 160
sinusitis and 102-3
theophylline and 519
topical nasal steroids for 492
see also infant(s); pediatric allergies
childhood allergies
see pediatric allergies
childhood asthma 52-53, 54t, 451-52
childhood atopic dermatitis 106, 155,
160-61, 245-51
allergic reaction in
symptoms of 249
tests for 250
elimination diet and 250-51
food allergy and 245-51
histamine-releasing factor in 248
immune system in 246-48
itching in 248
without food allergy 250
chimera, defined 533
chimney 174
chloramphenicol, and allergic drug
reactions 123
chlordiazepoxide, and drug-induced
photosensitivity 120
chlorine, and sinusitis 101
chlorpheniramine (Chlor-Trimeton)
496

chlorpropamide (Diabinese), as photosensitizer 137t
Chlor-Trimeton (chlorpheniramine)
496
chocolate 178
anaphylactic reaction to 167
avoidance of in food preparation 267
at Easter 177
chocolate chips, milk-free 267
cholera vaccine, anaphylaxis and 165
cholinergic urticaria 110
Christmas trees 175-76
artificial 176
chromates, and allergic contact
dermatitis 107
chromosomes, defined 533
chronic bronchitis
in elderly 454
over-the-counter antihistamines
contraindicated in 504
chronic hives 207-8
chronic inflammatory neuropathy
183
chronic obstructive pulmonary disease (COPD), air pollution and 342,
343t
chronic sinusitis 467
prevalence of 49t
socioeconomic impact of 49
chrysanthemums, and contact
dermatitis 403
Churg-Strauss syndrome, as cause of
asthma 84
cigarette smoke
and chemical sensitivity 393
formaldehyde in 394
and sinusitis 101
cinnamates, in sunscreens 138
cinnamon 178
Cladosporium (Hormodendrum) 315
clarithromycin (Biaxin), second-generation antihistamines
contraindicated with 497
Class I, II, and III molecules, defined
533
Class I/II restriction, defined 534
cleaning 332, 487
in allergen control 321, 326

clemastine (Tavist) 497, 504
climate, and asthma 141
climbing sumac 377
Clone, defined 534
clonidine, and contact dermatitis
400
closets 21, 86-87, 321, 331
clothing
and allergy 21, 87, 321, 331, 512
choice of
in prevention of insect sting 231,
358-59
in prevention of poison ivy 371
and contact dermatitis 404
contaminated, by poison ivy 371,
386, 476
"coal-tar" colors 222
coal-tar dyes 134
defined 224
cockroaches 354
affect of on children's allergies 159,
469
allergenic extract for 513
extract for 514t
perennial (year-round) allergies to
20, 318
codfish allergy 258
in Scandinavia 197
coffee beans, green 142
coffee creamer
color additives in 217
lactose in 238
coffee worker's lung 147, 148t
cold-induced anaphylactoid reaction
229
cold-induced urticaria 110, 168-69
defined 534
colds
and asthma 81, 84, 174
rhinitis from 19
sinusitis in 99
vs. allergy 309-11, 319
colic, food allergy and 203
colitis, ulcerative
defined 553
fiber and 303
socioeconomic impact of 179
colon *234*

color additives 217-25
  certifiable, defined 224
  in cosmetics 427-28
  exempt, defined 224
  FDA batch certification program for
    218-19
  FD&C Orange No. 1 223
  FD&C Red No. 2 220-21
  FD&C Red No. 3 219-20
  FD&C Yellow No. 5 (tartrazine) 218
  history of 221-23
  on ingredient list 300
  terms for 224-25
color lakes 223
color manufacturers, FDA requirements for 218-19
Colorado, pollen calendar for *65*
combination drugs 125
  antihistamine/decongestant 497, 505
  containing aspirin 122, *122,* 505
comforters 332
common cold 99, 103-4
  see also colds
common poison ivy *(Rhus radicans)*
  377-78, *379*
  see also poison ivy
complement, defined 534
complement cascade, defined 534
complement system 5, 11-13, *12*
  alternative pathway of 12, *12,* 13
    in asbestosis 147
    in hereditary angioedema 170
  classic pathway of *12,* 12-13
  defined 534
compresses, hot, for sinusitis 102
concealed milk proteins 241-43
condiments, maximum sulfite levels
  for 215
condoms, latex in 416, 419
conjunctivitis
  in airborne allergy 311
  allergic 123
Connecticut, pollen calendar for *65*
constant region, defined 534
constipation, fiber and 303
contact dermatitis 397-405
  allergic 107-9
    see allergic contact dermatitis

contact dermatitis, continued
  common sensitizers to 403-4
  cosmetic 425
  drug-induced 120
  finding source of 398-99
  irritant (nonallergic) 398
  from medications 400
  mild 402-3
  prevalence of 49t
  prevention of 404-5
  rash of 398
  severe 403
  socioeconomic impact of 401
  treatment of 402-3
  types of 397-98
contact eczema
  allergic
    see allergic contact dermatitis
  see contact dermatitis
contact lenses, color additives in 217,
  218
contaminants, in drugs, allergic reaction to 118, 126
contrast dyes
  and anaphylactic reactions 168, 229
  and pseudoallergic reactions 121,
    122
Cooked Salad Dressing *276*
cookies, for person with food allergy
  281, 283, 288, 291
cooling system 512
  see also air conditioning
coral sumac *(Metopium toxiferum)* 384
Cordarone (amiodarone)
  as photosensitizer 137t
  and phototoxicity 136
corn 258
  anaphylactic reaction to 167
  avoiding in food preparation 267
  foods containing 259, 261t
  technical names for 259, 259t
corn flour 261
  contains no gluten 258
corn syrup 258
  sulfites in 83
cornstarch 262
  contains no gluten 258
coronaviruses 99

corticosteroids 74
  adverse effects from 89, 520-21
  for allergic rhinitis 482
  for asthma 89
  for atopic dermatitis 409
  for cat-induced asthma 340
  for child's allergic
    gastroenteropathy 161
  defined 534
  for eczema 107
  for farmer's lung 149
  for hives 110
  for infant with food allergy 204
  long-term effects of 28
  oral, for allergic bronchopulmonary
    aspergillosis 153
  topical
    see topical corticosteroids
cortisones (adrenal steroids), for insect sting 360
Cosmetic, Toiletry, and Fragrance Association 432
cosmetic allergies 425-33
  cosmetic ingredients and 428t, 428-
    29
  incidence of 425, 431
  parts of body affected by 429t
  patch tests for 429-30
  types of cosmetics causing 427t
Cosmetic Fragrance Association Review Panel 431
cosmetic labels 429-31, 433
cosmetics
  and allergic contact dermatitis 107
  causing allergic reactions 427t
    reporting 431-32
  color additives in 217, 218, 222-23
  and contact dermatitis 399, 404
  ingredients in, causing allergic re-
    actions 428t
  new, first use of 432
  photoallergic reaction to 135
  and stinging insects 359
  testing of 427-28
co-stimulation, defined 534
cotton dust 142
cotton industry 139
cottonseed 69

cowpox 4
cow's milk 27, 157-58, 258
  children and 203-4
  concealed 241-43
crab 197, 254, 258
crackers
  filled, maximum sulfite levels for
    216
  recipes for 277-80
cranberries 178
Cranberry-Apple Sorbet *285*
Cranberry-Apple Tapioca with Pears
  285
crayfish 197, 254
Crohn's disease (regional ileitis) 182-
  83
  defined 534
  fiber and 303
  socioeconomic impact of 179
cromolyn sodium (Nasalcrom) 493t,
  498t
  adverse effects from 494t, 522
  for allergic rhinitis 22, 482
  for asthma 87
  in topical nasal sprays 494t
  in treatment of allergic disease 323
  in treatment of seasonal allergic
    rhinitis 20
Crooks, Donald M. 389
cross-reactivity
  and aspirin 130
  and cosmetic ingredients 428
  defined 126, 198, 535
  and nuts 206-7
  and peanuts 206-7
  and photosensitivity 136-37
  and poison ivy 403
  and shellfish 254
  to similar foods 198
Cryptostroma corticale 151
Crystodigin (digitoxin)
  and photophobia 136
  as photosensitizer 137t
C-type viruses 186
curds 238
Curran, Maureen 243
Current Dermatologic Therapy
  (Maddin, ed.) 400

curtains 21, 86, 321, 332, 512
Cushing syndrome 520
"cutaneous hyper-reactivity" 248
cutaneous necrotizing angiitis 112
  defined 535
cyclosporine (cyclosporin A), defined
  535
cyproheptadine
  for cold-induced urticaria 169
  for hives 110
cystic fibrosis, pediatric allergies and
  162
cytokines
  and asthmatic inflammation 469
  defined 535
  research on 462
cytotoxic, defined 535
cytotoxic T cells, defined 535
cytotoxicity testing 205

D

Dacron bedding 331
Daily Values 302
dairy products
  calcium in 239t
  lactose in 239t
  maximum sulfite levels for 215
dander 438, 512
  cat 337
  defined 535
dark skin, and photosensitivity 137
Date Bread 277
Daul, Carolyn 253
D&C, defined 222, 224
death
  from anaphylaxis 163, 164, 196,
    228, 229, 467
  from asthma 327, 437, 444, *444,*
    445, 446
  from insect sting 349, 363
deCastro, J. L. 136
decongestants
  before air travel 101
  for allergic rhinitis (hay fever) 496-
    97
  and blood pressure 504

decongestants, continued
  over-the-counter 504
  for sinusitis 102
  in topical nasal sprays 494t, 495-96
decorations for holidays, and allergy
  175
deer fly 353
degranulation, defined 535
dehumidifier 321
dehydrated potatoes, maximum
  sulfite levels for 216
dehydrated vegetables, maximum
  sulfite levels for 216
dehydration, in elderly asthmatic 456
Delaney anti-cancer clause (Food,
  Drug, and Cosmetic Act amendment) 219-20, 223
Delaware, pollen calendar for *65*
delayed hypersensitivity 5-6
dendritic cells, defined 535
deodorants 134
  color additives in 217
  and contact dermatitis 399
depilatories (hair removers) 431
dermatitis 407
  atopic
    see atopic dermatitis (eczema)
  contact
    see contact dermatitis
  contact, allergic
    see allergic contact dermatitis
  exfoliative, drug-induced 120
  of hand 411-13
  occupational 401
dermatitis herpetiformis 111-12
  defined 535
dermatologic allergy(ies) 105-13
  allergic contact dermatitis 107-9
  atopic dermatitis (eczema) 105-7
  drugs and 117t
  urticaria/angioedema 109-10
  vesiculobullous diseases 110-12
dermatomyositis 184
dermographism 110
  white 106
desensitization
  to allergic drug reaction 131, 232
  defined 535

desensitization, continued
ineffective for food allergy 203
to insect bites 361
for poison ivy 372, 477-78
schedule for 509-10
for sinusitis 101
desserts, recipes for 280-90
detergent industry, and occupational asthma 141, 145
dexamethasone
inhaled 74
in older nasal sprays 491
diabetes, oral decongestants contraindicated in 504
diabetes insipidus, and allergic drug reaction 121
diabetes mellitus (insulin-dependent), hospitalizations (U.S.) for *46*
Diabinese (chlorpropamide), as photosensitizer 137t
diagnostic allergens (skin test)
anaphylactic reactions to 166
see also skin test
diagnostic techniques, controversial 205-6
diaper rash 402
diaphragms, latex in 416
dibucaine, and contact dermatitis 400
diesel fuel 394
diet(s)
elimination, defined 536
special, and food labels 298-99, 302-3
dietary avoidance, for food allergy 202
Diflucan (fluconazole), second-generation antihistamines contraindicated with 497
digestive tract *234*
digitoxin (Crystodigin)
and photophobia 136
as photosensitizer 137t
digoxin, allergic reaction to 116
Dimetapp (brompheniramine) 496
diphenhydramine (Benadryl) 405, 477, 497
and contact dermatitis 400
diphtheria vaccine, anaphylaxis and 165

dirt, and mold 174
disability, caused by asthma 51, 52t
discoid lupus 112
"dishpan hands," and contact dermatitis 402
disodium EDTA 209
District of Columbia, pollen calendar for *65*
diuretics 124
and drug-induced photosensitivity 120
diverticulosis, fiber and 303
DNA (deoxyribonucleic acid), defined 535
doctor gum *(Metopium toxiferum)* 384
doctor office visits
for allergic rhinitis 18, 48-49, 54t
for allergy immunotherapy 54t
for anaphylaxis 49
for asthma 50-51, 54t, 78, 442, *442*
for chronic sinusitis 49
for insulin-dependent diabetes mellitus 54t
pediatric, for immunologic diseases 54t
for skin allergies 49, 54t
Doepel, Laurie K. 333
dog(s) 20, 318, 321
allergen control for 322
allergenic extract for 514t
and asthma sufferers 86
avoiding 326
breed of 326
double-blind food challenge 201, 250
down-filled blankets 321
doxepin (Sinequan), as photosensitizer 137t
doxycycline (Vibramycin), as photosensitizer 137t
dried fruits
maximum sulfite levels for 216
mold allergy and 315
sulfites and 213
sulfites in 83
dried potatoes, sulfites and 213
Dristan Allergy (brompheniramine) 496
Dristan (oxymetholone) 495

drowsiness
  anti-allergy medicines and 205, 323
  and antihistamines 504
drug(s)
  see medication(s)
drug fever, drug-induced 120
drug reaction, adverse, defined 115
drug reactions
  allergic 115-31
    see also allergic drug reactions
  idiosyncratic 125
  non-allergic 124-25
  paradoxical 125
drug-induced illness, socioeconomic
  impact of 115-16
dry foods, BHA in 212
dry milk solids 238
dry soup mixes, maximum sulfite levels for 216
Duraquin (quinidine), and
  photophobia 136
dust 64, 317-18, 481, 487
  affect of on children's allergies 159
  allergies to 20, 317-18
  in bedroom 21, 331-33
  defined 317-18
dust filters 331
dust mask 321
dust mite 15, 20, 86, 317, 328, 331, 354
  affect of on children's allergies 159
  and asthma sufferers 86-87
  desensitization to 510
  extract for 513, 514t
  as major cause of allergy worldwide
    15
  perennial allergic rhinitis and 317-
    18, 487
dust-free bedroom 321, 331-33
dusting, in allergen control 321
dwarf sumac (Rhus copallina) *383,*
  384
dye(s)
  coal-tar, defined 224
  and contact dermatitis 399
  contrast
    anaphylactic reactions to 168, 229
    and pseudoallergic reactions 121,
      122

food
  see color additives
  straight, defined 224

E

ear(s)
  and allergies 7
  ringing in 124, 125
Easter, allergies at 177
eating away from home, and food allergy 173-74
ECF (eosinophil chemotactic factor),
  defined 536
ECF-A
  see eosinophil chemotactic factor of
    anaphylaxis (ECF-A)
eczema
  atopic 105-7, 407-10
    see also atopic dermatitis (ec-
      zema)
  contact
    see also contact dermatitis
  defined 536
  hand 411-13
  infantile 408
  nummular 407
  seborrheic 407
  types of 407
edema, defined 536
effector cells, defined 536
eggs 178, 197, 302
  allergy to 243
  anaphylactic reaction to 167
  avoidance of 202
  and childhood atopic dermatitis
    245, 249
  at Easter 177
  foods containing 259, 260t
  technical names for 259, 259t
egg-whites 178, 258
Eiermann, Heinz 426, 432
elastic materials, and contact
  dermatitis 399
elderly
  air pollution and 342, 343t
  and allergic drug reactions 126-27
  asthma in 453-57

elderly, continued
  differential diagnosis of 453-54
  education of patient and 457
  medications for 455-56
  prevalence of 453
  treatment of 455-56
  blistering disorders in 111
  with contact dermatitis 402
  contact dermatitis in 402
electrostatic air precipitators 322-23
  in treatment of allergy-induced
    asthma 87
electrostatic filters
  for animal allergens 336
  for sinusitis 101
elemental formula 204
elimination diet
  defined 536
  in diagnosis of food allergy 200-201,
    257
  for food-related childhood atopic
    dermatitis 250-51
ELISA, in diagnosis of food allergy
  201
Ellis, Elliot 523
elm 313
emotional rhinitis 62
emotions, as asthma trigger 27-28, 85
emphysema
  asthma and, myths about 91
  over-the-counter antihistamines
    contraindicated in 504
endocrine-metabolic system, corticosteroids and 521
endotoxin, defined 536
English ivy, and contact dermatitis 403
environmental factors
  in asthma 467
  of atopic dermatitis (atopic eczema)
    409
  in food allergy 205
  in pediatric allergies 158-59
  research on 42
Environmental Protection Agency
  (EPA) 325
  on pesticides 388-89
  standards on particulate air pollu-
    tion 341-44, 343t

enzyme(s)
  in allergies 10-11
  asthma and 81
  bacterial 69, 145
  defined 536
  and occupational asthma 141
  see also specific enzyme, e.g., lac-
    tase
eosinophil(s) 8, 35
  in allergic lung reactions 459-62
    research on 459-62
  in allergic rhinitis 19
  in asthma 79
  defined 536
eosinophil chemotactic factor of anaphylaxis (ECF-A) 8
  defined 536
eosinophil granule proteins 459
eosinophil peroxidase 460
ephedrine, in nasal decongestants 102
Epicoccum 316
epinephrine (Adrenaline) 517
  defined 536
epinephrine inhalers, over-the-
  counter 505
epinephrine injection kit 231-32
  for food allergy 174, 203, 231
  for insect sting 231-32, 360-61, 366
  for latex allergy 420, 422
Epi-Pen, Epi-Pen Jr. 366
epitopes 32, 536
epsilon aminocaproic acid, for hereditary angioedema 170
erythroblastosis fetalis (Rh factor disease) 184-86, *185*
  defined 536
erythromycin, second-generation antihistamines contraindicated with
  497
erythrosine, defined 224
esophageal reflux, as asthma trigger
  84
ethanolamines 504
ethmoid sinuses *96, 97*
  pain in 98
ethylenediamine 404
eustachian tubes 61, 101
  defined 536

evergreen trees 175-76
examination gloves, latex in 416
exempt color additives, defined 224
exercise
  asthma and 174
    myths about 91
  and food allergies 202
  recommendations for asthmatics
    26, 83
exercise-induced anaphylactoid reaction 229
exercise-induced asthma 80, 83, 91
  cromolyn sodium for 87
exercise-induced food allergy 202
exfoliative dermatitis, drug-induced
  120
exhalation, in asthma 23, 78, 85-86
expiration, in asthma 23, 78, 85-86
Ext. D&C, defined 222, 224
external analgesics 477
extrinsic asthma, defined 537
eye(s)
  and allergies 7, 27, 504
  corticosteroids and 521
eye allergies, complications of 505
eye drops 123, 504
eyeglasses, and contact dermatitis 399
eyelid, and contact dermatitis 399
eyeliner, color additives in 217

F

fabric finishes, and contact
  dermatitis 399
face, and contact dermatitis 399
face mask 21, 320, 321
facial cleansers, allergic reaction to 426
facial makeup, allergic reaction to 426
fair skin, and photosensitivity 137
family recipes, adapting 266-67
farmer's lung 147-53, 148t, 317
  defined 537
Fc, defined 537
Fc receptor, defined 537
FDA
  see Food and Drug Administration
    (FDA)
FD&C, defined 222, 224

FD&C Orange No. 1 223
FD&C Red No. 2 220-21
FD&C Red No. 3 219-20
FD&C Red No. 40 223
FD&C Yellow No. 5
  see yellow color additive (FD&C No.
    5 [tartrazine])
feather pillows 86, 321
feathers 333
Federal Food, Drug, and Cosmetic Act
  (1958) 210
Federation of American Societies for
  Experimental Biology (FASEB)
  on use of BHA 212
  on use of sulfites 213
feet, and contact dermatitis 399
Fel d 1 337
Feldene (piroxicam)
  and photosensitivity 137
  as photosensitizer 137t
fetus, immune system of 157
fiber
  and kidney disease 302
  nutrition claims for 304
filled crackers, maximum sulfite levels for 216
film developers, and allergic contact
  dermatitis 107
filtering devices 87, 322-23, 487
finfish 258
fire ant 352-52
  anaphylactic reaction to 167, 229
  extracts for 514t
  venom of 167
firecracker fumes 178
firefighters, and poison ivy 478
fireplace, and allergy 174-75
firewood 174
first aid, for allergy symptoms
  see the subentry "treatment of" under specific topic, e.g., poison ivy,
    treatment of
fish 178, 197, 198
  anaphylactic reaction to 167, 228
  calcium in 239t
  and childhood atopic dermatitis 249
  natural histamines in 198
  questions about reaction to 200

Fisher, Alexander 400
Fish-Rice Casserole *271*
flavorings
 alcohol in 303
 hidden milk proteins in 241, 242
flaxseed 69
fleas 353
Flieger, Ken 487
floaters 317
floors 86, 331
Florida, pollen calendar for *65*
Florida poison tree *(Metopium
 toxiferum)* 384
flounder 258
flours, nonwheat 261-62, 266t
 baking with 264-65
flowers 178, 313
 of Pacific poison oak 381
 of poison ivy and oak 376, 378, *379*
 of poison sumace 383
flu shot, and asthma 176
fluconazole (Diflucan), second-
 generation antihistamines
 contraindicated with 497
flunisolde (Nasalide) 493t
fluticasone 489, 492
fluxes, soldering 142
fly 353
Focus on Food Labeling (FDA Consumer), order information for 297
folic acid, and liver disease 302
food(s)
 anaphylactic reaction to 227-32
 anaphylactic reactions to 167-68
 asthma and, myths about 92
 avoidance of
  during pregnancy 207
  in recipes 263
 calcium in 237, 239t
 color additives in 217-25
 containing corn 259, 261t
 containing eggs 259, 260t
 containing gluten 259, 261t
 containing milk 259, 260t
 containing wheat 259, 261t
 ingredients, mandatory nutrition
  labeling for 298-300
 lactose in 237-38, 239t

food(s), continued
 preservatives in
  see food preservatives
 snack, preservatives in 209
 sulfites in 82-83
 technical names for 259t-261t, 259-
  61
 thickening of, with nonwheat flours
  and starches 265
Food, Drug, and Cosmetic Act (1938)
 219, 222-23
 Delaney anti-cancer clause (1960
  amendment) 219-20, 223
food additives 162
 and hyperactivity 205
food allergens 197
 elimination of 242
 most common 302-3
Food Allergy Network 177, 302
food allergy/food hypersensitivity, defined 537
food allergy(ies) 195-208, 257-58
 anaphylactic reactions and 167-68,
  196, 201, 203, 227-32
 and atopic dermatitis (atopic eczema) 408-9
 and childhood atopic dermatitis
  245-51
 in children 203-4, 467
 common 197, 302-3
 to concealed milk proteins 241-43
 controversial 204-5
 cooking for people with 257-95
 cross-reactivity and 198
 diagnosis of 26-27, 199-202
  controversial techniques for 205-6
  diagnostic tests in 200-201
  elimination diet in 200-201
  patient history in 200
 differential diagnosis of 198-99
 eating away from home 173-74
 exercise-induced 202
 during holidays 173-74
 identification of 26-27
 and immune system 195, 196-97
 and infantile asthma 161
 in infants 157-58, 203-4
 mechanism of 196-97

food allergy(ies), continued
  multiple 202
  research on 42
  severe 202-3
  to shrimp 253-55
  symptoms of 196
  treatment of 26-27, 202-3
    controversial 206
  vs. food intolerances 195
Food and Drug Administration (FDA)
  Adverse Reaction Monitoring Sys-
      tem (ARMS) 213, 214, 225
    address 214, 225
  and drug safety 116
  and hydrocortisone products 402
  and latex allergy 416, 417, 419-20
  Office of Cosmetics and Colors 217
    address 225
  on over-the-counter drugs for poison
      ivy exposure 476-77
  regulation of color additives 217-19
    Orange No. 1 223
    Red No. 2 220-21
    Red No. 3 219-20
    Yellow No. 5 (tartrazine) 218
  regulation of food preservatives
      209-16
    butylated hydroxyanisole (BHA)
        211-12
    safety questions in 210-11
    sulfites 213-14
  research in trial methods 221
  on standardized allergen extracts
      482-84, 508, 513-15, 514t
food colorings
  see color additives
food hypersensitivity
  see food allergy
food ingredients, mandatory nutri-
    tion labeling for 298-300
food intolerance(s) 258-59
  defined 537
  psychological trigger of 199
  vs. food allergies 195, 198-99
food labels 259t-261t, 259-61, 297-305
  benefits of 298
  health claims 301
  "hidden milk" in 238

food labels, continued
  ingredient list 299-300
  nutrient claims 300-301, 304-5
  nutrition facts panel 298-99
  serving size information 299-300
  special diets 302-3
food pests 354
food preparation
  and care of asthmatic child 452
  omitting basic ingredient during
      263
food preservatives 209-16
  and aspirin intolerance 122
  butylated hydroxyanisole (BHA) as
      211-13
  safety regulations for 210-11
  sulfites as 213-14, 215-16
food sensitivities
  diagnosis of 168
  special diet for 302-3
food-dependent exercise-induced ana-
    phylaxis 230
foods, extracts for 514t
forced-air heating systems 87, 151
forced-air system's lung 151
  defined 537
Forest Service, and poison ivy 478
formaldehyde 142
  and chemical sensitivity 394
  and contact dermatitis 404
formula, infant 204
Foulke, Judith E. 216
foundation, allergic reaction to 426
Fourth of July, allergies and 178
fragrances
  allergic reaction to 426, 429
  and contact dermatitis 399
  and labeling claims 430
frappe, for person with food allergy
    286
french fries, sulfites and 214
fresh potatoes, sulfites and 214
fresh produce, sulfites and 213
Freund, Vicki 423
frontal sinuses *96,* 97
  pain in 98
fruit(s)
  anaphylactic reaction to 167

fruit(s), continued
  dried
    maximum sulfite levels for 216
    mold allergy and 315
    sulfites and 213
  glacé, maximum sulfite levels for 216
  at Passover 177
  poisonous
    of Metopium 384
    of Pacific poison oak 381
    of poison ivy and oak 376, 378
    of poison sumac 383
  raw, sulfites and 213
  sulfites and 213
fruit crisps 267
fruit juices, maximum sulfite levels for 216
fruit topping, sulfites in 83
fumes, and rhinitis 69
fungal infections 405
  and sinusitis 99-100
fungus, defined 537
"fungus ball" 316
fungus spores 64
  in mold allergy 314
  in pulmonary mycotoxicosis 152
fur 333
furnace filters 175
furniture 332
  and pet allergens 318
furniture makers, and contact dermatitis 401
furrier's lung 148, 148t
Fusarium 316

G

galactose 235
Galant, Stanley P. 508, 509, 510, 511, 513
Gambia, IgE levels in 157
garbanzo beans (chickpeas) 258
garden plants, and contact dermatitis 403
garlic, and contact dermatitis 403, 405
gasoline 394

gastroenteropathy, allergic 161
gastroesophageal reflux, as asthma trigger 84
gastrointestinal cancer, *vs.* food allergy 199
gastrointestinal (GI) diseases and disorders 182-83
  in child with food allergy 161-62
  in dermatitis herpetiformis 111
gastrointestinal (GI) tract
  adrenergics and 518
  and allergies 7
  corticosteroids and 521
  cromolyn sodium and 522
  defined 537
  effect of food allergy on 196
  theophylline and 519
Gehrig's disease (amyotrophic lateral sclerosis) 184
gelatin, maximum sulfite levels for 215
gene(s), defined 537
generally recognized as safe (GRAS) regulations 211
genetic association, defined 537
genetic factors 324-25
  allergy and 13, 14
  and asthma 156
  and food allergy 196
  in pediatric allergies 156-57
  and skin reactions 411
genetic markers
  for allergic disorders 14
  defined 537
  of self 33
geographic location, and asthma 438
Georgia, pollen calendar for *65*
geraniums, and contact dermatitis 403
gerbils 318
German measles (rubella) vaccine, anaphylaxis and 165
Gern, James E. 242
GI
  see under gastrointestinal (GI)
giant hives
  see angioedema (giant hives)
ginger, and contact dermatitis 403, 405
ginko trees 403

glacé fruit, maximum sulfite levels
   for 216
glaucoma, over-the-counter antihistamines contraindicated in 504
Gleich, Gerald J. 459-62
gliadin, and celiac disease 303
glomerulonephritis 13, 187
   defined 538
glomerulus *188*
gloves
   latex 417, 420, 468
      brands of 423-24
      recommendations for use of 420
   latex-free 420, 423-24
glucose 235
gluten
   foods containing 258-59, 261t
   function of 264
gluten intolerance 208, 258-59
gluten products, technical names for
   259, 260t
gluten-free diet, for dermatitis
   herpetiformis 111
gluten-sensitive enteropathy (celiac
   disease) 208
glyceryl monothioglycolate 426
glycoproteins, defined 538
glycosylation, of IgE 249
Gonzalez, Ernesto 418
grain(s)
   anaphylactic reaction to 167
   nonwheat 262
grain dust exposure 152
"grain fever" 152
grain products, maximum sulfite levels for 215
granule proteins, eosinophil 459
granulocytes, defined 538
grape(s), sulfites in 83
Grape Frappe *286*
grape juice, sulfites in 83
GRAS *(generally recognized as safe)*
   regulations 211
grass pollen 64, 69, 312, 313
   allergenic extract for 514t
   desensitization to 510
gravies, maximum sulfite levels for
   215

grinder's disease (sandblaster's
   silicosis) 146
griseofulvin, and drug-induced photosensitivity 120
Guillain-Barré syndrome 165-66, 183
   defined 538
guinea pigs 318
Gundel, Robert H. 459-62

H

Hageman factor (HF) systems 13
   defined 538
hair, of allergic person 512
hair dyes
   allergic reaction to 426
      prevention of 432
   and contact dermatitis 404
hair preparations, allergic reaction to
   426
   prevention of 432
hair removers (depilatories) 431
hair spray, and contact dermatitis
   399
hair straighteners 431
hairdressers, and contact dermatitis
   401
Halloween, allergies at 177
hand eczema (hand rash) 411-13
   diagnosis of 397, 398-400, 412
   prevention of 413
   stress and 412
   treatment of 412-13
hand tremors, adrenergic drugs and
   518
haplotype, defined 538
hardwood floors 86
harvester (agricultural) ant 352
hashish smoking 159
"hay fever"
   defined 538
   as term for allergic rhinitis 61, 479,
      484
health care products, color additives
   in 217
health claims, on food label 301
Health Industry Manufacturers Association 423

Health Research Group 220
heart
  see also under cardiac
heart problems, oral decongestants
  contraindicated in 504
heat registers 21, 331
heating systems 87, 151, 328, 331,
  512
heating vents 175, 321
Hecht, Annabel 478
Helminthosporium 315
helper factors, defined 538
helper T cells, defined 538
hematopoiesis, defined 538
Hemophilus influenzae, and sinusitis
  99
Henkel, John 225
heparin 35
hepatitis 181-82
  serum, transmission of 181-82
herbicides, for control of poison ivy/
  oak 370, 387-88
herbs, as natural preservatives 214
hereditary angioedema 170-71
  defined 538
heredity 324-25
  and allergy 13, 14
  and asthma 156
  and food allergy 196
  and pediatric allergy 156-57
  and skin reaction 411
heterologous, defined 539
Hevea brasiliensis 416
HF systems
  see Hageman factor (HF) systems
hiatus hernia, in elderly asthmatic
  456
hickory 313
high blood pressure, oral decongestants contraindicated in 504
high-efficiency particulate activating
  (HEPA) filters 321, 333
  in treatment of allergy-induced
    asthma 87
Hirschel, L. Anne 463
histamine(s)
  in allergic reaction 6, 8, *10,* 16, 35,
    71, 310, 486

histamine(s), continued
  defined 539
  in food-related childhood atopic
    dermatitis 247
  naturally occurring 198
  platinum salts and 143
histamine challenge 446
histamine toxicity 198
histamine-release test 72-73
  defined 539
histamine-releasing factor (HRF)
  248, 249, 251
histocompatibility (HLA) antigens 14
  testing for 189-90
histocompatibility (MHC) restriction
  33
HIV
  see human immunodeficiency virus
    (HIV)
hives 109-10
  chronic 207-8
  cold-induced 168-69
  drug-induced 120
  giant
    see angioedema (giant hives)
  rare with sulfites 208
  seasonal 109
  see also urticaria (hives);
    angioedema
HLA antigens *see* histocompatibility
  (HLA) antigens
  see histocompatibility (HLA) antigens
HLA histocompatibility antigens, defined 539
Hodgkin's disease 405
holiday allergies 173-78
holiday decorations, and allergy 175
home, air pollution sources in *70,*
  141, 141t
home heating system 175
homologous, defined 539
honey bee 229, 351, 352
hookworm 190
Hormodendrum (Cladosporium) 315
hormones
  allergic reactions to 126
  for hereditary angioedema 170
  for hives 110

hornets 167, 351, 352
  anaphylactic reaction to 167, 229
hospitalization
  for allergic drug reactions 115, 116-
    18
  for asthma 78, 327-28, 443, *443,*
    446, 466, 467
  drug side effects during, monitoring
    of 116
  for immunologic diseases *46,* 48
hot compresses, for sinusitis 102
hot dogs, hidden milk proteins in 241
hot forced-air heat 87, 321, 331
hot-water heat 87
house air conditioning 21
house dust 64, 317-18, 481, 487
  affect of on children's allergies 159
  defined 317-18
house dust mite
  see dust mite
house plants, and contact dermatitis
  403
housecleaning 332, 487
  in allergen control 321, 326
  and care of asthmatic child 452
household allergens
  affect of on children's allergies 159
  color additives in household items
    217
household gloves, latex in 416
household pets
  see pets
HRF
  see histamine-releasing factor
    (HRF)
human blood
  see blood
human immunity
  see immunity
human immunodeficiency virus (HIV)
  defined 539
  latex gloves as protection against
    423, 468
  and photosensitivity 137
human leukocyte antigens (HLA), defined 539
Human Nutrition Information Service 268

humidifier(s), for sinusitis 101
humidifier lung 148t, 151, 317
humidity levels, and mold 174
humoral, defined 539
humoral immunity, defined 539
hybridoma, defined 539
hydralazine, and allergic drug reaction 121
hydrocortisone
  in older nasal sprays 491
  over-the-counter
    for contact dermatitis 402-3
    for cosmetic allergic reaction 426
    for poison ivy exposure 372, 373,
      476-77
hydrogen breath test 235
hydrolysates, on ingredient list 300
hydroxyzine, for hives 110
Hymenoptera 351
  and anaphylactic death 229, 349
  feeding areas of 359
  nests of 359
hyperactivity 162
  and food allergy 205
hyperirritability of airways, in
  asthma 79
hypersensitivity
  defined 540
  delayed 5-6
  immediate (anaphylactic-
    hypersensitivity reaction) 4, 5
  see also allergy(ies); allergic
    reaction(s)
hypersensitivity pneumonitis (allergic pneumonia) 147-51, 148t, 315,
  317, 394
  defined 539
  drug-induced 121
  prevention of 153
  symptoms of 317, 394
hypertension
  see high blood pressure
hyperthyroidism, as asthma trigger
  85
hyperventilation 83
hyphae 314
hypogammaglobulinemia, defined 540
hyposensitization, defined 540

I

ibuprofen 82
  and aspirin intolerance 122
  photoallergic reaction to 135
  as photosensitizer 137t
ice, for insect sting 358
ice cream 178
ICGN
  see immune complex
      glomerulonephritis (ICGN)
Idaho, pollen calendar for *66*
idiopathic angioedema 207
idiotopes, site-associated, defined 550
idiotypes, defined 540
IFN, defined *see* interferon
IgA
  see immunoglobulin A (IgA)
IgE
  see immunoglobulin E (IgE)
IgG
  see immunoglobulin G (IgG)
IgM
  see immunoglobulin M (IgM)
Illinois, pollen calendar for *66*
immediate hypersensitivity
  (anaphylactic-hypersensitivity reaction) 4, 5, 17
  antihistamines for 22
  research on 39-40
immune complex(es) 5, *12,* 12-13
  in cutaneous necrotizing angiitis
      112
  defined 5, 540
immune complex assay 205-6
immune complex glomerulonephritis
  (ICGN) 187
immune reaction or response, defined
  540
immune system 31-32, 485-86
  in airborne allergy 310-11
  in allergic reaction 485-86
  in childhood atopic dermatitis 246-
      48
  communication network of 32
  corticosteroids and 521
  defined 540
  of fetus 157

immune system, continued
  and food allergy 195, 196-97
  in hypersensitivity pneumonitis
      149-50
  importance of 3
  in occupationally caused respira-
      tory diseases 139-40
  research on 471
  role of in allergic reactions 31-35,
      34
immune system diseases and disorders 179-91
  asthma as 445, 471
  blood disorders 184-86, *185*
  cancer 191
  gastrointestinal disease 182-83
  kidney diseases 187-88, *188*
  liver diseases 181-82
  neurological diseases 183-84
  by organ site 47t
  organ transplants 189-90
  parasitic diseases 190-91
  rheumatoid arthritis as 180-81
  socioeconomic impact of *45-54*
  systemic lupus erythematosus as
      186-87
  U.S. hospitalizations for *46*
immunity 3-4, 485
  active, defined 527
  defined 3, 540
  fundamental concept of 4
  historical assessment of 3-4
  humoral, defined 539
  importance of 3-4
immunization
  for poison ivy 372
  see immunotherapy (allergy shots)
immunoassay, defined 540
immunocompetent, defined 540
immunodeficiency, defined 540
immunogens, research on 42
immunoglobulin(s) (antibodies) 4, 6
  defined 540
immunoglobulin A (IgA) 182
  defined 541
  in dermatitis herpetiformis 111
  in transfusion reactions 169
immunoglobulin D (IgD), defined 541

immunoglobulin E (IgE) 4, 6, *8, 9, 11,* 16
  in allergic reaction 6, *9,* 33-34, 33-35, *34,* 80, 468, 486, 509
  in anaphylaxis 229
  defined 541
  duration of in body 16
  and fetus 157
  in food allergy 196-97
  function of 16
  genetics and 13-14
  in occupational asthma 142
  and parasitic infestation 156-57
  person's total level of 13
  prevalence of 327
  and ragweed pollen 16, *34,* 80
  research on 39-40
  in shrimp allergy 254
immunoglobulin E+ (IgE+) 249
immunoglobulin G (IgG) 5
  allergy shots and 21, 324, 361
  defined 541
  function of 16
  in hepatitis 181
  in hypersensitivity pneumonitis 149
  in transfusion reactions 169
immunoglobulin G (IgG) subclass assay 206
immunoglobulin M (IgM)
  defined 541
  as rheumatoid factor 180
immunologic diseases
  see immune system diseases and disorders
immunologic response
  in allergic rhinitis 69-71
  research on 69
immunosuppression, defined 541
immunotherapy (allergy shots) 21
  adverse reactions to 166
  allergen avoidance and 512-13
  for allergic asthma 25
  for allergic disease 324
  for allergic rhinitis 21, 74-75, 482, 484, 497-99
  for asthma 52-53, 89
  and atopic dermatitis (atopic eczema) 409

immunotherapy (allergy shots), continued
  candidates for 508-9
  for cat-induced asthma 340
  defined 541
  for eczema 107
  incidence of 48
  ineffective for food allergy 203
  for insect sting allergy 232, 361, 363-66
  length of 511-12
  prevalence of 49t
  results from 511-12
  "rush" 511
  for seasonal allergic rhinitis 20, 497
  shot schedule for 509-11
  for sinusitis 101
  standardizing extracts for 513-15, *514*
  venom extracts for 167
immunotherapy/immune modulation, for allergic rhinitis (hay fever) 497-99
immunotoxin, defined 541
impetigo 405
imported fire ant 352
impurities
  in color additives, FDA restrictions on 219
  in drugs, allergic reaction to 118, 126
in vitro, defined 541
in vivo, defined 541
Indiana, pollen calendar for *66*
indigotine, defined 224
indomethacin 82
  and aspirin intolerance 122
indoor allergens 327-29, 393-94, 399, 512-13
  asthma and 467
  color additives in household items 217
  mold as 174, 315
  socioeconomic impact of 327-28
  sources of 327, 393, 394
  see also specific allergen, e.g., dust mite
Indoor Allergens: Assessing and Controlling Adverse Health Effects (Institute of Medicine) 327

indoor tanning products 138
industrial activities, and rhinitis 69
industrial exposure, as cause of
asthma 24, 81
industrial materials, causing allergies 140t, 143t
industrial plants, proximity to 141
industrialized nations, asthma in 140
industry, and allergic respiratory disease 139
see also occupational asthma
infant(s)
and allergic drug reactions 126-27
atopic dermatitis in 407-8
contact dermatitis in 401-2
cow's milk and 157-58
food allergies in 157-58, 203-4
introduction of foods to 27
lactose intolerance in 235, 236
Rh factor and 184-86, *185*
see also children; pediatric allergies
infantile asthma 161
infantile eczema 106, 408
infections, as cause of asthma 23, 81,
158
infectious mononucleosis 123
inflammation
of airways, in asthma 78, 79
in asthma, *in vivo* analysis of 448
defined 541
produced by allergic reaction 6-8,
446, 471, 484
inflammatory bowel disease 182
inflammatory diseases, research on
40-41, 462
inflammatory neuropathy, chronic
183
inflammatory response 468
defined 542
influenza type A 158
influenza vaccines 165-66
Inform 214
ingredient list
and avoidance of foods 263
on food label 299-300
ingredient names 259t-261t, 259-61
inhaled allergens
see airborne allergens

inhaled bronchodilators 88
inhaled corticosteroids 89
for allergic asthma 25
inhaled cromolyn
for allergic asthma 25
for cat-induced asthma 340
inhaled steam, for sinusitis 102
inhaled steroids 89
inheritance
see heredity
injected dyes, anaphylactic reactions
to 168
injection therapy, defined 542
inner-city children, asthma in 469-70
insect(s)
allergy-causing 351, 353-54
biting 353-54
food pest 354
smaller 354
stinging 352-53
preventing attack by 358-59
insect allergy(ies) 349-61, 363-66
defined 350-51
diagnosis of 363
diagnostic tests for 356-57
insects causing 351
occurrence of 363
prevalence of 363
symptoms of 354-56
insect bites
allergic
avoidance of 358-59
treatment of 358-61
venom immunotherapy for 363-66
non-allergic, treatment of 358
insect sprays 322
insect stings
allergic reaction to 355-56, 366
anaphylactic reactions to 166-67,
228, 356, 366
avoidance of 231
death from 349, 363
delayed response to 356
identification of 356-57
multiple, toxic reaction to 355, 356
normal reaction to 354-55
instant potatoes, sulfites in 83
instant tea, sulfites in 82

insulin, zinc-free 124, 130
insulin intolerance 124, 130
Intal (cromolyn sodium) inhaler 482, 522
intercellular, defined 542
interferon (IFN)
   for common cold 104
   defined 542
interferon (IFN)-α, defined 542
interferon (IFN)-ß, defined 542
interferon (IFN)-γ, defined 542
interleukin (IL)
   defined 542
   in IgE synthesis 39
interleukin (IL)-4 471
   defined 542
interleukin (IL)-1, defined 542
interleukin (IL)-2, defined 542
interleukin (IL)-3, defined 542
International Fragrance Association 431
intestines, and allergic drug reaction 121, 127
intolerance
   food
      see food intolerance
   gluten
      see gluten intolerance
   lactose
      see lactose intolerance
intracellular, defined 542
intracutaneous test 357
intrinsic asthma, defined 542
intrinsic rhinitis 62
Iowa, pollen calendar for 66
ipratropium (Atrovent) 490t, 493t, 495
   for asthma 26
irritable bowel syndrome 208
   fiber and 303
irritant contact dermatitis 398
irritants, in contact dermatitis 398-400
isocyanates 392
isolated IgA deficiency 182
isoproterenol (Isuprel) 517
Isuprel (isoproterenol) 517
Italian Ground Beef with Rice 272

itch mite 405
itching
   in airborne allergy 311
   in anaphylaxis 119
   causes of 405
   in childhood atopic dermatitis 248
   in eczema 106
   of poison ivy 476

J

jams, maximum sulfite levels for 215
Japanese lacquer-tree *(Rhus verniciflua)* 384
jellies, maximum sulfite levels for 215
jelly beans 177
Jenner, Edward 4, 485
Johns Hopkins School of Medicine 364-66, 470
Johnson (grass) 313
joints, inflammation of
   see rheumatoid arthritis
July Fourth, allergies and 178

K

Kaliner, Michael A. 29, 93, 231, 331
Kansas, pollen calendar for 66
kaolin, for poison ivy blisters 476
Kentucky, pollen calendar for 66
Kentucky bluegrass 313
ketoconazole (Nizoral), second-generation antihistamines
   contraindicated with 497
kidney(s) 188
   and allergic drug reaction 121, 127
kidney disease, special diet for 207-8, 302
Kiechel, Frederic, III 501, 502
kinins 13
kissing bug 353
Klingman, Dayton L. 389
knick-knacks 86
Kobayashi, Ai Lan D. 501, 502
Kobayashi, Roger 501, 502
Kupffer cells, defined 542

Kurtzweil, Paula 305
Kurumaji, Yuko 135
Kwan, Jacki 227

L

label(s)
  cosmetic 429
  cosmetic claims 429-31
  food
    see food labels
  food industry claims 301
lacquer 384
lactase 233, 236, 258
lactase deficiency 198-99
  diagnosis of 208
lactose, hidden 237-38
lactose intolerance 208, 233-39, 258
  and balanced nutrition 236-37
  defined 233-34
  diagnosis of 234-35
  populations affected by 234
  prevalence of 234
  symptoms of 233
  treatment of 235-36
lactose tolerance test 234
LAK cells, defined 542
lakes
  color 223
  defined 224
lamb's quarters 313
lamina propria 79
Langerhans cells, defined 542
lanolin 431
late-phase inflammatory reactions
  (late-phase response) 17, 468
  in allergic rhinitis 491
  in atopic dermatitis 246
  in cat-induced asthma 338, 339
  research on 40-41, 468-69
latex
  allergenic extract for 514t
  vs. vinyl 423
latex allergies *415-24*
  extract for 513
  history of 416-17
  medical care and 419-22, *422,* 468
  in patient history 419-20

latex allergies, continued
  people at risk for 421-22
  self-testing for discouraged 418-19
  testing for 418-19
latex gloves
  need for 423, 468
  recommendations for use of 420
laundry products 69
  and contact dermatitis 399, 402,
    404
lawn 321
learning disabilities 162
leather, and contact dermatitis 399
leather gloves 413
leaves 321
  of Metopium 384
  of Pacific poison oak 381
  of poison ivy and oak 378, *379,* 404-
    5
  of sumac 383, 384
  wet, and mold 174
"leaves of three, let them be" *368,*
  370, 373, 374, 376
legumes 258
Lehrer, Samuel B. 253
Lemon Dessert Sauce *293*
lemon juice, bottled, sulfites in 83,
  216
Lemon Pudding *286*
leukocytes, defined 543
leukotrienes 35, 310
  defined 543
Lichtenstein, Lawrence M. 228, 232
licorice 177
lidocaine 477
Life Sciences Research Office
  (FASEB), on use of BHA 212
lifestyle, and allergies 512-13
light, sensitivity to
  see photosensitivity
lilacs, and contact dermatitis 403
Lim, Henry 136
Lin, Lawrence 211
line, defined 543
linoleum 86, 331
lips
  and contact dermatitis 399
  swelling of 207

lipstick
  color additives in 217
  and contact dermatitis 399
liver, and allergic drug reaction 121, 127
liver disease 181-82
  second-generation antihistamines contraindicated in 497
liver disorders, special diet for 302
lobster 197, 254, 258
  frozen, maximum sulfite levels for 215
local anesthetics, and allergic drug reactions 120
location, geographic, and asthma 438
Lockwood, Sue 415
loratadine 497
Lou Gehrig's disease (amyotrophic lateral sclerosis) 184
Louisiana, pollen calendar for *66*
Loveless, Mary 364
"low sodium" 301
lox 178
LPR (late-phase response)
  see late-phase inflammatory reactions (late-phase response)
lung
  see also entries at pulmonary
lung challenge test, for occupational asthma 144
lung involvement, in allergic drug reactions 120-21
lung reactions, allergic
  see allergic lung reactions
lupus erythematosus of the skin 112-13
  defined 543
lymph, defined 543
lymph cells, and allergic drug reaction 121
lymph nodes, defined 543
lymphatic vessels, defined 543
lymphocytes
  in asbestosis 146
  defined 543
  see also T lymphocytes (T cells)
lymphoid organs, defined 543
lymphokines tolerance, defined 543
lympholines, defined 544

M

mackerel, natural histamines in 198
macrolide antibiotics, second-generation antihistamines contraindicated with 497
macrophages 146
  defined 544
magnolias, and contact dermatitis 403
Maimonides 156
main dishes, recipes for 270-73
Maine, pollen calendar for *66*
major basic protein (MBP) 459-62
  and bronchial hyperactivity 460
  toxic effects of, prevention or reversal of 461-62
major histocompatibility complex (MHC) 33
  defined 544
major histocompatibility complex (MHC) restriction 33
makeup
  allergic reaction to 426
  and contact dermatitis 399
malabsorption syndromes 182
malt worker's disease 148t
mango 403
maple bark stripper's disease 147, 148t, 151
  defined 544
maraschino cherries 220
  maximum sulfite levels for 216
margarine, milk-free 267
marijuana smoking 159
markweed 377
Maryland, pollen calendar for *66*
mascara, color additives in 217
mask(s)
  face 320, 321
  at Halloween 177
  nuisance 21
Massachusetts, pollen calendar for *66*
mast cells 6, *8-11,* 15-16, 35, 80
  in anaphylactoid reaction 229
  defined 544
  in food allergy 196, 197
  life of 16

mast cells, continued
  mediators released by 16, 17, 35, *39*
  triggering of, defined 552
mattress pads 331
mattresses 86, 328, 331
Maxaire (pirbuterol) 517
maxillary sinuses *96,* 97
maximum expiratory level 85
maximum inspiratory level 85
mayfly 354
Mayo Medical School 459
McCarthy, Jane 419
meal planning, and food allergy 268
meat accompaniments, recipe for 274
meat cutter's (meat labeler's) asthma
  143
Meatloaf *273*
mediators
  in allergic rhinitis 69-71, 486, 491
  defined 544
  in drug-induced serum sickness 119
  inflammatory, in asthma 446
  life of 11
  production of 6, *10,* 10-11, *11,* 17, 35
Medic Alert tags 131, 203, 360, 420
  address 131
medical devices
  color additives in 218
  containing latex 419, 422t
  and latex allergies 419-22, *422*
  latex in 416
medication(s)
  adverse effects from 517-23
  for allergic rhinitis 21-22
  in asthma treatment 87-89
  as cause of asthma 24
  color additives in 218, 222-23
  over-the-counter, for allergies 503-5
  patient's definition of 128
  substitutes for 131
  topical, and contact dermatitis 400
  in treatment of allergic disease 322-
    23
  in treatment of insect bites 359-60
Medium White Sauce *293*
mefenamic acid, and aspirin intolerance 122
Mellion, Morris B. 501, 502

melons, and ragweed allergy 198
Menes, King of Egypt 349
meningitis 123
menthol 477
mercurochrome, and contact
  dermatitis 400
mercury
  and allergic contact dermatitis 107
  and contact dermatitis 400
mercury (poison ivy) 377
merthiolate, and contact dermatitis
  400
metabolites, drug, allergic reaction to
  118, 127
metal-refining industry 139
metals, and allergic contact
  dermatitis 107
Metaprel (metaproterenol) 517
metaproterenol (Alupent, Metaprel)
  517
Metcalfe, Dean 26
methacholine challenge 446
methylxanthines, for asthma 88
Metopium toxiferum (poisonwood,
  doctor gum, Metopium, Florida poison tree, coral sumac) 384
mexenone, in sunscreens 138
MHC *see* major histocompatibility
  complex (MHC)
MHC antigens
  class I 33
  class II 33
MHC restriction 33
  defined 544
Michigan, pollen calendar for *66*
microbes, defined 544
microfungi 64
micro-organisms, defined 544
middle ear, inflammation of 160
midge, biting 353
migraine headaches 204
milk 197, 198, 302
  allergy to 243
  anaphylactic reaction to 167
  avoidance of 202
    in food preparation 264, 267
  and childhood atopic dermatitis 249
  children and 203-4, 241-43

milk, continued
  foods containing 259, 260t
  lactose-reduced 236
  substitutes for 264
  technical names for 259, 259t
milk by-products 238
milk proteins, concealed 241-43
milk sugar
  see lactose
Miller, Laurence H. 373
minerals
  and liver disease 302
  on nutrition facts panel 299
Minnesota, pollen calendar for *66*
minorities, asthma in 53, 466
Mississippi, pollen calendar for *66*
Missouri, pollen calendar for *66*
mite 354
moisturizers, allergic reaction to 426
molasses
  calcium in 239t
  maximum sulfite levels for 216
  sulfites in 83
mold(s) 64, 314-17
  allergenic 315-16
    avoidance of 321, 487
  allergenic extracts for 514t
  and allergy 174
  on Christmas trees, eliminating
    175
  defined 314
  desensitization to 510
  growth of 315
  in hay, and farmer's lung 147
  information sources for 325
  and perennial allergy 20
  perennial (year-round) allergies to
    20
mold allergy, defined 314-15
mold counts 316
mold-related disorders 151, 316-17
molecular biology, in allergic disease
  research 41-42, 471
molecule, defined 544
monoclonal, defined 545
monoclonal antibodies, defined 545
monocyte, defined 545
monokines, defined 545

mononuclear cells
  in childhood atopic dermatitis 247-
    48
  in late-phase response 246
monsodium glutamate (MSG), adverse reaction to 199
Montana, pollen calendar for *67*
mortality
  see death
mosquitoes 353
moth 354
mothballs (naphthalene) 134
Mother's Day, allergies and 178
Mothers of Asthmatics, Inc. 93
  address 472
Motrin (ibuprofen)
  photoallergic reaction to 135
  as photosensitizer 137t
mountain cedar 313
mouse (mice)
  SCID, defined 549
  transgenic, defined 552
mouth, and contact dermatitis 402
MSG
  see monsodium glutamate (MSG)
mucocele 98
Mucor 316
Mucoraceae, and sinusitis 99-100
mucous membranes
  in allergic rhinitis 18-19, 311
  in asthma 10
  defined 545
  of nose 63
mucus
  in allergic rhinitis 18-19, 311
  in asthma 78, 79
Muffins *278*
"multiple chemical sensitivities" 392,
  394
multiple sclerosis 184
  defined 545
  socioeconomic impact of 179
mumps vaccine, anaphylaxis and 165
Munoz-Furlong, Ann 177
murine, defined 545
muscle spasm, in asthma 78
musculoskeletal system, corticosteroids and 521

mushroom(s), mold allergy and 315

mushroom worker's disease 147, 148t, 150

musk ambrette 135

myasthenia gravis (MG) 183
defined 545

mycotoxicosis, pulmonary 152-53

myocardial infarction, *vs.* anaphylaxis 363

N

NADPH, defined 545

nail polish, and contact dermatitis 399

nail preparations, allergic reaction to 426

names, technical, for foods 259t-261t, 259-61

naphazoline (Privine) 495
in nasal decongestants 102

naphthalene (mothballs) 134

naproxen sodium (Aleve), photoallergic reaction to 135

narcissus, and contact dermatitis 403

Nasacort (triamcinolone acetonide) 492, 493t

NaSal 495

nasal allergies
see allergic rhinitis (hay fever)

nasal congestion
during allergic rhinitis 19
normal 19
of rhinitis 63

nasal decongestants
see decongestants

nasal discharge, of rhinitis 62-63

nasal physiology, in allergic rhinitis 62-63

nasal polyps (nasal polyposis) 71, 82, 103, 170

nasal sprays, topical 491-96, 494t, 498t
cost of 493t

nasal steroids 489

Nasalcrom (cromolyn sodium) inhaler 482, 493t, 498t

National Ambient Air Quality Standard 341

National Asthma Education Program (NAEP) 439
address 472

National Center for Health Statistics 480-81

National Cooperative Inner-City Asthma Study (NCICAS) 324, 469-70

National Health and Nutrition Examination Survey II (NHANES II) 48, 50, 480-81

National Health Interview Survey 342

National Institute of Allergy and Infectious Diseases (NIAID) 92, 103, 231, 324, 465, 468, 513-15

National Institute of Arthritis and Musculoskeletal and Skin Diseases 373

National Institutes of Health 206

Native Americans, lactose intolerance in 234

natural killer (NK) cells, defined 545

natural resins 142

NCICAS
see National Cooperative Inner-City Asthma Study (NCICAS)

Nebraska, pollen calendar for 67

neck, and contact dermatitis 399

necrotizing angiitis, cutaneous 112

neomycin
and allergic drug reactions 123
and contact dermatitis 400

neoplasm, defined 545

NeoSynephrine (phenylephrine hydrochloride) 495

nephron *188*

nervous system
adrenergics and 518
antihistamines and 523
autoimmune diseases of 183-84
corticosteroids and 521
theophylline and 519

neurological diseases 183-84

neuromuscular system, adrenergics and 518

neuropathy, inflammatory, chronic 183

neutrophils 35
  in asthma 79
  defined 546
Nevada, pollen calendar for 67
New Guinea lung 147, 148t
New Hampshire, pollen calendar for
  67
New Jersey, pollen calendar for 67
New Mexico, pollen calendar for 67
New York, pollen calendar for 67
NHANES II
  see National Health and Nutrition
    Examination Survey II
    (NHANES II)
NIAID
  see National Institute of Allergy
    and Infectious Diseases (NIAID)
nickel
  and allergic contact dermatitis 107
  and contact dermatitis 399, 403
nickel salts 142
Nicklas, Richard 231
nicotinamide-adenine dinucleotide
  phosphate (NADP) 545
*1990 Annual Review of Pharmacology
  and Toxicology,* on use of BHA 212
nitrites 211
nitrofurantoin, and allergic drug reaction 120
nitrogen dioxide, and chemical sensitivity 393
nitrogen oxide 394
nitroglycerin, and contact dermatitis
  400
nitrosamines 211
Nizoral (ketoconazole), second-generation antihistamines
  contraindicated with 497
non-allergic drug reactions 124-25
"nondairy" 241
nondairy frozen desserts, hidden milk
  proteins in 241
nonfat dry milk powder 238
nonsteroidal anti-inflammatory drugs
  (NSAIDs)
  and asthma 82
  photoallergic reaction to 135
  and phototoxicity 136

nonwheat flours 261-62
  baking with 264-65
  thickening with 265
nonwheat starches 261-62
  thickening with 265
non-Whites, asthma in 466
North American Contact Dermatitis
  Group 425
North American Contact Dermatitis
  Group Standard Patch Test Series
  401
North Carolina, pollen calendar for
  67
North Dakota, pollen calendar for 67
Northwestern University Medical
  School (Chicago) 230
nose
  crease in, allergic rhinitis and 62
  physiology of, in rhinitis 62-63
Novocain (procaine), and allergic
  drug reactions 120
NSAIDs
  see nonsteroidal anti-inflammatory
    drugs (NSAIDs)
Nucleic acids, defined 546
nuisance masks 21
nummular eczema 407
Nuprin (ibuprofen), photoallergic reaction to 135
nut(s) 197, 258, 303
  anaphylactic reaction to 167, 228
  cross-reactivity and 206-7
  at Easter 177
  at Passover 177
  see also specific nut, e.g., pistachio
nut products, maximum sulfite levels
  for 216
nutrient claims, on food label 300-
  301, 304-5
nutrition, balanced, and lactose intolerance 236-37
nutrition facts panel, on food label
  298-99
nutrition information 297-305
Nutrition Labeling and Education
  Act (1990) 218

O

oak 313
oat(s), gluten in 258
oat flour 262
oatmeal, for poison ivy exposure 371, 476
Obstetrics and Gynecology 230
occupational asthma 24, 81, 140-45
  development of 142-43
    allergic factors in 142, *143*
    inhaled irritants and 142
    pharmacologic factors in 143
  diagnosis of 144
  lung challenge test for 144
  prevention of 145
  treatment of 145
  see also occupational/environmental respiratory diseases
occupational dermatitis 401
occupational illness, types of 139
occupational/environmental respiratory diseases 139-53
  allergic bronchopulmonary aspergillosis 153
  allergic pneumonia (hypersensitivity pneumonitis) 147-51, 148t
  asbestosis 146-47
  asthma 140-45
    see also occupational asthma
  berylliosis 147
  farmer's lung 147
  forced-air system's lung 151
  grain dust exposure 152
  maple bark stripper's disease 151
  pulmonary mycotoxicosis 152-53
  silicosis 146
  see also occupational asthma
Ocean Nasal Mist 495
office building, hypersensitivity pneumonitis and 394
Office of Cosmetics and Colors 217
  address 225
office visits
  see doctor office visits
Ohio, pollen calendar for *67*
oil, preservatives and 215

oil glands
  of cat 336
  of cats 337
Oklahoma, pollen calendar for *67*
OKT3, defined 546
Old-Fashioned Rice Pudding *287*
oleanders, and contact dermatitis 403
oleoresins 477-78
olfactory awareness 392
onions, and contact dermatitis 403, 405
opium 481
opportunistic infection, defined 546
opsonize, defined 546
orchard (grass) 313
Oregon, pollen calendar for *67*
organ transplants, rejection responses, types of 189-90
organic phosphorus 142
organism, defined 546
Orinase (tolbutamide), and photophobia 136
ornaments, holiday, and allergy 175
osteoarthritis, and food allergy 204
osteoporosis, special diet for 303
otitis media, serous, in child with allergic rhinitis 160
Otrivin (xylometazoline) 495
outdoors
  allergens 512
  mold 174, 315
  poison ivy/oak/sumac
    see poison ivy; poison oak; poison sumac
  pollen
    see pollen
pollutants 393
overdosage, *vs.* allergic reaction 124-25
over-the-counter medications
  for allergies 483t, 503-5
  antihistamines 29, 483t
  for asthma 92, 505
  color additives in 218
  combination 131
  containing aspirin 122, *122,* 131
  decongestants 481, 483t
  photoallergic reactions to 135
  see also specific drug, e.g., hydrocortisone

oxalates 237
oxtriphylline, for asthma 88
oxybenzone, in sunscreens 138
oxymetazoline, in nasal decongestants 102
oxymetholone (Afrin, Dristan) 495
ozone 322-23
and chemical sensitivity 393

P

PABA, in sunscreens 138
Pacific poison oak *(Rhus deversiloba)*
380-82
geographic range of 380, *381*
growth of 380
identification of 381-82
Page, Barry 423
paint, fresh 322
pancreatic extracts 142
paper wasp *(Polistes* wasp) 352
Pappert, Amy 137
paprika 222
para-aminosalicylic acid, and allergic
drug reaction 121
paracrine, defined 546
parainfluenza virus, as cause of
asthma 81
paraphenylenediamine 404
parasite, defined 546
parasitic diseases 16, 190-91
IgE response and 156-57, 486
socioeconomic impact of 180
parasympathetic (cholenergic) nervous system 63, 73
defined 546
paratyphoid vaccine, anaphylaxis
and 165
parents, caring for asthmatic child 452
parents' allergies, and children's allergies 196, 204
parents' smoking, affect of on
children's allergies 159
Parkinson's disease 184
parsnips, and contact dermatitis 403,
405
particulate air pollution, populations
at risk from 341-44

particulate matter, types of 344
passive immunity, defined 546
Passover, allergies at 178
Pasteur, Louis 4
patch test
for allergic contact dermatitis 108
for allergic drug reaction 128
for cosmetic allergies 429-30
defined 546
do-it-yourself, for cosmetics 432
for hand rash 412
for poison ivy 478
for skin allergy 400-401, 412
pathogen, defined 546
Paturas, Jim 417
Pauling, Linus 26
peak expiratory flow rate 24
peak flow, defined 24
peak flow meters
in asthma treatment 89-90, 469
for elderly 454
for home use 24
peanut(s) 27, 197, 198, 302
allergenic extract for 514t
allergy to 243
avoidance of 202, 267
and childhood atopic dermatitis
245, 249
cross-reactivity and 206-7, 487
mold spores on 487
peanut allergy, extract for 513
Peanut Butter Bars *288*
peanut oil, avoiding in food preparation 267
Pearson, Michele 417
pecan tree 313
pediatric allergies 155-62
allergic rhinitis as 159-60
atopic dermatitis 160-61
common 156
in cystic fibrosis 162
developmental aspects of 157-58
environmental factors in 158-59
gastrointestinal disorders 161-62
genetic factors in 156-57
infantile asthma 161
serous otitis media and 160
socioeconomic impact of 52-53, 54t
see also children; young adults

pemphigus vulgaris 111
  defined 546
penicillin
  and allergic drug reactions 118,
    120, 121, 123, 131
  anaphylaxis and 164, 228, 229, 467
  contaminants in, allergic reaction
    to 126
  desensitization to 232
  IgE antibodies to 164
  and mold allergy 487
  semisynthetic 164
  and serum sickness 119
  for subacute bacterial endocarditis
    131
Penicillium 315
Pennsylvania, pollen calendar for *67*
Peppermint Chiffon Cake *284*
peptide, defined 547
peptide-induced anergy 471
perennial allergic rhinitis 19, 20, 312,
  479
  from dust and dust mites 317-18
  from molds 314
  treatment of 20, 21-22
    immunotherapy in 497-98
perfume
  and contact dermatitis 399
  in cosmetic allergy 430
  and stinging insects 359
The Perils of Particulates (ALA) 344
permanent (hair treatment) 425, 433
  allergic reaction to, prevention of
    432
permanent listing, defined 224
pesticide(s) 388-89
Pesticide Enforcement Policy Statement (PEPS) 389
pet(s)
  allergen control for 322
  and asthma sufferers 86
  avoiding 326
  short-haired, and asthma 438
  washing 326
pet allergies 86, 335-40, 512
pet dander 337, 438, 512, 535
petroleum products 134
Peyer's patches, defined 547

phagocytes, defined 547
phagocytosis, defined 547
Phenergan (promethazine)
  and contact dermatitis 400
  as photosensitizer 137t
phenylbutazone 82
  and aspirin intolerance 122
phenylenediamine 404, 426
phenylephrine (NeoSynephrine) 495
  in nasal decongestants 102
phenytoin, and serum sickness 119
philodendrons, and contact
  dermatitis 403
phosphorus, and kidney disease 302
photoallergies 135
photophobia, drug-induced 136
photoreactions 133-34
photoreactive agents (photosensitizers) 133-34, 137t
  effect of on other diseases 137
"photo-recall" 137
photosensitivity 133-38
  common causes of 137t
  drugs causing 134, 137t
  history of 134-35
  long-term 134
  sunscreens and 138
  symptoms of 134
  tanning booths and 138
  variations in among individuals
    136-37
photosensitization, and contact
  dermatitis 399
phototoxicity (phototoxic reactions)
  135-36
physician, visits to
  see doctor office visits
picry 377
pie *282*
pillows 21, 86, 321, 328, 331
pine tree pollen 313
Pineapple Upside-Down Cake *289*
pink eye, allergic 123
pinworm 190
pirbuterol (Maxaire) 517
piroxicam (Feldene), and photosensitivity 137
pistachio nuts 227-28

pituitary preparations, and allergic
  drug reaction 121
pituitary snuff taker's disease 148t
pizza, for person with food allergy *270*
pizza dough, sulfites in 82
plague 485
plague vaccine, anaphylaxis and 165
Plain Cake *290*
plant(s)
  and contact dermatitis 403
  pollen and 313-14
plant arrangements, holiday 176
plant pollination 312-13
plant protein isolates, maximum
  sulfite levels for 216
plasma cells, defined 547
plasmapheresis 187
plastic masks, at Halloween 177
platelet(s), defined 547
platelet activating factor 10
platinum salts 139, 142, 143, 143t
Plaut, Marshall 513
pleiotropic, defined 547
pluripotent, defined 547
PM$_{10}$ (particulate matter less than 10m
  in diameter) levels 341-44, 343t
pneumonia, drug-induced 121
pneumonitis, hypersensitivity, defined 539
poinsettias, and contact dermatitis 403
poison ash
  see poison sumac *(Rhus vernix)*
poison creeper 377
poison dogwood
  see poison sumac *(Rhus vernix)*
poison elder
  see poison sumac *(Rhus vernix)*
poison ivy 367-74, *368,* 375-89, 475-
  78
  blisters of 371-72, 374, 385, 476
  common myths about 372-73
  contact with, treatment of 371-72,
    373-74, 475-76
  control of 386-88
  dead 388
  dermatitis of 403
    severe 477
  dissemination of 387

poison ivy, continued
  exposure to 370-71, 384-86, 385,
    386, 475-76
  geographic range of 367, 370, *376*
  growth of 375-76, 377
  identification of *368,* 370, 375-76, 377
  immunization against 372, 373,
    477-78
  ineffective remedies for 476
  of Pacific Coast states
    see Pacific poison oak *(Rhus
      deversiloba)*
  patch test for 478
  prevention of 370-71, 477, 478
  rash of 369
  removal of 386-87
  sensitivity to 369-70
  skin test for 478
  symptoms of 385
  treatment of 405, 475-78
poison oak 367-74
  see also poison ivy
poison oak *(Rhus toxicodendron)* 375-
  89, 378-80, *380*
  control of 386-87
  exposure to 384-86
  geographic range of 367, 370, *380*
  growth of 375-76
  identification of 375-76
  location of *380*
  Pacific
    see Pacific poison oak *(Rhus
      deversiloba)*
  treatment of 475-78
poison sumac *(Rhus vernix)* 367-74,
  375-89, *382,* 382-84, *383*
  geographic range of 367, 370, *382*
  identification of *383,* 383-84
  species introduced to United States
    384
  treatment of 475-78
poisonwood *(Metopium toxiferum)* 384
Polistes wasp (paper wasp) 352
pollen 312-13
  airborne 309
  and asthma sufferers 86
  avoidance of allergens 20-21, 487,
    512-13

pollen, continued
  defined 547
  from grasses 64, 312, 313
  from trees 64, 312, 313
  from weeds 64, 312, 313
pollen allergy (hay fever) 309, 312-14,
  467, 507
  information sources for 325
  see also allergic rhinitis (hay fever)
pollen calendar 313
  by state *65-68*
pollen counts 20-21, 69, 313-14
pollen extracts 482-84
  anaphylaxis and 228
pollutants
  air
    see air pollutants (air pollution)
  causing chemical sensitivity 393-94
polyclonal activators, defined 547
polymorph, defined 547
polymorphism, defined 33
polymyositis 184
  defined 547
polyps 103
  defined 547
polyurethane foam industry 139
Pope, Andrew M. 328
poppy seeds 178
Porcupine Meatballs *273*
portable air cleaners 175
postnasal drip, in airborne allergy 311
potassium
  and kidney disease 302
  on nutrition facts panel 299
potassium bisulfite 215
potassium metabisulfite 215
potato starch 262
  contains no gluten 258
potatoes
  anaphylactic reaction to 167
  sulfites and 83, 213, 214, 216
potpourri, holiday 176
poultry stuffing 267
prednisolone, in older nasal sprays 491
prednisone
  for allergic bronchopulmonary
    aspergillosis 153
  for cat-induced asthma 340

prednisone, continued
  oral
    for allergic rhinitis 74
    for eczema 107
pregnancy
  as asthma trigger 85
  and avoidance of foods 207
  calcium requirement during 236
  Rh factor and *185,* 186
  rhinitis during 62
  topical nasal steroids in 492
preservatives
  allergic reaction to 426
  see also food preservatives
prick test
  see skin test
primrose, and contact dermatitis 403
printing chemicals 142
prioxicam (Feldene), as photosensitizer 137t
Priviline (naphazoline) 495
procaine (Novocain), and allergic
  drug reactions 120
produce, fresh, sulfites and 213
product liability claims, chemical sensitivity issue in 395
progesterone, and idiopathic anaphylaxis 231
proliferate, defined 548
promethazine (Phenergan)
  and contact dermatitis 400
  as photosensitizer 137t
propylene glycol 426
prostaglandin synthetase 109
prostaglandins 10, 35, 310
  defined 548
  possible role in allergic disorders 10
prostate problems
  oral decongestants contraindicated
    in 504
  over-the-counter antihistamines
    contraindicated in 504
protein
  and kidney disease 302
  and liver disease 302
  milk
    see milk proteins
  nutrition claims for 304

protein hydrolysates, on ingredient list 300
proteins
  acute phase, defined 527
  defined 548
  IgE antibody reacts against 6, 126
protozoa, defined 548
Proventil (albuterol) 517
provisional listing, defined 224
PSBA, in sunscreens 138
pseudoallergic drug reactions 121-23
psoralens 134
psoriasis 134
psychological stress
  and asthma 90, 437
  and eczema 107
  and hand rash 412
puddings, for person with food allergy *286-87*
Pullularia (Aureobasidium) 316
pulmonary
  see also entries at lung
pulmonary fibrosis 13
pulmonary function tests 85
pulmonary mycotoxicosis 152-53
  defined 548
Pure Food and Drugs Act, and food additives 222
Purim, allergies at 178
puss caterpillar 353-54
pyrogenic, defined 548

Q

quindoxin 134
quinidine (Duraquin), and photophobia 136
quinolone antibacterials 135

R

rabies vaccine, anaphylaxis and 165
radiator heat 87
radioallergosorbent test (RAST) 319-20
  for allergic rhinitis 72-73
  for cat-induced asthma 338
  defined 548

radioallergosorbent test (RAST), continued
  for food allergy 201
  for insect sting 357
ragweed
  and cross-reactivity to melons 198
  efforts at eradication 29
  extract for 513, 514t
  geographic range of 487
ragweed pollen 479, 480-81, 487
  IgE antibodies and *9, 34*
  as major cause of U.S. allergy 14-15
  and process of allergic reaction 16, *34*
raisins, sulfites in 83
Rapp, Doris J. 177
rash
  of contact dermatitis 107, 398
  hand 411-13
  of poison ivy 371-72, 374
RAST
  see radioallergosorbent test (RAST)
rebound congestion, effect (rhinitis medicamentosa) 62, 74, 102, 481, 496, 504, 549
receptor, defined 548
receptor-blocking antagonists 449
recessive trait, defined 548
recipes
  and food allergy 268-93
    see also specific food to be avoided, e.g., wheat
  index to recipes 294-95
recommended dietary allowance (RDA), for calcium 236
rectum *234*
red color additives 219-21
  FD&C Red No. 2 220-21
  FD&C Red No. 3 219-20
  FD&C Red No. 40 223
redroot pigweed 313
redtop (grass) 313
Reeder, Jean 417
regional ileitis (Crohn's disease) 182-83
Reid, Craig 138
rejection, defined 548
rejection responses 189-90

relishes, maximum sulfite levels for 215
relocating
    for asthma 438-39
    ineffective in allergy treatment 320
renal
    see kidney
Report of the Working Group on the Toxicology and Metabolism of ANtioxidants, on use of BHA 212
resins, natural 142
resorcinol 477
respiratory infection
    in elderly asthmatic 456
    first asthma attack during 158
respiratory syncytial virus, as cause of asthma 81, 158
respiratory tract
    and allergies 7
    cromolyn sodium and 522
restaurants
    and food allergy 173, 268
    french fries in 214, 216
    use of sulfites 82-83
Reynolds, Adriana 419
Reynolds, Paul 419
Rh antigen, defined 548
Rh factor disease (erythroblastosis fetalis) 184-86, *185*
rheumatoid arthritis 13, 180-81
    defined 548
    and food allergy 204
    hospitalizations (U.S.) for *46*
    socioeconomic impact of 179
rheumatoid factor 180
    defined 548
Rh-immune globulin 186
rhinitis
    allergic
        see allergic rhinitis (hay fever)
    and aspirin intolerance 122t
    chronic 62
    defined 61, 549
    types of 19
rhinitis medicamentosa (rebound congestion) 62, 74, 102, 481, 496, 504, 549
rhinoviruses 99, 103

Rhizopus 316
Rhode Island, pollen calendar for *68*
Rhus deversiloba (Pacific poison oak) 380-82
Rhus radicans (common poison ivy) 377-78, *379*
    see also poison ivy
Rhus toxicodendron (poison oak) 378-80, *380*
    location of *380*
Rhus verniciflua (Japanese lacquer-tree) 384
ribonucleic acid (RNA), defined 549
rice, anaphylactic reaction to 167
rice allergy, in Japan 197
rice flour 261, 265
    contains no gluten 258
rice noodles 262
Rice Salad *275*
Rice Stuffing *274*
rings
    and contact dermatitis 404
    and hand rash 413
Rocky Mountain spotted fever 123
rodents, affect of on children's allergies 159, 318
room air filters, in treatment of allergy-induced asthma 87
rose 313
rose fever (hay fever) 312
rosemary 214
Rosh Hashanah, allergies at 178
Roy, Cynthia A. 419
rubber
    and contact dermatitis 399, 404
    see also latex allergies
rubber bands, latex in 416
rubber chemicals, and allergic contact dermatitis 107
rubella (German measles) vaccine, anaphylaxis and 165
rugs 21
    wall-to-wall 328
running, and asthma 26, 83
runny nose
    in airborne allergy 311
    antihistamines for 483t
    of rhinitis 62-63

601

"rush" immunotherapy 511
Russian thistle (tumbleweed) 313
rye, gluten in 258
Rye Crackers *279*
rye flour 262
ryegrass pollen 480-81

S

saffron 222
sage 214
sagebrush 313
salad, salad dressing, recipes for 275-76
salad bars, use of sulfites 82-83
salicylates, in sunscreens 138
saline nose sprays 495, 498t
SalineX 495
saliva
    animal, perennial (year-round) allergies to 20, 86, 318, 335-37
    cat 20, 318, 335-40, 336
Sampson, Hugh A. 241, 250, 251
sandalwood oil 134, 135
    in sunscreens 138
sandblaster's silicosis (grinder's disease) 146
Sanders, John 426
sauces
    arrowroot in 262
    maximum sulfite levels for 215
    for person with food allergy *292-93*
    recipes for 292-93
    sweet, maximum sulfite levels for 216
sauna taker's disease 147, 148t
scabies 405
scalp, and contact dermatitis 399
scavenger cells, defined 549
scent
    in cosmetics 430
    and stinging insects 359
scented candles, holiday 176
Schindler, Lydia Woods 35
schistosomiasis 190
    defined 549
school, latex allergy and 420

school absenteeism, asthma and 78, 155, 451, 466
Schwartz, Howard J. 457
SCID mouse, defined 549
scopolamine, and contact dermatitis 400
Scott, Glenn 212
scratch skin test
    see skin test
Scripps Clinic 470
Scripps Clinic and Research Foundation (California) 100
seafood, calcium in 239t
seafood products, processed, maximum sulfite levels for 215
season, poison ivy and 373-74
seasonal allergic rhinitis (hay fever) 18-20, 312, 479, 484
    from molds 314
    as most common allergic disease 484-85
    symptoms of 479
    treatment of 20-22, 481-82
    immunotherapy in 497-98
seasonal hives 109
sebaceous glands, of cats 337
seborrheic eczema 407
second messengers, defined 549
sedatives, and drug-induced photosensitivity 120
seeds 69
    anaphylactic reaction to 167
Segal, Marian 232
Seldane (terfenadine) 481
self, altered, defined 528
self and nonself 4, 31, 32-33, 485
    genes and 33
    in hepatitis 181
    histocompatibility matching and 189
self-tolerance 32
sensitive skin, dermatitis and 404-5
sensitivity, measures to reduce 131, 361
    see also immunotherapy (allergy shots)
sensitization *38*
    to cosmetics 426
    to poison ivy 369-70

sensitize, defined 549
sequoiosis 148t
serotonin 11
defined 549
serous otitis, defined 549
serous otitis media, in child with allergic rhinitis 160
serum, defined 550
serum hepatitis, transmission of 181-82
serum sickness
after insect sting 356
defined 550
drug-induced 5, 119
serving size information, on food label 299-300
sex hormones, for systemic lupus erythematosus 180
shades 21, 86, 321
shag carpets 321, 331
shampoo
color additives in 217
and contact dermatitis 399
shaving cream
color additives in 217
and contact dermatitis 399
sheets 332
Shelley, Walter 399, 403
shellfish 258
allergy to 197, 228, 253
shock, anaphylactic, defined *see* anaphylactic shock
Shortbread Cookies *291*
shortening 267
shrimp 197, 198, 258
food allergy to 253-55
maximum sulfite levels for 215
sulfites in 83
shrimp peelers, and contact dermatitis 401
shrub
Pacific poison oak 380
poison ivy 377-78
poison oak 378
siblings
of asthmatic child 452
of child with asthma 452
silicosis 146
defined 550

silk 69
silo, uncapping of 152-53
silverfish 354
Sinequan (doxepin), as photosensitizer 137t
sinus attack 95, 97, 99
sinuses 95-97, *96*
pain in 97-99
transillumination of 98-99
sinusitis 95-104
acute 97
in allergic patients 71, 100
and allergies 28
as asthma trigger 84
chronic
persistent 98
prevalence of 49t
socioeconomic impact of 49
defined 95, 550
diagnosis of 98-99
in elderly asthmatic 456
infections as complication of 99-100
pain of 97-99
prevention of 100-101
research on 103-4
severe 102
symptoms of 97
treatment of 101-3
sister, of asthmatic child 452
site-associated idiotopes, defined 550
skin
and allergies 7, 397-98
and contact dermatitis 398
corticosteroids and 520
cromolyn sodium and 522
and food allergy 197
lupus erythematosus of 112-13
skin allergy
see also contact dermatitis
skin color, and photosensitivity 137
skin glands
of cat 336
of cats 337
skin inflammation, prevention of 404-5
skin medications
and contact dermatitis 400
and ultraviolet (UV) light 135
see also photosensitivity

603

skin patches, and contact dermatitis 400

skin rashes, prevalence of 49t

skin reactions
allergic, prevalence of 49t
allergic drug reactions and 117t, 120
nonallergic 123, 398

skin test 17-18, 201, 319
allergen increase in 510-11
for allergic drug reaction 127
for allergic rhinitis 72, 480
in allergy diagnosis 17-18
and anaphylaxis 510-11
and atopic dermatitis (atopic eczema) 409
for cat-induced asthma 338
for childhood atopic dermatitis 250
defined 550
for food allergies 27, 168
for food allergy 201
before immunotherapy 508-9
for insect sting 357
for latex allergy 418
for occupational asthma 144
patient history and 509
for poison ivy 478
positive, and development of allergic disease 71, 106, 481
reaction to 510
for shrimp allergy 254
statistics on 480-81

skin-care products, allergic reaction to 426

Slater, Jay E. 230-31, 417, 419-20

SLE
see systemic lupus erythematosus (SLE)

sleepiness 323
and antihistamines 504, 522

slow reacting substance of anaphylaxis (SRS-A) 8
defined 550

small intestine *234*

smallpox 4, 485

Smith, Sydney 481

smoke
from burning poison ivy 387, 403
and rhinitis 69

smoke, continued
tobacco, and chemical sensitivity 393

smoking
affect of on children's allergies 159
asthma and 26
myths about 92
and grain dust exposure 152
and sinusitis 101

smooth sumac (Rhus glabra) *383, 384*

snack foods, preservatives in 209

sneezing
in airborne allergy 311
antihistamines for 483t

soaps
antibacterial 134
for poison ivy exposure 476

social bee 352

socioeconomics of allergy 45-54

sodium, and kidney disease 302

sodium ascorbate 211

sodium benzoate, and aspirin intolerance 122

sodium bisulfite 215

sodium caseinate, in processed meats 242, 243

sodium cromoglycate 145

sodium cromolyn 162

sodium erythorbate 211

sodium metabisulfite 215

sodium nitrite 211

sodium sulfite 215

solar urticaria 110

soldering fluxes 142

solitary bee 352

sorbet, for person with food allergy *285*

soup mixes, dry, maximum sulfite levels for 216

South Carolina, pollen calendar for *68*

South Dakota, pollen calendar for *68*

soy, soybean 198, 303
anaphylactic reaction to 167
and childhood atopic dermatitis 249
children and 203-4

soy flour 261

soy sauce, mold allergy and 315

soybean flour, contains no gluten 258

soybean formula, for infants 158
soybean products 258
spacer device, for oral asthma medication 456
special diets, and food labels 302-3
specificity, defined 550
sphenoid sinuses *96,* 97
  pain in 98
spice(s) 178
Spice Cake *290*
spices 178
spina bifida, incidence of latex allergy with 417, 421
spinach, anaphylactic reaction to 167
spinners (cotton) 139
spirometer
  in asthma diagnosis 24
  defined 550
spleen, defined 550
sporadic asthma 81
spores
  defined 551
  fungal 314
sputum, defined 551
squash 178
SRS-A
  see slow reacting substance of anaphylaxis (SRS-A)
stable fly 353
staghorn sumac (Rhus typhina) *383, 384*
Staphylococcal infection, and sinusitis 99
starches, nonwheat 261-62, 266t
state, pollen calendar by *65-68*
steam
  inhaled, for sinusitis 102
  for nasal congestion 495
Stehlin, Isadora B. 424, 433
stem cells, defined 551
steroids
  in allergic rhinitis 74
  anabolic 323
  for atopic dermatitis 410
  defined 551
  nasal, topical 491-96, 494t, 498t
  oral, for elderly asthmatic 456

stinger
  ant 353
  honey bee 358
  insect 351
stinging insects
  allergy-causing 351
  behavior of 352-53
  preventing attack by 358-59
stomach *234*
stomach acid preparations, lactose in 238
stool acidity test z235
straight dye, defined 224
Streptococcus
  and immunoglobulin IgG 16
  and sinusitis 99
streptomycin
  and allergic drug reactions 123
  and contact dermatitis 400
stress
  and asthma 90
  and hand rash 412
stress rhinitis 62
stuffed toys 332
stuffing, rice *274*
stuffy nose
  decongestants for 483t
  of rhinitis 63
  of sinusitis 102
subacute bacterial endocarditis 131
subcutaneous provocative challenge 205
suberosis 148t
sublingual provocative challenge 205
submucous glands
  in allergic rhinitis 18
  in asthma 79
subunit vaccine, defined 551
sugar(s)
  maximum sulfite levels for 216
  on nutrition facts panel 299
Suleiman, Orhan H. 417, 418, 423
sulfa drugs
  and allergic drug reaction 121
  and drug-induced photosensitivity 120
sulfasalazine (Azulfidine)
  and allergic drug reaction 121
  as photosensitizer 133

sulfites 213-14
  adverse reaction to 199
  as cause of asthma 24, 82-83, 92
  and meats 210
  names of 215-16
  regulations for 208
  sensitivity to, symptoms of 216
sulfonamides
  and allergic drug reactions 121,
    123-24
  and serum sickness 119
sulfur dioxide 199, 215, 393
sulfur oxide 394
sulfuric acid, and asthma 24
sumac, poisonous *vs.* nonpoisonous 383
sunlight, sensitivity to
  see photosensitivity
sunscreen(s)
  bergamot oil in 134
  as cause of photosensitivity 138
  and contact dermatitis 399
  as protection against photosensitiv-
    ity 138
superantigens, defined 551
superoxide radical
  defined 551
  possible role in asthma 10
suppressor T cells, defined 551
Suprofen, photoallergic reaction to 135
surgical equipment, latex in 416
surgical sutures, color additives in
  218
swamp sumac
  see poison sumac *(Rhus vernix)*
sweet vernal (grass) 313
sweeteners
  artificial 134
  on ingredient list 300
swelling of airways, in asthma 78, 79
swimming
  and asthma 26, 83
  and sinusitis 101
sympathetic (adrenergic) nervous
  system 63, 73
  defined 551
sympathomimetic(s) 73-74
  defined 551
syrups, maximum sulfite levels for 216

systemic lupus erythematosus (SLE)
  113, 186-87
  defined 550, 551
  hospitalizations (U.S.) for *46*
  sex hormones for 180
  socioeconomic impact of 179-80

T

T lymphocytes (T cells)
  antigen recognition and 33
  cytotoxic, defined 535
  defined 551, 552
  and eosinophils 461-62
tachyphylaxis 496
tanning booths 138
tapioca 262
  for person with food allergy *285*
tapioca flour, contains no gluten 258
tar, fresh 322
tartrazine (yellow, FD&C No. 5)
  see yellow color additive (FD&C No.
    5 [tartrazine])
tattooing 134, 402
Tavist (clemastine) 497
tea
  instant, sulfites in 82
  maximum sulfite levels for 215
technical names, for foods 259t-261t,
  259-61
teenagers
  see young adults
Tennessee, pollen calendar for *68*
terbutaline (Bricanyl, Brethine) 517
terfenadine (Seldane) 481, 497
tetanus vaccine 130
  anaphylaxis and 165
tetracaine 477
tetracylines
  and drug-induced photosensitivity 120
  and phototoxicity 136
Texas, pollen calendar for *68*
Thanksgiving, allergies at 178
theophylline
  adverse effects from 518-20
  for asthma 25, 26, 88
    in elderly 455-56
  for cat-induced asthma 339-40

theophylline-ephedrine combination drugs, over-the-counter 505
therapeutic allergens, anaphylactic reactions to 166
thiamin, and liver disease 302
thiazides, and drug-induced photo-sensitivity 120
thickening foods, with nonwheat flours and starches 265
thimerosal 136-37
thiouracil, and serum sickness 119
three-leaved ivy 377
throat, angioedema in 119
throw rugs 21, 86, 321, 331
thunderwood
  see poison sumac *(Rhus vernix)*
thymic epithelial cells, defined 552
thymus, defined 552
thyroid disease, oral decongestants contraindicated in 504
thyroid gland, and asthma 85
thyroiditis, autoimmune, hospitalizations (U.S.) for *46*
tidal volume 85
timothy (grass) 313
tissue-typing techniques 189
titanium dioxide, in sunscreens 138
tobacco smoke 322
  affect of on children's allergies 159
  and chemical sensitivity 393
  second-hand, and asthma 467
tocopherol (vitamin E), as natural preservative 214
tofu, calcium in 239t
tolazamide (Tolinase), and photophobia 136
tolbutamide (Orinase), and photophobia 136
tolerance, defined 552
Tolinase (tolazamide), and photophobia 136
Tollefson, Linda 218
toluene di-isocyanate (TDI) 81, 141, 142
tomatoes
  anaphylactic reaction to 167
  and contact dermatitis 403, 405
tonsils, defined 552

toothpaste
  color additives in 217
  and contact dermatitis 399
topical corticosteroids, in treatment of seasonal allergic rhinitis 20
topical medications, and contact dermatitis 400
topical nasal sprays 489-99, 498t
  for chronic allergic rhinitis (hay fever) 497
  cost of 493t
  types of 491-96
topical steroids
  inhaled, few side effects from 28
  nasal 491-96, 494t, 498t
    for allergic rhinitis 22
    in treatment of allergic disease 323
torsade de pointes 497
tourniquet
  in epinephrine emergency kit 231-32
  and stinging insects 359-60
Toxicology Advisory Committee (FDA) 220
toxins, defined 552
toys 332-33
  latex in 416
transdermal patches, and contact dermatitis 400
transfusion(s), Rh factor in 184-86
transfusion reactions 5, 169
transgenes, defined 552
transgenic mice, defined 552
transillumination, of sinuses 98-99
transplantation
  189-190
  hospitalizations (U.S.) for *46*
transplanted tissues, as antigens 32, 33
tree(s), Christmas 175-76
  artificial 176
tree nuts 197
tree pollen 64, 312, 313, 479, 484
  allergenic extracts for 514t
triamcinolone, for allergic rhinitis 74
triamcinolone acetonide (Nasacort) 492, 493t

triggering of mast cells, defined 552
trimellitic anhydride(s) 81, 142
trimethoprim (Bactrim), as photosensitizer 137t
tripedane 489, 492
tripelennamine hydrochloride 477
tropomyosin protein, in shrimp 254-55
trout 258
TSH, defined 552
tuberculosis vaccine, anaphylaxis and 165
tulip bulb, and contact dermatitis 403
tumbleweed (Russian thistle) 313
tuna, natural histamines in 198
tuna fish, hidden milk proteins in 241, 243
Turkeltaub, Paul C. 480, 513
turmeric 222
"twentieth century disease" 392
typhoid fever 123
typhoid vaccine, anaphylaxis and 165

U

ulcer, *vs.* food allergy 199
ulcerative colitis 182-83
  defined 553
  fiber and 303
  socioeconomic impact of 179
ultraviolet (UV) light
  in photoallergies 135
  in phototoxicity 135-36
  sensitivity to
    see photosensitivity
  sunscreens and 138
  therapy with, for atopic dermatitis 409
ultraviolet (UV) sunlamps, in photoallergies 138
underwear, latex in 416
United States
  allergies and asthma in, socioeconomic impact of 45-54
  causes of allergy in 15
  particulate air pollution in, populations at risk from 341-44
  risk of occupation-induced asthma in 141

United States Department of Agriculture (USDA), on vegetable and animal proteins 242
United States Department of Health and Human Services 325
United States Food and Drug Administration (FDA)
  see Food and Drug Administration (FDA)
United States Forest Service, and poison ivy 478
United States Hospital Discharge Survey *46,* 48
University of California, Irvine 513
upholstered furniture 332
upper respiratory tract infection, as cause of asthma 81
urban minorities, asthma in 53
urinary tract
  antihistamines and 523
  theophylline and 520
urticaria (hives) 109-10
  and aspirin intolerance 122t
  cholinergic 110
  cold-induced 110
    defined 534
  defined 553
  solar 110
  symptoms of 109
  see also hives; angioedema
urushiol (from poison ivy sap) 369, 371, 372, 373, 385, 477
  preventing spread of 371, 373, 386
Utah, pollen calendar for *68*

V

vaccination
  defined 553
  Edward Jenner and 4, 485
vaccine(s)
  anaphylactic reactions to 165-66
  defined 553
vaccine therapy, future of 471
vacuuming 321, 328
vagus nerve 142
Valentine, Martin 366

Van Metre, Thomas E. 340
Vancenase AQ (beclomethasone) 492, 493t
Vancenase Pockethaler (beclomethasone) 492, 493t
variable region, defined 553
vasculitis, as cause of asthma 84
vasomotor rhinitis 19, 62, 480t
vegetable(s)
  anaphylactic reaction to 167
  calcium in 239t
  canned
    maximum sulfite levels for 216
    sulfites in 83
  and contact dermatitis 403, 405
  dehydrated, maximum sulfite levels for 216
  raw, sulfites and 213
  sulfites and 213
vegetable juice, maximum sulfite levels for 216
vegetable oil 267
venetian blinds 21, 86, 321, 332
venom
  extract for 514t
  honey bee 358
  insect 351
    extract for 513
venom extracts, for immunotherapy 167, 357
venom immunotherapy 363-66
  length of 365-66
ventilation systems 328
Ventolin (albuterol) 517
Vermont, pollen calendar for 68
vesiculobullous diseases 110-12
  defined 553
Vibramycin (doxycycline), as photo-sensitizer 137t
vinegar 303
  maximum sulfite levels for 215
  mold allergy and 315
vines, of poison ivy 377
vinyl, vs. latex 423
vinyl gloves
  and contact dermatitis 404
  and hand rash 413
viral hepatitis 181

viral infections
  and asthma 448
  and sinusitis 99
viral vaccines, anaphylaxis and 165
Virginia, pollen calendar for 68
Virginia creeper, vs. poison ivy 377
virus(es)
  as cause of asthma 81, 158
  c-type 186
  defined 553
visiting, and allergy 176
vitamin B12, and liver disease 302
vitamin C, and allergies 26
vitamin D 237
  nutrition claims for 304-5
vitamin E (tocopherol), as natural preservative 214
vitamins
  color additives in 217
  and liver disease 302
  on nutrition facts panel 299
volleyball, rubber 415
von Pirquet, Clemens Freiherr 3

W

Waffles 280
wall-to-wall carpeting 86, 321, 328
walnuts 197
washing
  in allergen control 321
  in poison ivy exposure 371, 475-76, 478
Washington, D.C., pollen calendar for 65
Washington (State), pollen calendar for 68
wasp(s) 351
  anaphylactic reaction to 167, 229
  behavior of 352
wasp stings 167
weather conditions
  and allergy 174
  and Hymenoptera 359
  and molds 316
  and pollen 313
weed pollen 64, 312, 313, 479
  allergenic extracts for 514t

weevil 354
West Virginia, pollen calendar for *68*
wet leaves, and mold 174
wheal and flare reaction 319, 480
wheat 178, 258, 302
  anaphylactic reaction to 167
  avoiding in food preparation 267
  and childhood atopic dermatitis 249
  foods containing 259, 261t
  gluten in 258
  technical names for 259, 260t
wheat flour, substituting for 265-66, 266t
wheat weevil disease 148, 148t
wheezing, in asthma 79
whey 238
whipped topping, lactose in 238
White Americans, asthma in 439, 444, *444*
White children, asthma in 53
white dermographism 106
whooping cough vaccine, anaphylaxis and 165
wine 178
  maximum sulfite levels for 215
  natural histamines in 198
  sulfites in 82, 83, 199
wine vinegar, sulfites in 83
Wisconsin, pollen calendar for *68*
women
  rheumatoid arthritis in 180
  systemic lupus erythematosus 186-87
wood pulp worker's disease 148t
woodburning stoves 175
  and chemical sensitivity 394
woodwork 331
wool 332
  and contact dermatitis 404
work
  asthma and 452, 466
  latex allergy and 420-21
work areas, design of 145, 394
workers' compensation claims, chemical sensitivity issue in 395
workplace-related chemical sensitivity 394-96

workplace-related respiratory disease
  see also occupational/environmental respiratory diseases
  see occupational asthma
World Health Organization 103, 115
Wyoming, pollen calendar for *68*

X

xenografts, defined 553
x-ray study dyes
  and anaphylactic reactions 168
  and pseudoallergic reactions 121, 122
xylometazoline (Otrivin) 495
  in nasal decongestants 102

Y

yeara
  see Pacific poison oak *(Rhus deversiloba)*
yeast(s) 314
  mold allergy and 315
yeast breads 269
yellow color additive (FD&C No. 5 [tartrazine]) 218, 225
  and aspirin sensitivity 130
  and asthma 82
  and hives 109
  and pseudoallergic reactions 121, 122, 199
yellow fever vaccine, anaphylaxis and 165-66
yellow jackets 351, 352
  anaphylactic reaction to 167, 229
yogurt, calcium in 237
Yom Kippur, allergies at 178
Young, Stuart H. 511-12
young adults
  allergic diseases in 52-53
  allergic rhinitis in 71
  asthma in 53
  atopic dermatitis in 408
  use of marijuana by 159
  see also adolescents; teenagers
  see also pediatric allergies
Yunginger, John 508, 509, 511

Z

Zamula, Evelyn 405
zinc acetate, for poison ivy blisters
   476
zinc carbonate, for poison ivy blisters
   476
zinc oxide, for poison ivy blisters 476

zinc-free insulin 124
zirconium 405
   and allergic contact dermatitis 107
Zithromax (azithromycin), second-
   generation antihistamines
   contraindicated with 497
Ziyad, Joann 213, 214